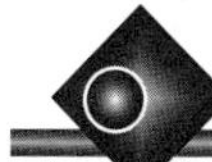

Gerontological Protocols for Nurse Practitioners

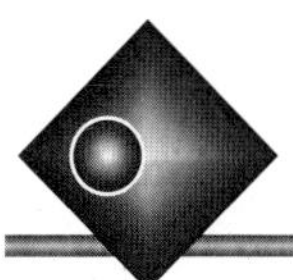

Gerontological Protocols for Nurse Practitioners

JERI B. BROWN, MSN, RNCS, GNP, CDE

Nurse Practitioner, Vanderbilt University Medical Center
Adjunct Instructor of Nursing, Vanderbilt University School of Nursing
Nashville, Tennessee

NANCY K. BEDFORD, MSN, RNCS, GNP, CRRN

Nurse Practitioner, Department of Veterans Affairs Medical Center
Adjunct Instructor of Nursing, Vanderbilt University School of Nursing
Nashville, Tennessee

SARAH J. WHITE, MSN, RNCS, GNP, FNP

Nurse Practitioner, Vanderbilt University Medical Center
Adjunct Instructor of Nursing, Vanderbilt University School of Nursing
Adjunct Faculty, Vanderbilt University School of Medicine
Nashville, Tennessee

Physician Consultant:

JAMES S. POWERS, MD

Assistant Professor of Medicine and Director, Senior Care Service
Vanderbilt University Medical Center
Chief of Geriatrics, Department of Veterans Affairs Medical Center
Nashville, Tennessee

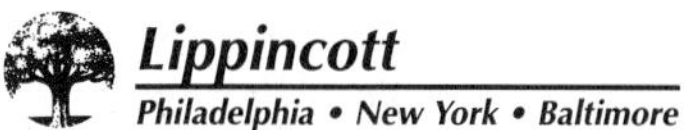

Editorial Assistant: Dale Thuesen
Senior Production Editor: Virginia Barishek
Senior Production Manager: Helen Ewan
Production Service: Berliner, Inc.
Printer/Binder: R. R. Donnelley & Sons Company/Crawfordsville

9 8 7 6 5 4 3 2 1

Library of Congress Cataloging-in-Publication Data

Brown, Jeri B.
Gerontological protocols for nurse practitioners / Jeri B. Brown, Nancy K. Bedford, Sarah J. White ; physician consultant, James S. Powers.
p. cm.
Includes bibliographical references and index.
ISBN 0-7817-1567-9
1. Geriatric nursing. 2. Nursing care plans. 3. Nurse practitioners. I. Bedford, Nancy K. II. White, Sarah J. III. Title.
[DNLM: 1. Geriatrics Nursing—standards. 2. Primary Health Care—standards Nurses' Instruction. WY 152 B878g 1999]
RC954.B76 1999
610.73'65—dc21
DNLM/DLC 99-24355
for Library of Congress CIP

Care has been taken to confirm the accuracy of the information presented and to describe generally accepted practices. However, the authors, editors, and publisher are not responsible for errors or omissions or for any consequences from application of the information in the book and make no warranty, express or implied, with respect to the contents of the publication.

The authors, editors, and publisher have exerted every effort to ensure that drug selection and dosage set forth in this text are in accordance with current recommendations and practice at the time of publication. However, in view of ongoing research, changes in government regulations, and the constant flow of information relating to drug therapy and drug reactions, the reader is urged to check the package insert for each drug for any change in indications and dosage and for added warnings and precautions. This is particularly important when the recommended agent is a new or infrequently employed drug.

Some drugs and medical devices presented in this publication have U.S. Food and Drug Administration (FDA) clearance for limited use in restricted research settings. It is the responsibility of the health care provider to ascertain the FDA status of each drug or device planned for use in clinical practice.

✦

For Jerry, Hughes, Clay, and my parents,
and for Elsie Nason
J.B.B.

To Barry, Andrea, my parents and grandmother
N.K.B.

To Bruce, Elizabeth, Meredith, Rebecca, and my mother;
and in memory of my father
S.J.W.

✦

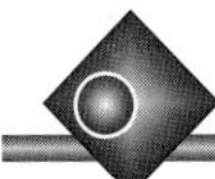

Preface

Gerontological Protocols for Nurse Practioners is designed for health care practitioners who find themselves caring for an ever-growing number of aging patients. The book has been developed as a compendium of clinical guidelines that focus on the assessment and management of age-specific problems. It is meant to augment available adult primary care protocols rather than to stand alone as a complete adult protocol text. The major focus is on care within the primary care setting, with specific issues related to acute care, extended care, and home care addressed at the end of each protocol. Subacute care, an expanding alternative level of care blending many aspects of acute and extended care, is not identified in the protocols as a separate setting; however, many of the recommendations listed under both the acute care and the extended care setting will be applicable to subacute care.

This book makes use of extensive cross-referencing between protocols. The authors consider this an important difference from other adult protocol manuals, but essential for this population. The elderly population is very heterogeneous with often complex and inter-related comorbidities. Recommendations for optimal care of any given condition must take into consideration co-existing problems. Cross-referencing between protocols is designed to emphasize this interrelatedness.

Preventive care is covered in detail in the **Protocol on Prevention and Health Maintenance.** These recommendations should be considered in the management of any acute or chronic problem in this population. In addition, preventive measures specific to a particular problem are listed in each protocol. The authors believe this emphasis on prevention is warranted in the care of the elderly.

Many references are made throughout the protocols to consulting with a physician. The assumption made by the authors is that the nurse practitioner is practicing in a collaborative relationship with a physician. The frequency and timing of physician consultation are individualized and should be based upon the nurse practitioner's level of expertise, practice situation, state regulations, NP/physician collaborative agreement, and practice-specific guidelines or protocols.

Due to the complexity of issues for this population, the authors advocate an interdisciplinary approach to care. Nurse practitioners in all settings are encouraged to develop strong working relationships with colleagues in other disciplines and to build an effective team. References are made throughout the protocols to the input of other team members in the care of a specific problem.

In regard to laboratory and radiological testing, an effort has been made to use generic terminology and to avoid regional differences. Nurse practitioners are encouraged, however, to confirm the correct name of a test in their own setting and to consider the availability, coverage, and cost.

The **Chapter on Medication Issues** deals in detail with medication usage in this age group. Throughout the protocols, the doses given are recommended ranges and care should be taken to individualize. Again, nurse practitioners are encouraged to check availability with their specific formularies and to take into account the cost associated with the medication.

The authors believe that the elderly are a very special group who teach us all a great deal every day. The goal of this book is to help other health care providers better meet the unique health care needs of seniors in a variety of settings and situations.

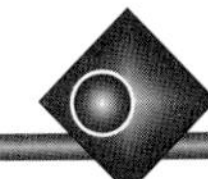

Acknowledgments

The authors wish to acknowledge our patients along with their families and caregivers who have shared their lives and unique experiences with us and who have enriched our practices over the years. We also wish to recognize the invaluable contributions of the interdisciplinary team members and the many health professions students who have taught us to look beyond a single perspective and to adopt a broader, more holistic approach to care of seniors.

Specifically, the authors wish to thank the following individuals for their time and input in the development of this work:

Anita Arline, BSN, RN, CETN
Brandy Basham Cox, Nutritionist
Michael G. Carlson, MD
Debbie Croley, MSN, RNCS, GNP
Stephen N. Davis, MD
Kelly Floyd, OTR/L
Debbie Harrell, D.Ph., CGP
Kathryn Kidd, MSW
Bobby Knight, PT
William J. Kovacs, MD
James M. May, MD
Alvin C. Powers, MD
Linda Varnell, RD, LDN
Bruce D. White, DO, JD
Kimber Zuplo, CCC-SLP

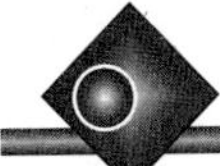

Contents

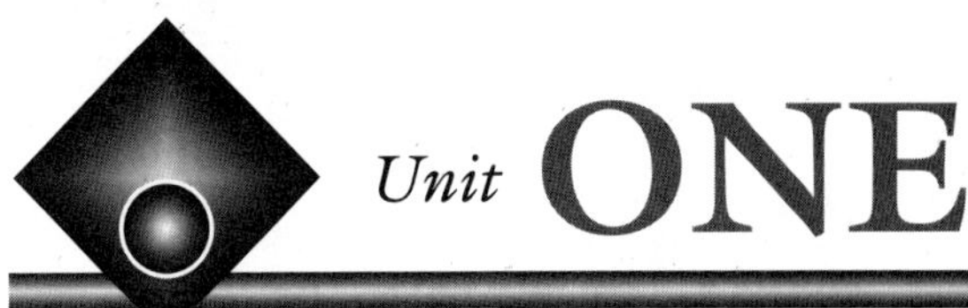

Prevention and Health Maintenance

Chapter 1

Prevention and Health Maintenance

SCREENING GUIDELINES

✦ Screening guidelines have been established by the Canadian Task Force on Periodic Health Examination, the U.S. Preventive Services Task Force, and others for use in the elderly population. **See References.**

✦ **Given the increase in the elderly population, there is a critical need for continued research to better define the efficacy of specific preventive measures.**

✦ Selection of screening services should be based on patient's risk profile, risks versus benefits of screening, and patient's acceptance.

✦ **Some clinicians may not initiate appropriate screening and interventions in the elderly due to ageism.**

✦ Screening establishes baseline for future interventions, may help to reduce use of acute-care services, and facilitates coordination of services.

✦ Goals of screening in the elderly are to: (1) maximize functional status, (2) minimize morbidity and limit disease progression, (3) maintain independence, and (4) increase life satisfaction. **Preservation of independent functioning is the key issue for the elderly, with the following areas of utmost concern: mobility, bowel-bladder status, mental status, self-care ability, environmental safety, and social support.**

✦ **Activities to prevent decline and preserve function may be more appropriate than costly and arduous screening for new disease in the elderly.**

✦ Screening is most cost-effective and beneficial for the following high-risk groups: (1) history of recent hospital discharge; (2) recently bereaved; (3) socially isolated; (4) financially stressed.

✦ Numerous **geriatric screening tools** are available (functional status, depression, caregiver burden). Use screening tools selectively, according to particular needs to be addressed. Use of screening tools facilitates a standardized approach to the elderly patient's needs. Literacy, cognitive status, and cultural limitations must be considered. Patients may overstate their abilities to avoid loss of independence or institutionalization. Caregivers may understate the elderly patient's abilities.

HISTORY

✦ **The elderly may under-report symptoms.**

✦ **Sex? Race? Based on ethnicity and gender, the following groups have increased risk for given health care problems as compared to their cohorts:**

Ethnicity/gender	*Health care problem*
White females	Osteoporosis
White males	Suicide
African American females*	Hypertension Diabetes mellitus
African American males	Stroke Cirrhosis Diabetes mellitus Lung cancer
Native American males	Diabetes mellitus Alcohol (EtOH) abuse
Native American females	Diabetes mellitus
Asian females	Osteoporosis

✦ Sexual preference? Marital status?

✦ Urinary incontinence?

✦ Difficulty sleeping?

✦ Problems with bowel function?

✦ Tobacco, EtOH, and other drug use? Consider use of CAGE questionnaire (JAMA 1984;252:1905–1907) to assess EtOH use.

✦ Domicile: independent living; living with family member; assisted living; extended-care facility; boarding home or group home; homeless; migrant; recent immigrant; correctional institution?

✦ Support system? Caregivers? Dependents?

✦ Dietary intake? **5–15% of elderly suffer from nutritional deficiency. Restrictive diets designed for management of some chronic illnesses should be used cautiously.**

✦ Level of physical activity? Ability to perform activities of daily living?

*African American females > 65 years of age are at greater risk for hypertension than any other group in the United States.

- Medications: prescriptions/over-the-counter (OTC)?
- History of falls, fractures, burns?
- Past medical history: skin cancer or lesions; colorectal cancer, polyps, or inflammatory bowel disease; upper-body radiation for cancer; coronary artery disease; hyperlipidemia; cerebrovascular disease or transient ischemic attacks (TIAs); hypertension; atrial fibrillation; diabetes mellitus?
- Family history: skin cancer; first-degree relative with colorectal cancer; breast, ovarian, or endometrial cancer; diabetes mellitus; early-onset coronary artery disease?
- Previous or present occupation? Note risk for exposure to blood or blood products.
- Automobile driving? **By the year 2000, it is estimated that 28% of all drivers in the U.S. will be aged 65 or older.** History of motor vehicle accidents? **The elderly may withhold report of decreased performance for fear of losing driving privileges.**
- Health care services provided by specialty care (e.g., dentist, ophthalmologist, podiatrist)?
- Economic barriers to health care?
- Immunization status?
- Females: early menopause or history of oophorectomy before menopause; last Pap smear/results? Last breast examination/results? Last mammogram/results? History of gestational diabetes?
- Males: problems with urination? History of benign prostatic hypertrophy or prostate cancer?
- Losses: illness or death of spouse or other significant others; divorce or separation; change in economic/role status secondary to retirement, unemployment, or other income restrictions; recent relocation; presence of chronic pain; social isolation secondary to conditions such as urinary incontinence, chronic obstructive pulmonary disease (COPD)?
- Depression/history of depression? Anxiety?
- Memory loss? Change in cognition? Behavioral changes?
- Advance directives?

PHYSICAL EXAMINATION

- **See Appendix A, Common Changes of Aging.**
- Vital signs
    - Height; measure once between ages 65–75, then every 3 years to screen for kyphosis and loss of height secondary to osteoporosis.
    - Weight. **Obesity contributes to cardiovascular disease, Type 2 diabetes mellitus and difficulties with mobility/activities of daily living**

(ADLs). Malnutrition is a common problem in the older old; patient may be obese yet have protein malnutrition.

✧ Blood pressure (BP) every 2 years if normotensive; annually if diastolic 85–89. Maintaining BP < 160/90 in the 65–79-year-old age group decreases cardiovascular morbidity and mortality; if age > 80 years, there is high risk of falls or hip fracture with iatrogenic hypotension.

✦ Eyes: Visual acuity screening with Snellen or Rosenblum chart.

✦ Ears: Hearing ability screening with whisper test.

✦ Oral cavity: especially for current smokers/history of tobacco or EtOH use. Note tooth decay, loose teeth, gingivitis.

✦ Thyroid: Palpate for nodules in individuals with history of upper body radiation.

✦ Neuro: Evaluate gait. Screen for automobile driving safety risk by evaluating motor and sensory function.

✦ Skin: complete examination if family history of skin cancer, history of increased exposure to sunlight, skin lesions, or cancer. Be alert for signs of physical abuse or neglect in all elders.

✦ Cardiovascular: auscultate heart rate to screen for atrial fibrillation. Auscultate for carotid bruits if history of TIAs. Auscultation of carotid bruits in asymptomatic patients has low sensitivity and specificity.

✦ Abdomen: palpation for aneurysm has 80–90% sensitivity when aneurysm is large enough for surgery. Palpation not recommended for individuals not eligible for surgery or who would decline surgery based on personal choice.

✦ Rectal: Fecal occult blood testing reduces mortality but is not very sensitive or specific. Necessary pre-test dietary restrictions are difficult to accomplish resulting in a high false-positive rate. Detection of nodules on digital examination may lead to treatment that carries risk of significant morbidity. **Before testing, discuss potential follow-up with patient.**

✦ Genitalia: Females: annual breast examination; annual pelvic examination—not recommended for women older than age 60 unless history of abnormal Pap results. **Ovarian cancer occurs more frequently in women older than 60, but is not usually detected by pelvic examination.**

DIAGNOSTIC TESTS

✦ Mental status examination if cognitive changes.

✦ Tuberculosis screen for high-risk groups (malnourished, immunosuppressed, or residents of extended care facilities).

✦ Refer to ophthalmologist for glaucoma screen.

✦ Refer for audiometry if hearing reduced when canals are cerumen-free.

✦ Annual urinalysis to screen for asymptomatic bacteriuria, hematuria, or proteinuria.

✦ Thyroid function tests—recommended for women >50 because of higher risk.

✦ Some authorities recommend screening for high cholesterol every 5 years. However, adequate studies of efficacy of treatment in the elderly have not yet been conducted. Consider screening only those at high risk.

✦ Recommendations concerning flexible sigmoidoscopy screening in the elderly are controversial. Flex sig is an invasive procedure that may cause patient discomfort, pain, and embarrassment and detects more polyps than cancer.

✦ Females: annual mammogram to age 75. **Incidence of breast cancer increases with advancing age**—annual mammogram recommended by some authorities until age 85 and beyond for women who remain functionally intact; annual Pap smear not recommended over age 65 if previous smears have been negative and there is no other risk factor. Pap smear every 2–3 years until late life if history of abnormal smear or cervical cancer. Bone mineral densitometry (BMD) for high-risk groups (Caucasian and Asian females; sedentary lifestyle; smoking history).

✦ Males: Prostate-specific antigen (PSA) has high false-positive rate and follow-up of elevated levels may result in treatment-associated morbidity.

✦ Dementia and depression screens recommended for symptomatic elderly.

MANAGEMENT

Health Maintenance for All Elderly

IMMUNIZATIONS

✦ **Strongly encourage elderly patients to maintain up-to-date personal record of immunizations.**

✦ **Pneumococcal vaccination** at age 65. **Pneumonia is the leading cause of death in the elderly.** Patients who previously received the 14-valent vaccine should be revaccinated with 23-valent. High-risk patients (chronically ill, asplenic, health care workers, extended care residents) should be vaccinated before age 65 and revaccinated every 6 years. Debilitated and high-risk patients may not mount immune response to vaccine.

✦ **Annual influenza vaccination** for those > 65 years and younger than 65 in high-risk groups (as above for pneumonia). **95% of all influenza deaths occur among the elderly.**

✦ **Tetanus vaccination** every 10 years or when dirty wound occurs and no vaccination within previous 5 years.

EXERCISE

- Recommend walking 2–3 times per week (15–30-min sessions) if patient is capable.
- Activities (gardening, range-of-motion exercises) should be encouraged.
- Weight training to prevent falls by increasing muscle mass.

SEAT BELT USE

- **At all times while in automobiles or other vehicles.**

WEIGHT MAINTENANCE

- **Refer to nutritionist if 20% above or below ideal body weight.**

ADVANCE DIRECTIVES

- **Counsel regarding advance directives.**
- **Re-evaluate patient's desire on regular basis.**
- If indicated, screen with values assessment tool.
- Do not accept a wish to die as mere desire for advance directives. Consider possible suicide risk.

Management of Specific Risks

REDUCED ABILITY TO PERFORM ADLS/IADLS

- Refer to social worker for education and counseling regarding community resources.
- Refer for appropriate assistive services (home health). Medicare reimbursement only if there is a skilled need.
- Refer to occupational therapy (OT) for home assessment.
- Refer to physical therapy (PT) for assessment of gait, balance, and safety. Recommend for assistive devices (home or outpatient).

KNOWN CORONARY OR CEREBROVASCULAR DISEASE

- Acetylsalicylic acid (ASA, aspirin) 81 mg PO qd, if no contraindications.

FAMILY HISTORY OR PAST MEDICAL HISTORY OF COLON CANCER

- Stool guaiac, digital rectal examination.
- Consider endoscopy.

TOBACCO USE

- Smoking cessation.
- Consider nicotine supplement.

ETOH AND OTHER DRUG ABUSE

- Refer to mental health and community agencies.
- Review medications for possible interactions.
- Counsel families regarding injury risks; remove weapons from home.

POSTMENOPAUSAL, S/P HYSTERECTOMY

- Consider hormone replacement therapy (HRT) to reduce cardiovascular and osteoporosis risk. If history of breast cancer, consider risks vs. benefits of HRT.

OSTEOPOROSIS RISK

- Increased risk for Asian and Caucasian females, smokers, sedentary.
- Counsel regarding calcium supplementation, weight-bearing exercise, HRT, and prevention of falls.

URINARY INCONTINENCE

- Evaluate for underlying cause (infection, obstruction, pelvic relaxation, medications).
- Refer to urologist or gynecologist.

AUTOMOBILE ACCIDENT RISK

- Refer patients with cognitive, sensory, or motor deficits to OT for driver assessment and possible vehicle modification.
- Driver examinations and restrictions on impaired drivers vary from state to state.
- Counsel patient and families regarding safety of continued driving.
- Refer to social worker for resources to alleviate driving needs.
- Refer to mental health agencies for counseling regarding emotional loss of surrendering driving privileges.

RISK FOR CAREGIVER STRESS

- Refer to home health, volunteer organizations, adult day care, respite care, support groups.

ELDER ABUSE (PHYSICAL, EMOTIONAL, FINANCIAL)

- If indicated, refer to protective services (vary from state to state).
- Refer to legal services for financial protection.
- Refer to local area agency on aging.
- Refer to ombudsman if extended care resident.

SUICIDE RISK

✦ Immediate acute-care referral if indicated.

✦ Refer to mental health agencies or crisis intervention agencies.

✦ Counsel regarding removal of firearms and lethal drugs from home environment.

RISK FOR VIOLENT INJURY

✦ Counsel to remove firearms, avoid intoxication with EtOH and other drugs.

✦ Provide information regarding crisis center, shelters, protective services, and protection of dependents.

KEY ISSUES

Economic Considerations

✦ Third-party reimbursement may not be available for screening procedures. Discuss options with patient prior to scheduling.

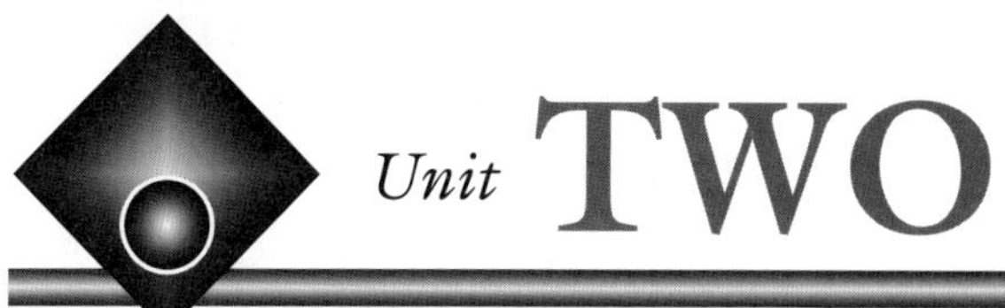

Unit TWO

Protocols in Primary Care Geriatrics

Chapter 2

Head, Ears, Eyes, Nose, and Throat

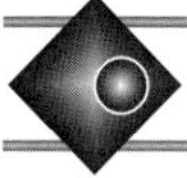

Tinnitus

HISTORY

✦ Describe the sound. The physiologic sound is generated within the auditory system and is louder than environmental sounds. Frequent descriptors are hissing, ringing, clicking, roaring, buzzing, ocean, or the sound of crickets.

✦ Is the sound constant or intermittent?

✦ Pitch? **Low frequency is associated with Meniere's disease.**

✦ Pulsatile? **Associated with blood flow through a narrowed vessel and is transmitted secondary to conductive hearing loss.**

✦ Onset/duration? **Sudden onset, short duration indicative of acute process such as otitis media, traumatic head injury, labyrinthitis, and noise exposure.**

✦ Frequency? Setting?

✦ Location? Head? One or both ears?

✦ Relieving factors? **Tinnitus may disappear in recumbency or when leaning over.**

✦ Dizziness? **See Protocol on Dizziness.**

✦ Hearing loss? **Can be related to conductive or neurosensory loss; not necessarily related to hearing loss.**

✦ Visual changes? Headaches or increased tension? **Due to impairment of posterior circulation.**

✦ Pressure in head/ears? Pain? Location? Character?

✦ Associated factors such as fatigue, stress, anxiety?

✦ Drainage from ear?

✦ Hearing aid(s)?

- Allergies: seasonal, food, drugs?
- Other medical conditions: multiple sclerosis, head trauma, vascular disease, valvular heart disease?
- History of frequent or prolonged noise exposure?
- Medications: prescription/OTC? Offending medications include aspirin, NSAIDs, quinine, furosemide, tricyclic antidepressants, cisplatin, ototoxic antibiotics such as gentamicin, and antimalarials. Caffeine-containing foods/beverages?
- Smoker? EtOH intake?
- Family history?
- Does the sound affect normal daily function or sleep?
- Is the sound distressing?
- Weight change?

PHYSICAL EXAMINATION (see Table 2-1)

- Vital signs/weight—check blood pressure in both arms, and supine, sitting and standing to rule out autonomic neuropathy of postural hypotension. **Tinnitus has been associated with hypertension and orthostasis. Rapid, extreme weight loss/diuresis can lead to a widely patent eustachian tube causing tinnitus described as rushing air, ocean roar, echo, or click accentuated with nasal breathing.**
- Assess cranial nerves.
- Examine nares for polyps, swelling, occlusion.
- Assess mouth and pharynx for lesions and postnasal drainage.
- Observe palate for myoclonus.
- Assess hearing acuity/determine conductive hearing loss:
  - Asymmetric/retrocochlear or central tinnitus.
    - Associated with CNS lesions in the cerebellopontine area.
    - May be associated with pulsation in involved ear.
  - Symmetric/cochlear loss or inner ear or peripheral tinnitus.
    - Most common type can be associated with presbycusis.
- Assess external ear canal for impacted cerumen, foreign bodies. **See Protocol on Cerumen Impaction.**
- Assess tympanic membrane for perforation/cholesteatoma/fluid in middle ear.
- Palpate temporomandibular joint (TMJ) for crepitus during chewing motion; ascultate for click.
- Palpate for lymph nodes and neck masses, enlargement/nodularity of thyroid.

TABLE 2-1. Differential Diagnosis of Tinnitus

External tinnitus	Middle ear tinnitus
Impacted cerumen	Allergy
Infection	Infection
Foreign body	Injury
Fibrosis	

✦ Assess optic disc for changes suggesting increased intracranial pressure.

✦ Assess for nystagmus in the presence of vertigo.

✦ Auscultate for carotid/temporal bruits/venous hums.

✦ Auscultate heart sounds/rule out valvular heart disease.

✦ Evaluate gait, observe for cerebellar ataxia.

DIAGNOSTIC TESTS

✦ Audiometry to rule out need for hearing aid/benefit of a masker–fits like hearing aid, has a competing noise.

✦ Consider assessing drug levels to rule out toxicity.

✦ Consult otolaryngologist for additional procedures/testing.

Consider:

✦ CBC, erythrocyte sedimentation rate (ESR), to rule out anemia, polycythemia, inflammation.

✦ Thyroid function studies.

✦ Lipid profile.

✦ Electrolytes, blood urea nitrogen (BUN), creatinine, blood glucose.

✦ Albumin, prealbumin to assess nutritional state.

✦ Consider rapid plasma reagin test (RPR, to rule out CNS syphilis).

✦ MRI (rule out tumors such as acoustic neuroma/other lesions/signs of multiple sclerosis). Consult physician.

✦ Referral to psychiatry to rule out auditory hallucinations of psychiatric origin.

✦ Referral to neurologist.

✦ Referral to psychologist for counseling, if appropriate.

PREVENTION

✦ Appropriate dosing/monitoring of ototoxic medications.

✦ Cerumen management. **See Protocol on Cerumen Impaction.**

✦ Early treatment of ear infections.

✦ Proper hearing aid cleaning and care.

✦ **See Protocol on Prevention and Health Maintenance.**

MANAGEMENT

✦ Correct underlying pathology (impacted cerumen, drug toxicity, nutritional deficiencies, uncontrolled diabetes mellitus, hypo- or hyperthyroidism, anxiety/depression, renal failure).

✦ Refer to audiologist for potential "noise-masker" (best used when there is no hearing loss) and/or hearing aid to override noise.

✦ Suggest white noise at night (fan or other noise-producing equipment) or relaxation tapes to be played during the night to aid insomnia.

✦ Suggest setting the radio dial between two FM stations to override tinnitus.

✦ Consider mild hypnotic such as Xanax (alprazolam) 0.25–1 mg or Ativan (lorazepam) 0.25–0.5 mg for resistant insomnia.

✦ Meditation/relaxation exercises to reduce tension.

✦ Instruct or refer for biofeedback techniques.

✦ Reduce/discontinue use of stimulants such as coffee, tea, caffeine-containing sodas, and EtOH.

✦ Encourage smoking cessation (nicotine often exacerbates condition).

✦ Refer to smoking cessation group.

✦ Consider nortriptyline, alprazolam, or oxazepam. The anticonvulsant, carbamazepine, has also been used with success. Dosing is up to half the usual dose for seizure control. Monitor closely for side effects. Benzodiazepines have been shown to increase fall risk.

✦ Instruct to avoid noise exposure, ototoxic agents.

KEY ISSUES

Patient/Caregiver Education

Patient/caregiver should be able to:

✦ Demonstrate proper use of "noise masker" and/or hearing aid.

✦ Identify stressful factors contributing to tinnitus.

✦ Identify psychologic distress secondary to tinnitus.

✦ Demonstrate appropriate use of prescribed medications. Observe for overuse of benzodiazepines and carbamazepine.

- ✦ Demonstrate proper use of biofeedback techniques.
- ✦ Identify proper measures to protect against noise exposure.

Economic Considerations

- ✦ Consider elder's resources prior to detailed work-up.
- ✦ Audiometry evaluation, noise-maskers, and hearing aids can be costly.

Psychosocial Considerations

- ✦ Assess for suicidal ideation (has accompanied severe tinnitus).
- ✦ Quality of life and perception of well-being are important factors in adaptation.
- ✦ Assess for safety issues related to decreased concentration.
- ✦ Depression is common, assess early. Consider antidepressant therapy. **Tricyclic group can cause, as well as treat, tinnitus.** Monitor patient response.
- ✦ Consider referral to support groups.

Extended Care Setting

- ✦ Consider implementation of cerumen management team.
- ✦ Encourage use of hearing aids/amplification system.
- ✦ Encourage proper cleaning and care of hearing aids; address issues while grooming.
- ✦ Tinnitus may be present in the patient thought to be experiencing auditory hallucinations. Consider tinnitus as a contributor to agitation/acting out in the elderly patient with dementia.
- ✦ Plan scheduled review of prescribed medications, eliminating causative agents when possible.
- ✦ Refer as appropriate.

Home Setting

- ✦ Observe for alteration in activities of daily living (ADLs) and instrumental activities of daily living (IADLs) associated with tinnitus.
- ✦ Environmental safety checks to prevent falls.
- ✦ Reinforce instructions provided for noise-maskers, hearing aids, biofeedback devices, relaxation methods.
- ✦ Assess early for signs/symptoms of depression.
- ✦ Assess for social isolation/withdrawal.

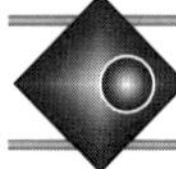

Cerumen Impaction

HISTORY

✦ Onset and duration of symptoms?

✦ Decreased hearing? Onset and duration? **Hearing loss secondary to cerumen obstruction is usually insidious. Sudden loss can occur with expansion of cerumen to complete obstruction following swimming, bathing, or initial irrigation.**

✦ Pruritus? Pain? Fullness? **May also suggest infection, foreign body obstruction.**

✦ Dizziness? Ringing in ear? **See Protocols on Dizziness and Tinnitus.**

✦ Drainage? **May suggest infection.**

✦ Are hearing aids worn?

✦ History of previous cerumen impactions? Ear hygiene?

✦ History of tympanic membrane perforation? Ear surgery?

✦ Effect on daily life: social isolation or withdrawal, depression, paranoia, inappropriate acting out?

PHYSICAL EXAMINATION

✦ Otoscopic examination to determine quantity, color, and consistency of cerumen. **Cerumen accumulation is increased in the elderly due to increased keratin production and decreased cerumen secretions.**

✦ Examine external ear canal for excessive hair growth (especially in males) and foreign objects (especially in presence of cognitive impairment).

✦ Assess canal for anatomic variation.

✦ Assess canal for erythema, edema, tenderness and pain. **Long-standing cerumen impaction is commonly complicated by external otitis.**

✦ Assess hearing acuity before and after cerumen removal. **Cerumen impaction impairs low frequency hearing.**

DIAGNOSTIC TESTS

✦ Consider audiometry if hearing acuity is subnormal following cerumen removal.

PREVENTION

- Avoid swabs to remove cerumen. **Promotes further cerumen packing.**
- Prevent trauma to canal by avoiding use of sharp objects such as hair pins, keys, and toothpicks to remove cerumen.
- Clip excessive hairs from ear canal when barbers are unavailable.
- Perform appropriate maintenance of hearing aids.
- **See Protocol on Prevention and Health Maintenance.**

MANAGEMENT

- Instill 5–10 gtts ceruminolytic agents such as Debrox (carbamide peroxide 6.5%), 3% hydrogen peroxide, mineral or baby oil, or docusate sodium liquid to fill the canal, wait at least 10 min, preferably 15–30 min prior to irrigation or bid 1–5 days prior to irrigation. **Ceruminolytic agents and irrigation are contraindicated in the presence of perforated tympanic membrane or infection.**
- Irrigate using tepid tap water, adjust to patient's comfort, using auto-fill utility syringe with rounded tip or pulsating dental irrigation system at lowest pressure. Direct irrigation upward toward the posterior wall adjacent to cerumen plug (10 o'clock position right ear and 2 o'clock position left ear).
- Curette removal using Buck size 0–00 or cerumen spoon or loop. While immobilizing head, pass curette beyond the impaction on the posterior wall of canal and pull medially, outward. Must be done under direct visualization of canal. With good lighting, occasionally forceps may be required for debris, cornified epithelium. Avoid in presence of infection/history of tympanic rupture. **Tympanic membrane and canal are fragile. Canal can be easily macerated/excoriated by any technique.**
- Dry canal following irrigation with alcohol or low heat hair dryer.
- Consider steroid/antibiotic otic solution (Cortisporin Otic) 4 gtts tid–qid for 5–7 days following prolonged lavage and following trauma to canal.
- Consider ceruminolytic instillation bid for 5 days monthly in recurrent and resistant cases. Duration of treatment to be determined during suggested 3-month follow-up. Set schedule for compliance such as first or last week of the month.
- In elderly with mild-to-moderate dementia, cue to assist by placing hand on ear basin against side of face, simply inform, ask for feedback, and reassure frequently during irrigation. Limit procedure time (may need several short sessions to complete). Consider premedication with mild anxiolytic when appropriate. Consider ceruminolytic instillation alone in the presence of comprehension deficits or agitation.

✦ Refer treatment resistant cases or those with history of perforated tympanic membrane to otolaryngologist.

KEY ISSUES

Patient/Caregiver Education

Patient/caregiver should be able to:

✦ Demonstrate safe ear hygiene (washcloth over index finger).

✦ Describe and demonstrate proper use of ceruminolytic agents.

✦ Demonstrate proper instillation of ear drops.

✦ Demonstrate proper cleaning and care of hearing aid.

Economic Considerations

✦ Consider expense of ceruminolytic agents.

✦ Consider coverage of irrigation/curettage as a separate procedure by HMO, Medicare, Medicaid.

Psychosocial Considerations

✦ Observe for behavioral changes associated with impaired hearing such as social withdrawal/isolation, depression, paranoia, confusion, or acting out.

✦ Quality of life is negatively affected by hearing impairment.

Acute/Inpatient Setting

✦ Assess routinely on admission, intervene as appropriate; hearing deficit can negatively impact compliance and rehabilitation process.

Extended Care Setting

✦ Assess routinely on admission, semi-annually, and with behavioral change such as withdrawal, depression, headache/otalgia, paranoia, or inappropriate acting out. **High incidence of cerumen impaction exists among residents of extended care.**

✦ Implement interdisciplinary cerumen management teams (medicine, nursing, audiology) for routine screening, surveillance, and treatment.

Home Setting

✦ Perform routine assessment for cerumen impaction.

✦ Evaluate techniques of ear drop instillation and self-ear irrigation.

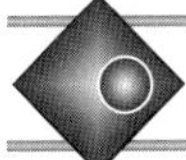

Orofacial Pain

HISTORY

- ✦ Onset, location, duration of pain? Radiation of pain?
- ✦ Character of pain: sharp or dull, superficial or deep, burning or aching?
- ✦ Intensity of pain? **Use of a pain scale to quantify pain may be helpful.**
- ✦ Is pain constant or intermittent?
- ✦ Aggravating or ameliorating factors?
- ✦ Effect of pain on activities such as talking, chewing, yawning, swallowing?
- ✦ Change in sensation or motor function, hyperesthesia, falls?
- ✦ Headache? Onset, location, duration? Character of pain?
- ✦ Presence on ocular symptoms: tearing, redness, edema, change in vision? History of glaucoma?
- ✦ Presence of ear pain, tinnitus, drainage?
- ✦ Presence of nasal symptoms: congestion, drainage? History of sinusitis?
- ✦ Presence of cutaneous symptoms: change in color, temperature, sweating?
- ✦ Presence of oral symptoms: bruxism, clenching, halitosis, dental caries or abscess, periodontal disease, missing teeth, poorly fitting dentures, xerostomia? When was last dental examination? **More than 50% of elderly are edentulous.**
- ✦ History of trauma, infection, allergies, weight loss, systemic illness (i.e., diabetes mellitus, cancer, rheumatic conditions)?
- ✦ History of arthritis? Presence of neck pain or stiffness?
- ✦ History of nutritional deficiencies or anemia?
- ✦ Recent stressors? Change in sleep patterns?
- ✦ Change in balance or gait? History of falls?
- ✦ History or symptoms of depression or anxiety?
- ✦ Medications: prescription/OTC?

PHYSICAL EXAMINATION

- ✦ Vital signs.
- ✦ Assess for signs of inflammation in head and neck.
- ✦ Palpate site of pain and surrounding area including adjacent salivary glands and lymph nodes.

✦ HEENT: examine all structures including dentition, gingiva, tongue, and oral mucosa; examine area underneath tongue.

✦ Neck: assess for range of motion, tenderness on palpation, auscultate for crepitus with movement of neck.

✦ Palpate TMJ for crepitus; auscultate for clicking.

✦ Assess cranial nerves as appropriate.

DIAGNOSTIC TESTS

✦ Customize to rule out underlying systemic illnesses.

✦ CBC if infection a possible cause.

PREVENTION

✦ Annual and prn dental examinations and cleaning.

✦ Good oral hygiene.

✦ Reassess dentures for fit with weight loss or gain. **There is often resorption of the gum ridge with normal aging resulting in poorly fitting dentures.**

✦ Annual eye examination.

✦ Regular cleaning and care of hearing aids; ear examinations for impacted cerumen. **See Protocol on Cerumen Impaction.**

✦ Avoid tobacco products and other oral irritants.

✦ Relaxation techniques and stress management.

✦ **See Protocol on Prevention and Health Maintenance.**

MANAGEMENT

Somatic Pain

Somatic pain is related to underlying structures; may be superficial (sharp pain precisely located and constant in location, duration, and intensity) or deep (dull sensation, less precisely located, frequently associated with hyperalgesia or referral of pain).

SUPERFICIAL SOMATIC PAIN

Superficial somatic pain arises from the skin of the lips, face, outer nares, external auditory canal, and from mucogingival tissues of the mouth.

✦ **See Protocols on Mouth Lesions and Cerumen Impaction.**

✦ Consider Xylocaine (lidocaine HCl 2%) viscous solution or analgesic lozenges for palliative relief.

✦ Consider oral analgesics.

✦ For xerostomia: eliminate or decrease saliva-depressing drugs such as tricyclic antidepressants, antipsychotics, antihistamines, antiarrhythmic drugs, antihypertensives, anticonvulsants, diuretics; recommend chewing gum or sour, sugarless, hard candies to stimulate salivary flow; keep water available, or recommend saliva substitutes.

DEEP SOMATIC PAIN

Deep somatic pain arises from dental, musculoskeletal, or visceral structures, i.e., teeth, gums, TMJ, pharynx, tonsils, sinuses, eyes, or ears.

✦ Treat underlying cause if etiology determined. **See Protocols on Nasal Congestion, Mouth Lesions, and/or Degenerative Joint Disease.**

✦ Refer to specialist when appropriate, i.e., dentist, ophthalmologist, or otolaryngologist.

✦ Consider oral analgesics or antiinflammatory agents for palliative treatment.

Neuropathic Pain

Neuropathic pain is characterized by burning pain that is spontaneous, triggered, or ongoing and unremitting; occurs disproportionately to stimuli; accompanied by other neurological symptoms; can be episodic or continuous.

EPISODIC NEUROPATHIC PAIN

Episodic neuropathic pain may be neurovascular as characterized by migraine or cluster headaches. **See Protocol on Headache.** Trigeminal neuralgia is a classic type of episodic neuropathic pain.

✦ Trigeminal neuralgia or **tic douloureux**: episodic, unilateral, intermittent, lancinating, triggerable, shock-like facial pains over the distribution of the 5th cranial nerve. **There is an increased incidence in the elderly and in females.**

✦ Trial of Tegretol (carbamazepine) 100 mg bid, maximum 600 mg bid. Available in suspension 100 mg/5 ml. **Improvement of symptoms with carbamazepine suggests pain is due to trigeminal neuralgia.** May need to be taken long term (<3 years). Can cause leukopenia, agranulocytosis, and aplastic anemia. Obtain pretreatment laboratory values of blood count and platelets and monitor weekly to biweekly for 2 months, then monitor monthly. Begin at low dose and titrate slowly to minimum dose required to control symptoms. **Onset of skin rash is early indication to stop the therapy.** May cause confusion and agitation in the elderly.

✦ Consider trial of Lioresal (baclofen) 5 mg tid, maximum 80 mg daily. Not as effective as carbamazepine but fewer side effects. **Taper dose to discontinue.** Monitor closely with renal impairment.

✦ Other possible medications: Dilantin (phenytoin) 100–300 mg at bed time; or Elavil (amitriptyline HCl) 10–25 mg daily. **Consider contraindications; monitor Dilantin levels.**

✦ Consider referral to a neurosurgeon for rhizotomy or microvascular decompression. Consult with physician before referral.

CONTINUOUS NEUROPATHIC PAIN

Continuous neuropathic pain includes neuritis pain, i.e., herpes zoster and post-herpetic neuralgia **(See Protocol on Herpes Zoster)**, traumatic neuralgia, and toothache of unknown origin (atypical odontalgia).

✦ Consider topical analgesic such as Zostrix (capsaicin) cream, which may cause an increase in pain initially, but repeated applications provide relief. Apply five times daily to affected area for the first week, three times daily for the next 3 weeks. Capsaicin can be mixed with 5% lidocaine ointment.

✦ Consider low dose of a tricyclic antidepressant or a selective serotonin reuptake inhibitor (SSRI). **See Protocol on Depression.**

✦ Consider trial NSAIDs or Ultram (tramadol HCl) 50–100 mg q 4–6 hr; maximum 400 mg daily. **See Protocol on Degenerative Joint Disease.**

✦ Consider referral to a Pain Management Center if available.

✦ **See Protocol on Pain Management.**

KEY ISSUES

Patient/Caregiver Education

Patient/caregiver should be able to:

✦ Maintain a pain diary if indicated.

✦ Verbalize treatment regimen.

✦ Identify precipitating factors and avoid when possible.

✦ Verbalize importance of preventive strategies.

Economic Considerations

✦ Pain can be debilitating, lead to costly treatments, result in inability to perform normal activities.

✦ Laboratory monitoring can be costly in terms of the testing itself and in transportation to obtain testing.

Psychosocial Considerations

✦ Pain may have a psychogenic component; evaluate carefully.

✦ Assess for depression or anxiety. **Neuropathic pain can exacerbate depressive symptoms. See Protocols on Depression and Anxiety.**

✦ Assess for sleep disturbances.

✦ Consider biofeedback techniques or relaxation therapy as adjuncts to treatment regimen.

✦ Consider referral for counseling if needed.

Acute/Inpatient Setting

✦ Be alert to orofacial pain in nonverbal or demented patients.

✦ Include careful orofacial assessment in admission examination.

Extended Care Setting

✦ Be alert to orofacial pain in nonverbal or demented patients; include in differential diagnosis when evaluating behavioral problems.

✦ Mobile dental services are often available for nursing home patients. Dental maintenance should be a routine part of care.

Home Setting

✦ Enlist family/caregivers in monitoring pain and complying with pain management regimen.

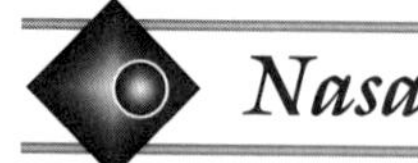

Nasal Congestion

HISTORY

✦ Recent upper respiratory illness? **Signs and symptoms of a cold persisting beyond 7–10 days with purulent nasal secretions is suggestive of sinusitis.**

✦ Sneezing? **Usually present in rhinitis; uncommon with sinusitis.** Drippy/runny nose? Characteristics of nasal secretions, such as thin/thick, clear/purulent/bloody? **Secretions of allergic rhinitis are clear, thin, and watery; infectious rhinitis may be thick or thin and white; and sinusitis is usually thick and green/yellow.**

✦ Nasal congestion/blockage? **Rule out foreign body, especially in patient with dementia.**

✦ Fever? Fatigue/malaise? Dizziness?

✦ Headache? Facial discomfort when bending over? Maxillary teeth pain? Postnasal drip and/or frequent clearing of throat? **May suggest chronic sinusitis. Facial pain and pressure may be present with allergic and nonallergic rhinitis.**

✦ Cough? **Common with sinusitis; may or may not be present with rhinitis.** Wheezing? Sputum production? Characteristics?

✦ Decreased hearing, smell, or taste? Bad breath? Loss of appetite?

✦ Insomnia? Mood or cognitive changes? Sinusitis is a cause of delirium in the elderly. Hallucinations may be presenting symptom. **Central nervous system effects of allergic rhinitis and antihistamines can have negative effect on mood and cognition especially in the elderly. These effects include: fatigue, sedation, decreased alertness, impaired physical/cognitive performance, all of which predispose to safety concerns. Consider use of second-generation nonsedating antihistamines to decrease these effects.**

✦ When did symptoms first begin? **Allergic rhinitis rarely has onset after the age of 40.**

✦ Are symptoms episodic or continuous? If episodic, when do symptoms occur, how often? **Episodic symptoms suggest reaction to trigger(s). Episodic daily symptoms suggest perennial allergies, anatomic problems, or environmental/occupational etiology.**

✦ Duration of symptoms?

✦ Provoking or exacerbating factors such as: activities, environment, weather, emotions, OTC/prescription/recreational drugs, occupation/hobby related? **Grass, pets, fallen leaves, and dampness aggravate allergic rhinitis. Odors, occupational or hobby-related irritants, emotions, exercise, and changes in weather or sudden changes in environmental temperatures may suggest nonallergic rhinitis such as vasomotor instability.**

✦ Recent dental work?

✦ History of respiratory allergies or asthma? History of hypertension, diabetes mellitus, glaucoma, coronary artery disease, or HIV?

✦ How have symptoms affected ADLs/quality of life?

✦ What interventions/home remedies have been tried? What has helped?

✦ What OTC/prescription drugs have been used? What has/has not helped? **Poor response to nasal decongestants is common with sinusitis.**

✦ How important is it to the patient that symptoms be treated?

PHYSICAL EXAMINATION

✦ Vital signs; observe for oral breathing when checking respirations. **Pulse and blood pressure elevation may be secondary to sympathomimetic use. Fever suggests infection; lack of fever in elderly does not exclude infection. Temperature is normal in allergic and nonallergic rhinitis; fever may or may not be present in infectious rhinitis and may come and go in sinusitis.**

✦ Assess eyes for excess tearing, exudate, and conjunctival/scleral injection. **See Protocol on Red Eye**.

✦ Assess for periorbital venous congestion and periorbital edema. **Common in allergic rhinitis. Allergic shiners (dark rings under the eyes) may not be seen as often in the elderly.**

✦ Inspect ear canals for inflammation, exudate. Assess tympanic membrane for scarring, rupture, retraction, bulging, erythema, movement, and fluid levels behind membrane.

✦ Assess ability to smell.

✦ Assess nose "allergic salute," a transverse crease over bridge caused by chronic wiping of nose. Assess turbinates/mucosa for color, edema, type/color of drainage. **Intranasal membranes are pale, swollen, boggy, and lighter in color than the lips in noninfectious rhinitis. Reddened mucosa suggest acute infectious rhinitis or abuse of topical drugs. Purulent secretions from the middle meatus is predictive of maxillary sinusitis.**

✦ Assess for nasal polyps, obstruction, and foreign objects. **Polyps appear as clear turbinates with glistening/sheer surface and are usually located near the middle or superior tubinates. Patients with nasal polyps may be sensitive to nonsteroidal antiinflammatory agents, including aspirin.** Assess septum and nares for structural abnormalities. **Any of these abnormalities may contribute to recurrent sinusitis.**

✦ Assess pharynx for adenoid/tonsilar enlargement/inflammation and presence/color of postnasal drainage. Assess voice for hoarseness/nasal quality.

✦ Tap and palpate areas over frontal, maxillary sinuses. **Tenderness is specific for sinusitis.**

✦ Assess for decreased transillumination over frontal/maxillary sinuses.

✦ Palpate lymph nodes for tenderness/enlargement.

✦ Auscultate lungs for wheezing/crackles. **Suggest asthma vs. secondary infection such as bronchitis/pneumonia. See Protocol on Pneumonia.**

DIAGNOSTIC TESTS

✦ Diagnosis of allergic/nonallergic, noninfectious rhinitis can be made from history and clinical findings.

✦ Consider CBC with differential if infection is suspected.

✦ Consider posterior/anterior and lateral x-ray of chest if there are abnormal pulmonary findings.

✦ Consider sinus CT if history and clinical findings are suggestive that sinusitis or rhinitis is refractory to treatment, chronic, or severe. **Dementia patients may require sedation prior to scanning.** Plain sinus films are often unrevealing. Consult physician.

✦ Consider referral to otolaryngologist for sinus aspirate, biopsy, culture, and sensitivity in refractory cases.

PREVENTION

✦ Prescribe adequate decongestants/nasal medication refills for patients who have allergic symptoms. **Avoid overuse of topical nasal decongestants.**

✦ Suggest air conditioning/air filtering to reduce dust and removal of damp/moldy carpets/furniture.

✦ Avoid known triggers when possible.

✦ **See Protocol on Prevention and Health Maintenance.**

MANAGEMENT

Rhinitis

See Display 2-1 for differential diagnosis of rhinitis.

✦ Etiology of rhinitis determines treatment. **May be due to allergens, microbial pathogen, anatomic/structural problems, vasomotor instability system disease or medication use.**

✦ Presence of purulent discharge prompts consideration of antibiotic therapy.

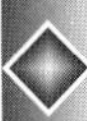

DISPLAY 2-1. *Classification of Rhinitis*

Allergic rhinitis
- Seasonal
- Perennial

Infectious rhinitis
- Viral
- Bacterial

Noninfectious/nonallergic rhinitis
- Vasomotor rhinitis
- Rhinitis medicamentosa or rebound rhinitis
- Occupational/hobby-related rhinitis

✦ Refer to otolaryngologist when: etiology is anatomic/structural; patient has immune deficiency; uncertain diagnosis, concomitant comorbidities such as upper respiratory infection, asthma, otitis media with effusion, chronic sinusitis, or nasal polyps; and failure to respond to allergen avoidance and pharmacologic protocols. Consult physician.

CHRONIC ALLERGIC/NONALLERGIC/NONINFECTIOUS RHINITIS

✦ Antigen avoidance is most effective treatment. Provide written list of common environmental triggers and discuss those most appropriate to patient. May include: dust; animal dander; molds; pollen; cockroaches; irritants such as odors, smoke, paint fumes, or dirty furnace filters; and dramatic changes in environmental temperatures to a lesser degree.

✦ The bedroom and bathroom need to be the most allergen-free rooms in the house.

✦ Consider referral for allergy testing. Radioallergosorbent (RAST) testing is reserved for those in whom skin testing is contraindicated. Consult physician.

✦ Consider referral to otolaryngologist for chronic or resistant rhinitis/sinusitis for possible polypectomy/other surgical intervention.

✦ Determine patient's understanding of and intention of compliance prior to initiation of intervention.

✦ Drug therapies: See Display 2-2.

✧ Oral antihistamines treat itching/sneezing, runny nose, eye symptoms, and possibly nasal congestion.

✧ Topical corticosteroids are usually less effective than antihistamines and antihistamine/decongestant combinations in treating itching/sneezing, runny nose, nasal blockage, impaired smell, and eye symptoms.

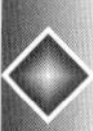

DISPLAY 2-2. *Medications to Treat Rhinitis*

ANTIHISTAMINES

H1-receptor antagonists work by antagonizing histamine, relieving sneezing, runny nose, nasal, ocular, and palatal itching. Sedating antihistamines in the elderly may increase the risks of falls, decline in cognitive and functional status. Metabolism occurs more slowly, increasing serum levels and the potential for adverse drug–drug interactions. Oral vasoconstrictors can elevate blood pressure, cause urinary retention, have CNS effects, and promote arrhythmias.

Nonsedating

Hismanal (astemizole) 10 mg daily
Zyrtec (cetirizine HCl) 10 mg daily, 5 mg daily if creatinine clearance is 31 mL/min or less.
Claritin (loratadine) 10 mg daily, 10 mg qod if creatinine clearance is <30 mL/min.

QT prolongation and arrhythmias have occurred with astemizole when used with erythromycin, clarithromycin, ketoconazole, or itraconazole. **Caution:** Avoid use of listed nonsedating antihistamines in presence of hepatic dysfunction.

Sedating

Chlor-Trimeton (chlorpheniramine maleate) 8–10 mg bid
Tavist (clemastine fumarate) 1 mg bid–tid
Periactin (cyproheptadine HCl) 4 mg tid, maximum dose 0.5 mg/kg daily
Benadryl (diphenhydramine HCl) 25–50 mg tid–qid
Atarax (hydroxyzine HCl) 25 mg bid–tid

ORAL DECONGESTANTS

Oral alpha-adrenergic agonists decrease nasal congestion by constricting nasal mucosa blood vessels. Agents do not affect itching, sneezing, or runny nose. Peripheral blood vessels are also constricted with side effects of hypertension, palpitations, tachycardia, insomnia, and nervousness. Use cautiously in presence of cardiovascular disease, thyrotoxicosis, or glaucoma.

Sudafed (pseudoephedrine HCl) 30–60 mg qid; timed-release 120 mg q 12 hr
Entex (phenylephrine, phenylpropanolamine, and guafenesin) 1 cap qid or sustained release 1 cap every 12 hr

(continued)

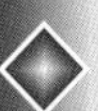

DISPLAY 2-2. *Continued*

COMBINATION ANTIHISTAMINE/ORAL DECONGESTANT

Claritin-D (loratadine/pseudoephedrine sulfate) 1 tablet daily; decrease to 1 tablet every other day if creatinine clearance < 30 mL/min.

Allegra-D (fexofenadine HCl/pseudoephedrine HCl) 1 tab bid; decrease to 1 tab daily in presence of renal insufficiency.

Use cautiously in the elderly. Pseudoephedrine-containing drugs are contraindicated with narrow angle glaucoma, severe hypertension, coronary artery disease, and urinary retention.

Dimetapp (brompheniramine maleate/phenylpropanolamine HCl) 1 cap q 4–6 hr. Dimetapp Extentab 1 tab bid.

NASAL CORTICOSTEROID SPRAYS

Beconase AQ or Vancenase AQ (beclomethasone dipropionate) 2 sprays nasally bid

Nasalide or Aerobid (flunisolide) 2 sprays nasally bid

Nasacort AQ (triamcinolone acetonide) 2 sprays nasally daily

All corticosteroid sprays may take up to 2 weeks to become effective.

TOPICAL DECONGESTANTS

Afrin/Dristan/Neo-synephrine 12 hour (oxymetazoline HCl)

Neo-Synephrine (phenylephrine HCl)

Otivan (xylometazoline HCl)

Privine (naphazoline HCl)

All topical decongestants relieve nasal congestion rapidly. Limit use, tolerance develops rapidly. Overuse can cause rebound nasal congestion and rhinitis medicamentosa. All may aggravate hypertension and cardiac arrhythmias.

INTRANASAL ANTICHOLINERGICS

Atrovent (ipratropium bromide) 0.03%, 0.06% solution, 2 puffs nasally bid

Anticholinergic bronchodilator derived from atropine. Controls excessive runny nose. Effects felt within 30 min and last 8–12 hr. Has drying effect; effective treatment for allergic/nonallergic rhinitis such as gustatory or vasomotor rhinitis or "dripping" seen in the elderly. Agent has no effect on sneezing, itching, or nasal congestion.

(continued)

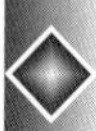

DISPLAY 2-2. ***Continued***

MOISTURIZING AGENTS

Saline or propylene glycol and polyethylene glycol sprays. Use for perennial rhinitis. Use just prior to topical corticosteroid to help prevent drug-induced local irritation.

PRINCIPLES OF COMBINATION THERAPY

Antihistamine/decongestant + topical nasal corticosteroid: moderately severe ocular/nasal symptoms.
Topical nasal corticosteroids: used on continuous basis for patient with perennial rhinitis; during seasonal exacerbations consider adding antihistamine.
Topical nasal corticosteroid + bronchodilator: for patients with allergic rhinitis plus asthma.

✧ Oral decongestants treat runny nose, nasal blockage, impaired smell.

✧ Combination antihistamine/decongestants treat itching/sneezing, runny nose, nasal blockage, impaired smell, and eye symptoms.

✧ Limit topical decongestant to 3–7 days, while beginning topical corticosteroid.

✧ Cromolyn sodium is less effective than other agents and requires compliance for response.

✧ Intranasal anticholinergics are most effective for runny nose.

✧ Oral corticosteroids are very effective in treating itching/sneezing, runny nose, nasal blockage, impaired smell, and eye symptoms, but should be reserved for temporary use in severe cases.

Sinusitis

See Display 2-3 for classification of sinusitis.

✦ Predisposing factors include allergic rhinitis, upper respiratory infections, and obstruction. **Nasogastric feeding tubes act as obstruction; be alert to acute sinusitis. See Protocol on the Management of the Enterally Fed Patient.**

✦ Sinus CT demonstrates opacification, air-fluid levels, or mucosal thickening of at least 5 mm.

✦ Common causative pathogens: *Streptococcus pneumoniae*, *Hemophilus influenzae*, Beta lactamase + *Hemophilus influenzae* (resistant to amoxicillin and ampicillin), *Moraxella catarrhalis*, *Staphylococcus aureus*. Fungi are often seen in patients with diabetes, HIV, or immunosuppression.

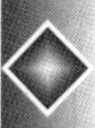

DISPLAY 2-3. ***Classification of Sinusitis***

Acute:	Symptoms last < 1 month
Subacute:	Symptoms last 1–3 months
Chronic:	Symptoms last > 3 months

✦ In chronic sinusitis, less pneumococcus is seen. There are increased anaerobes; staphylococcus, oral anaerobes, and gram-negative organisms.

✦ Treatment for acute sinusitis consists of decongestant and/or antihistamine and antibiotic. Treatment for chronic sinusitis: decongestant and antibiotic. Steroids and surgical intervention may be indicated. **Decongestant/antihistamine use is controversial: decongestants may dry secretions/antihistamines may contribute to tenacious secretion. Both may prevent sinus drainage. Consider trial, if patient does not improve, stop the decongestant/antihistamine, continue the antibiotic. See Management of Rhinitis for guidelines—Entex is often useful if patient is compliant with increased fluid intake.**

✦ Empiric antibiotic therapy goals:

✧ Prevent secondary intracranial/orbital complications.

✧ Avoid chronic infection.

✦ Antibiotic choices:

✧ Amoxil (amoxicillin) 250–500 mg q 8 hr (first line drug in acute sinusitis). May fail in purulent sinusitis due to beta lactamase + organism. **Adjust dose per creatinine clearance.**

✧ Augmentin (amoxicillin-clavulanate) 250–500 mg q 12 hr (beta lactamase inhibitor). **Adjust dose per creatinine clearance.**

✧ Bactrim or Septra (sulfamethoxzole-trimethoprim) one regular-strength tab bid to one double-strength tab bid. **Follow renal function closely; acute renal failure is common in the elderly.**

✧ Ceftin (cefuroxime axetil) 250 mg bid.

✧ Vibramycin (doxycycline hyclate) 100 mg bid day one, 100 mg daily thereafter.

✧ Zithromax (azithromycin) comes as Z-Pak: 500 mg day one, then 250 mg × 4 days.

With the exception of Zithromax, treatment guidelines suggest 7–10 days of antibiotic for acute sinusitis; subacute/chronic sinusitis may require 2–3 weeks.

✦ Saline spray, prn. Warm, moist compresses to the face provide comfort and enhance drainage. **Crock pots (slow cookers) set on lowest setting are convenient when using compresses but may be safety hazard depending on functional status of patient. Water should be changed at least daily.**

✦ Restrict vasoconstricting drugs such as Afrin to 3 days. **Rhinitis medicamentosa or rebound rhinitis is common.**

KEY ISSUES

Patient/Caregiver Education

Patient/caregiver should be able to:

✦ Identify pharmaceutical agents by name and describe why it is given and potential side effects requiring notification of health care provider.

✦ Verbalize awareness of possible drug–drug interactions.

✦ Verbalize the need to report any unusual signs/symptoms to health care provider.

✦ Verbalize symptoms of secondary infection requiring additional treatment.

✦ Demonstrate proper technique in use of nasal inhalers.

✦ Identify changes in ADLs/IADLs requiring health care provider notification.

✦ Verbalize understanding in avoiding identified allergens.

✦ Verbalize understanding not to mix household cleaning agents.

✦ Verbalize the importance of beginning medication before the beginning of spring, summer, or fall seasonal allergies.

✦ Verbalize the importance of taking medication regularly in advance of allergen exposures to prevent perennial rhinitis.

✦ Verbalize understanding of transmission of infection and need for proper hand washing and tissue disposal.

Economic Considerations

✦ Financial constraints may prevent management compliance, especially with long-term treatment needs.

✦ Indoor climate control provides optimal management; however, this may be prohibitive. Other sources of heat/cooling may compromise management.

✦ Change in residence to decrease triggers may impose financial drain.

✦ Replacement of items such as feather pillows, down comforters, or carpeting can be costly.

✦ Baseline functional status may prevent client from vacuuming, dusting, etc. Hired help may be financially prohibitive.

✦ Nonsedating antihistamines are more expensive than sedating antihistamines.

✦ CT sinus x-rays cost same as plain films.

✦ Immunotherapy ("allergy shots") may be inconvenient, costly, yet should be offered if other treatment is unsuccessful.

Psychosocial Considerations

✦ Be alert for grieving/depression due to alteration in body image due to symptoms.

✦ A "drippy nose" is a common complaint leading to embarrassment and potential social isolation and alteration in ability to read or participate in activities requiring forward head tilts.

✦ Monitor for changes in cognitive status due to pharmaceutical agents.

Acute/Inpatient Setting

✦ Be alert for household cleaners as allergen triggers.

✦ Screen for immunizations.

✦ Severe sinusitis with fever and headache may require inpatient care, IV antibiotics.

Extended Care Setting

✦ Be alert for environmental allergens, especially household cleaning agents.

✦ Educate staff to monitor resident hand washing and proper tissue disposal.

Home Setting

✦ Assist patient/caregiver with environmental assessment for possible allergens, especially in bedroom and bathroom.

✦ Suggest routine air filter changes.

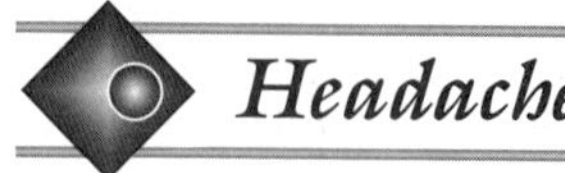

Headache

HISTORY

✦ Age? **Incidence of new onset of migraine headache decreases with age, but the risk of headache due to a serious medical problem increases 10-fold after age 65.**

✦ Gender? **Migraine and tension-type headaches predominate in females; cluster headaches occur more frequently in males.**

✦ Time of day headache usually occurs? Any pattern?

✦ Frequency?

✦ Duration?

✦ Location and severity of pain?

✦ Associated signs/symptoms: Fever, visual disturbances (diplopia), sinus congestion or drainage, nausea, vomiting, weakness, paresthesia, aphasia, vertigo, syncope, insomnia, disturbed sleep, daytime somnolence, neck pain or stiffness, teeth grinding, jaw tenderness, eye pain?

✦ Presence of prodromal symptoms (mood change, food cravings, visual changes, irritability, yawning, speech difficulties) or aura (scotomata, numbness in hands, dysphasia)?

✦ Alleviating treatment?

✦ Co-existing conditions: menopause, fasting, depression, history of head trauma, hypertension, rheumatoid arthritis, asthma, Raynaud's phenomenon, systemic lupus erythematosus (SLE)?

✦ Last dental examination? Last eye examination? Glasses or contacts? Changes in visual acuity?

✦ Medication review: note use of medications that may induce headache—hormone replacement therapy (HRT), nitrates, nitroglycerine, indomethacin, atenolol, captopril, griseofulvin, nifedipine, ranitidine, cimetidine. Note use of analgesics/OTC preparations for headache treatment.

✦ Family history of migraine headache?

✦ Intake of possible dietary triggers: excess caffeine; tyramine-containing foods; monosodium glutamate (Chinese foods); aspartame; yeast-containing foods; cheese (except for cottage cheese); chocolate; citrus; onions; chili; cinnamon; pickled, processed, or fatty foods; dairy products; EtOH?

✦ Extent to which headaches limit job performance, ability to perform ADLs/IADLs, or social interaction?

✦ Psychosocial stressors?

PHYSICAL EXAMINATION

✦ Vital signs.

✦ Head: inspect for signs of trauma; palpate scalp, sinuses, and TMJ for tenderness; inspect nose for deviated septum; inspect temporal arteries for enlargement and palpate for tenderness or induration.

✦ Eyes: inspect cornea, sclera; visual acuity screen; funduscopic examination for hypertensive retinopathy, papilloedema.

✦ Mouth: inspect for tooth erosion, which may indicate teeth grinding, or improper fit of dentures.

✦ Lymph: assess for adenopathy.

✦ Neuro: assess cranial nerves, especially pupil reactivity, extraocular movements, reflexes, motor strength, and sensation.

✦ Musculoskeletal: assess range-of-motion of neck; palpate posterior neck muscles for tenderness or contraction; palpate cervical vertebrae.

DIAGNOSTIC TESTS

✦ CBC with differential if suspect infectious process, systemic disorder, or meningitis.

✦ ESR—elevation may indicate temporal arteritis, multiple myeloma, hidden malignancy, or bacterial endocarditis.

✦ Urinalysis to screen for infection.

✦ Liver function tests.

✦ Consider x-ray of sinuses, although often low yield. Consider CT of sinuses.

✦ Consider thyroid function tests.

✦ *Normal aging changes may reduce predictive value of cervical x-rays.*

✦ Therapeutic drug levels as indicated.

✦ CT scan provides assessment of intracranial lesions or bleeding. MRI provides better interpretation of brain structures but not bleeding.

✦ If CT/MRI normal, analysis of cerebrospinal fluid with lumbar puncture. Lumbar puncture is contraindicated in presence of space-occupying lesion (seen on CT).

MANAGEMENT

✦ Begin with search for serious underlying etiology. **See Headache as Symptom of Increased Intercranial Pressure** (below). **See Protocol on Transient Ischemic Attack (TIA)/Cerebrovascular Accident (CVA).**

✦ See Table 2-2 for differential diagnosis of headache.

✦ Advise patient who presents with history of repetitive headaches to keep a headache diary for 6–8 weeks, recording:

✧ Date, time headache begins and ends.

✧ Location of pain.

✧ Rating of pain intensity (using scale 1–10).

✧ Possible trigger sources (foods, emotional stress, posture, sleep loss, hunger, eye strain, activity prior to onset).

Headache as Symptom of Increased Intercranial Pressure (Brain Mass, Subarachnoid Hemorrhage, Subdural Hemorrhage, Cerebral Aneurysm)

✦ Immediate referral to physician/emergency department if elderly patient presents with complaint of headache accompanied by any of the following:

✧ Sudden onset of severe pain.

✧ Slow progression of worsening pain.

✧ Onset with exertion, cough, sexual activity.

✧ Loss of balance.

✧ Nuchal rigidity.

✧ Papilloedema or fundal hemorrhage.

✧ Unequal or poorly reactive pupils.

✧ Sensory loss.

✧ Asymmetrical reflex or abnormal plantar reflex.

✦ Death rate is higher in the elderly when headache occurs as result of cerebral insult. **CT scan or MRI is indicated if severe headache of recent onset (especially if described as "worst headache of life" accompanied with neurological signs/symptoms, fever, or signs of meningitis).**

Migraine

✦ **Elderly rarely present with new onset of migraine. Be aware of atypical manifestation of migraine with aging. Migraine may present as complaint of slow progression of a neurological deficit over an extended period of minutes with or without pain. TIA/CVA must be excluded. See Protocol on Transient Ischemic Attack (TIA)/Cerebrovascular Accident (CVA).**

✦ Pain is usually unilateral but may be bilateral; pulsating pain of moderate to severe intensity; duration of 4–72 hr.

✦ 80% of patients have family history of migraine.

TABLE 2-2. Differential Diagnosis of Headache

	Characteristics	Management
Cluster headache	More prevalent in males 20–50 years of age; severe pain in orbit occurs during night, lasts approximately 1 hr for a few nights to weeks. Exacerbated by EtOH.	Treatment with propanolol, verapamil, or lithium.
Temporal arteritis	More common in elderly. Headache combined with pain in the temporal area, jaw pain with chewing, visual abnormalities, polymyalgia, weight loss, or fever. Markedly elevated ESR (>50 mm/hr Westergren method).	Prompt treatment with prednisone 40–60 mg PO qd to prevent permanent blindness. Refer to physician for biopsy to confirm diagnosis and establish long-term maintenance (steroid titrated to ESR and clinical symptoms).
Sinus headache	Pain at forehead or orbital area; may be accompanied by nasal congestion or discharge. Location of pain may change with change in position of head.	**See Protocol on Nasal Congestion.**
Acute glaucoma	Severe pain around orbit; nausea/vomiting; fixed and semidilated pupils with scleral injection.	**See Protocol on Glaucoma.**
Psychogenic headache	Associated with symptoms of depression or anxiety. Dull pressure; may occur with constant frequency and extended duration.	**See Protocols on Depression and Anxiety.**
Eye-strain headache	Occurs only during or after reading or other close work	Refer to ophthalmologist if indicated by acuity screen.
Herpes zoster/ post-herpetic headache	May occur up to 10 days before vesicles occur.	**See Protocol on Herpes Zoster.**
Sleep apnea	Frequent morning headache with daytime somnolence and insomnia.	Refer to pulmonologist for diagnosis/treatment of sleep apnea.
Trigeminal neuralgia	Brief, unilateral, shock-like pain. May be provoked by shaving, talking, washing face, or brushing teeth. Often accompanied by facial muscle spasm.	**See Protocol on Orofacial Pain.**

✦ May be associated with nausea/vomiting, photophobia, phonophobia.

✦ Frequency usually decreases with aging but may increase during menopause.

✦ Prodromal symptoms may occur 24 hr before onset.

✦ Usually preceded by aura 5–60 min before headache onset followed by neurological signs.

✦ Possible 24-hr postdrome of weakness, fatigue, sore muscles, or euphoria (secondary to relief).

✦ Treatment should be initiated at first sign. Prophylactic therapy is indicated if headaches occur more than two times per month.

✦ Management plan should include avoidance of triggers: loud noise, strong smells, flashing lights, missed meals, stress, foods.

✦ Acute treatment options:

✧ Anacin (aspirin/caffeine) 1–2 tablets 400 mg PO q 4 hr; maximum 10 tablets qd; contraindicated in renal or hepatic impairment.

✧ Tylenol (acetaminophen) 325–650 mg PO every 4 hr; maximum five doses qd; use cautiously to avoid hepatic impairment.

✧ Midrin (isometheptene mucate 65 mg, dichloralphenazone 100 mg, and acetaminophen 325 mg) two capsules at onset; may repeat in 1 hr; maximum dose five capsules every 12 hr.

✧ NSAIDs: Advil (ibuprofen) 200–400 mg every 4–6 hr, maximum dose 1,200 mg qd. May produce GI upset. Cautious use in hypertension, history of ulcer disease. Monitor renal function.

✧ Imitrex (sumatriptan) **oral form:** usual adult dose 25–50 mg at onset; geriatric dose 25 mg at onset; may be repeated at same dose in 1 hr; maximum of six doses; **subcutaneous form:** 6 mg at onset; may be repeated in 1 hr; **nasal spray preparation:** available as 5 mg and 20 mg preloaded doses; response varies widely with dose size; may repeat after 2 hr; maximum dose 40 mg qd. **Alert: clinical trials excluded patients > 65 years. Contraindicated in ischemic heart disease, Prinzmetal's angina, hemiplegic or basilar migraine, uncontrolled hypertension, concomitant MAOI therapy. Cardiovascular evaluation in patients with risk factors should be completed prior to initiation of therapy.**

✧ Ergostat (ergotamine tartrate): usual adult dose 2 mg sublingually, geriatric dose 1 mg sublingually; may repeat every 30 min until relieved; maximum dose 6 mg qd. **Ergotamine preparations are not initial choice for use in elderly because of potential side effects of nausea, vomiting, diarrhea, paresthesia. Use with caution in patients with peptic ulcer or hypertension. Contraindicated in liver disease, vascular disease.**

✧ Ergotamine inhaler (Medihaler-Ergotamine) one spray immediately; repeat q 5 min as needed; maximum dose six inhalations qd.

✧ Cafergot (ergotamine tartrate 2 mg and caffeine 100 mg) suppository; one suppository followed by one suppository in 1 hr if needed; maximum dose two suppositories qd.

- ✧ Concomitant antiemetic therapy may be needed.

✦ Prophylactic treatment options:

✧ Beta-blockers: Inderal (propanolol HCl) 20 mg qd. Contraindicated in asthma, heart failure, chronic obstructive pulmonary disease (COPD), or atrioventricular (AV) conduction disorders, concomitant MAOI therapy.

✧ Calcium channel blockers: verapamil, diltiazem, nifedipine. Selection of agent based on site of action.

✧ Depakote (dilvalproex sodium) 250 mg PO bid; maximum dose 1,000 mg qd. Contraindicated in hepatic disease.

✧ Elavil (amitriptyline HCl) effective dose ranges from 10 to 175 mg PO; beginning geriatric dose 10 mg PO every night with increase of 10 mg at 2-week intervals. **Side effect of sedation increases risk of injury for elderly patient.** Anticholinergic effects of dry mouth or urinary retention may be bothersome. SSRI agents may be alternatives to tricyclics in migraine prophylaxis.

Tension or Muscular Contraction Headache

✦ 90% of all headaches occurring in the elderly are tension headaches.

✦ Characterized by bilateral pain, often located in the headband region, with a tightening, not throbbing, quality.

✦ Not aggravated by physical activity.

✦ Have slow progression but last for extended periods.

✦ May be associated with muscle spasms.

✦ Not associated with nausea, vomiting, prodrome or aura, or neurological deficits.

✦ Begin treatment with identification and reduction of triggers: lack of sleep, emotional stress, poor posture, eye strain, hunger, foods.

✦ Recommend relaxation therapy as indicated:

✧ Deep breathing.

✧ Meditation.

✧ Exercise.

✧ Massage.

✧ Biofeedback.

✦ Avoid remaining in same position for long periods and reading in insufficient light or glare.

✦ Cold therapy (ice pack) or warm therapy (warm shower) may be useful for acute onset.

✦ Acute therapy options include aspirin, acetaminophen, and NSAIDs (**see Migraine**).

✦ Many elderly patients treat tension headache with OTC medications such as combinations of analgesic and caffeine.

✦ Prophylaxis if headaches occur more than twice a week. Tricyclic antidepressant is drug of choice.

Mixed Headache

✦ Characterized by chronic, daily tension-type headache with intermittent migraine headaches.

✦ If headaches are severe, tricyclic antidepressant: amitriptyline or nortriptyline given at bed time. Consider combination with a beta-blocker, verapamil, or Depakote (divalproex sodium) usual adult dose 250–1,000 mg qd in divided doses. Side effects nausea, sedation.

Drug-Induced Rebound Headache

✦ Common with withdrawal from many analgesics (NSAIDs, acetaminophen, narcotics).

✦ Occur as result of treating headache with ergotamine preparations, aspirin, acetaminophen, barbiturates, or caffeine for prolonged periods (> 30 days) more frequently than qod. **Use of NSAIDs does not usually cause rebound.**

✦ More common in females.

✦ Psychological or physiological dependence on medication usually present.

✦ Onset on waking of headache (caused by drug-free overnight period) that persists throughout the day; mild-to-moderate, dull pain; bilaterally diffuse or frontal-occipital location.

✦ No accompanying visual or autonomic disturbance, but superimposition of migraine may occur.

✦ History of medication q 3–4 hr with transient, incomplete relief.

✦ **Treatment must include withdrawal from current headache regimen.** If non-narcotic use, withdrawal should be abrupt. If narcotic, gradual withdrawal and use of neuroleptic is indicated. **See Acute/Inpatient Setting** (below).

✦ With medication withdrawal, severe headache will occur. With previous ergotamine use, onset of headache may be delayed, but duration will be prolonged. Headache will last 72 hr.

✦ **Critical management issue is to remain off medication.** Following wean, patients should be advised to maintain headache diary for 2 months. Management then proceeds based on identification of headache type.

Menopausal Headache

✦ Common among women taking HRT. Nonfluctuating levels of estrogen may be less likely to cause headache. Consider use of low-dose transdermal estradiol 0.0375 mg/day or ethinyl estradiol 0.02 mg/day.

✦ May be secondary to menopausal changes rather than HRT. Consider prophylaxis with Calan (verapamil) usual adult dose 240 mg qd; maximum dose 600 mg qd.

KEY ISSUES

Patient/Caregiver Education

Patient/caregiver should be able to:

✦ State purposes for medications and appropriate dosing.

✦ State potential side effects of therapy.

✦ Verbalize importance of headache diary and use of results to avoid triggers.

✦ Rate pain on a continuum. Select and work toward a target level of symptom relief.

Psychosocial Considerations

✦ Chronic pain, frequent headaches may produce psychologic reactions, medication dependency.

✦ Provide emotional support during withdrawal period of rebound headache treatment. Elderly may interpret withdrawal of medication as punitive.

✦ Manage associated anxiety or depression.

Acute/Inpatient Setting

✦ Severe headache may require hospitalization for diagnosis and management.

✦ Patients admitted for drug-induced rebound headache may require IV fluids, sedatives, hypnotics, and antiemetics for up to 14 days if severe withdrawal symptoms occur.

Home Setting

✦ Medications prescribed for other members of residence may be misused. Potential for drug–drug interactions should be emphasized.

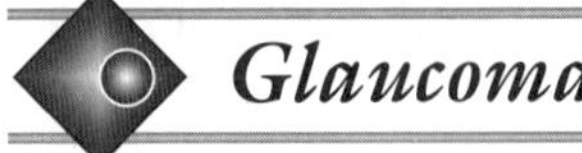

Glaucoma

HISTORY

✦ Blurred vision?

✦ Perception of colored haloes around lights?

✦ Ocular pain? Onset, duration, character? **Acute closed angle glaucoma presents as a painful inflamed eye; an ophthalmologic emergency.**

✦ Subjective visual field defects? **Most patients are unaware of their visual field defects until disease is advanced. Glaucoma is third leading cause of blindness after cataracts and macular degeneration.**

✦ Decreased visual acuity?

✦ Loss of color vision?

✦ Complaints of seeing flashes or floaters?

✦ Sense of "painless pressure" in the eye?

✦ History of blackouts, headaches, weakness, ischemic symptoms? **Neurological symptoms in the presence of low tension glaucoma are an indication for a neurological referral. Low tension glaucoma is considered in patients with progressive disc cupping and field loss with normal or mildly elevated intraocular pressure (IOP). 20–50% of all primary open angle glaucoma (POAG) fall into this category; more common in elderly.**

✦ History of hypertension, thyroid disease, diabetes mellitus? **Known association with POAG.**

✦ History of cataracts? Eye surgery? Macular degeneration? Other eye disorders or infections? **Secondary open angle glaucoma occurs in association with another eye disease or trauma. See Protocol on Age-Related Macular Degeneration.**

✦ History of trauma to eye/face? (Even distant trauma.)

✦ Last eye examination?

✦ Family history of glaucoma? **POAG is most common type of glaucoma; occurs insidiously with no identified etiology except genetic or hereditary predisposition. POAG is a diagnosis of exclusion.**

✦ Medications? Use of corticosteroids, beta blockers, calcium channel blockers? Eye drops?

✦ Functional status? Ability to self-administer eye drops?

✦ Race? (More prevalent in black population.)

PHYSICAL EXAMINATION

✦ Older patients should be encouraged to have an annual eye examination by an ophthalmologist.

✦ Assess visual acuity and visual fields

✦ Complete eye examination including fundoscopic. **Increased pallor and cupping on the temporal sides of the discs and asymmetry of the physiologic cup between eyes is suspicious for early glaucoma.**

✦ Complete neurological examination if symptoms warrant.

✦ Focused examination based on individual patient.

DIAGNOSTIC TESTS

✦ IOP by tonometry; several air-puff screening tonometers are available. IOP of ≥ 22 mm Hg is suspicious for glaucoma. **Approximately 15% of elderly have increased IOP, which may progress to vision loss. Goal of treatment is to prevent visual loss.**

✦ Elevated IOP should be confirmed by applanation tonometry and referred to an ophthalmologist for specialty eye examination.

✦ Formal visual field testing identifies optic nerve impairment.

PREVENTION

✦ Recommend and refer for annual eye examination for all patients.

✦ If glaucoma is suspected, more frequent examinations by an ophthalmologist are recommended.

✦ **See Protocol on Prevention and Health Maintenance.**

MANAGEMENT

✦ It is essential to know whether glaucoma is open or closed angle. Records may be obtained from ophthalmologist.

✦ Open angle glaucoma is often first treated medically. Laser trabeculoplasty (LTP) is usually used only when medical therapy fails or visual loss progresses.

✦ Closed angle glaucoma is primarily treated surgically with peripheral iridectomy.

✦ Reinforce education on correct instillation of ocular drugs. Nasolacrimal (NL) occlusion (finger pressure) for 3 min during and after drug instillation improves response of medications and may allow less frequent administration with lower concentrations.

✦ Reinforce compliance with ocular medications. **Patient may benefit from a drug card detailing medications and schedule. Consider preparing a card for each eye if schedules are different.**

✦ **Pharmacologic therapy will be initiated and adjusted by an ophthalmologist. However, the nurse practitioner (NP) may have many patients in his or her practice using these agents and should be knowledgeable of their usage and possible side effects.**

✦ The general strategy in medical management of POAG is to begin with a beta blocker or epinephrine compound or combination of the two, add a miotic, apraclonidine, or topical carbonic anhydrase inhibitors (CAI) if needed. LTP, oral CAI, or filtration surgery are additional treatment options (see Display 2-4).

KEY ISSUES

Patient/Caregiver Education

Patient/caregiver should be able to:

✦ Describe ocular medication regimen.

✦ Correctly instill eye drops and differentiate between prescriptions.

✦ Describe importance of consistent use of medications even after symptoms improve or if no symptoms are present.

✦ Identify and discuss functional limitations secondary to low vision.

✦ Demonstrate proper use of adaptive equipment and low-vision aids.

Economic Considerations

✦ **See Protocol on Age-Related Macular Degeneration.**

Psychosocial Considerations

✦ Assess for anxiety, depression, social withdrawal, and isolation secondary to visual changes.

✦ Visual loss greatly impairs functional status and life satisfaction.

✦ Fear of loss of vision adds to emotional stress; may exacerbate symptoms of depression.

Acute/Inpatient Setting

✦ Continue ocular medication regimen during hospitalization.

✦ Be alert to adverse effects of medications.

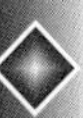

DISPLAY 2-4. *Medications to Treat Glaucoma*

Beta Adrenergic Blockers

Decrease intraocular pressure by decreasing aqueous humor formation. Nonselective beta blockers may produce systemic effects, i.e., slowed heart rate, decreased blood pressure (BP), exacerbation of asthma or congestive heart failure, altered mental status. Also may enhance effects of systemic beta blockers and digoxin. Usual dose is 1 gtt bid.

Nonselective

Timoptic (timolol maleate) 0.25% or 0.5%, also available in gel form
Betagan (levobunolol HCl) 0.25% or 0.5%
Ocupress (carteolol HCl) 1%
OptiPranolol (metipranolol) 0.3%

Selective

Betoptic (betaxolol HCl) 0.25% or 0.5%
Cardioselective beta blocker, which may have less effect on the respiratory system.

Sympathomimetics

Improve aqueous outflow.
Epifrin (epinephrine HCl) 0.5, 1% or 2%
Epinal (epinephrine borate) 0.5 or 1%
Propine (dipivefrin HCl) 0.1%, causes fewer systemic effects than epinephrine

Miotics

Parasympathomimetic agents that mimic the effect of acetylcholine within the eye. Consist of two categories: direct acting (cholinergic) and indirect acting (cholinesterase inhibitors).

Cholinergic

Isopto Carbachol (carbachol) 0.75%, 1.5%, 2.25%, or 3%
Ocusert-Pilo (pilocarpine): ocular inserts
Isopto Carpine (pilocarpine HCl) 0.25–10%, available in a wide variety of strengths and under different brand names.
Pilagan (pilocarpine nitrate) 2% or 4%

(continued)

DISPLAY 2-4. *Continued*

Cholinesterase inhibitors

Eserine ophthalmic ointment (physostigmine) 0.25%
Humorsol (demecarium) 0.125% or 0.25%
Phospholine Iodide (echothiophate iodide) 0.03%, 0.06%, 0.125%, or 0.25%

ALPHA-SELECTIVE AGONISTS

Increase aqueous humor outflow.

Iopidine (apraclonidine) 0.5% or 1%, available in single dose applicator for suppression of acute intraocular pressure spikes after laser treatments. Generally useful for short-term therapy, increased risk of tachyphylaxis within 3 months.
Alphagan (brimonidine) 0.2%, can be used on a chronic basis with reduced risk of tachycardia.

CARBONIC ANHYDRASE INHIBITORS (CAIS)

Used both topically and systemically to reduce aqueous secretion. Systemic agents are limited by side effects, i.e., paresthesias, anorexia, GI upsets, headaches, altered taste/smell, sodium/potassium depletion, ureteral colic, and a predisposition for renal calculi.

Azopt (brinzolamide) 1% ophth. suspension
Diamox or Diamox Sequels (acetazolamide) 125–250 mg tablets or 500 mg timed-release capsules
Daranide (dichlorphenamide) 50 mg tablets
Neptazane (methazolamide) 25–50 mg tablets
Trusopt (dorzolamide HCl) 2%

PROSTAGLANDINS

Increase aqueous humor outflow.
Xalatan (latanoprost) 0.005%

HYPEROSMOTIC AGENTS

Create an osmotic gradient between the blood and intraocular fluid, causing flow of aqueous humor into the bloodstream.

Osmoglyn (glycerin) 50% 1–1.5 g/kg PO
Ismotic (isosorbide) 45% 1.5 g/kg PO
Osmitrol (mannitol) 5–20% 0.5–2 g/kg IV
Ureaphil (urea) powder or 30% solution 0.5–2 g/kg IV

✦ Consider referral to occupational therapy (OT) for functional assessment and recommendations for needed adaptations related to low vision.

✦ Consider referral to physical therapy (PT) for assessment of gait, safety, use of assistive devices.

✦ Make written patient education materials available in large print.

Extended Care Setting

✦ Communicate ocular medication regimen on transfer to extended care facilities.

✦ **See Protocol on Age-Related Macular Degeneration.**

Home Setting

✦ Assist with strategies to help improve compliance with eye drops.

✦ Consider home OT evaluation for home adaptations to maintain independence with low vision.

✦ **See Protocol on Age-Related Macular Degeneration.**

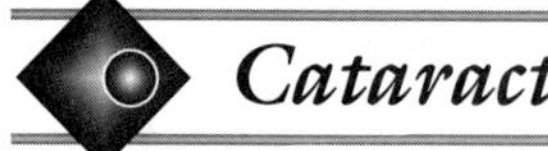

Cataract

HISTORY

✦ Age is the strongest risk factor for development of cataract. **95% of those > 65 years of age have some degree of lens opacity. The number of cases of senescent blinding cataract is expected to double by the year 2010.**

✦ Sex? Risk is slightly higher in females.

✦ Race? **In the U.S., discrepancies exist in access to care. African Americans are 30% less likely than whites to undergo surgical removal of cataract.**

✦ Normal aging of the eye results in loss of lens flexibility, loss of accommodation to changes in light intensity, and denaturation of lens proteins.

✦ Cloudy, filmy, or hazy vision? Change in way colors are seen? **Yellowing of lens with cataract may interfere with blue-green vision.**

✦ Problems driving at night because headlights seem too bright or glare from sunlight, lamps, or other lighting? With cataract, vision is worse in bright light because multiple opacities have light-scattering effect.

✦ Diplopia? Refractive changes of the lens that occur with cataract may not be uniform.

✦ **The elderly may attribute visual changes to "normal" aging and underreport.**

✦ Depression? May result from impaired vision.

✦ History of falls or injury as a result of decreased vision?

✦ Past medical history: Eye puncture injury or inflammation of eye? Frequent changes in eyeglass prescription? Diabetes mellitus (increased incidence of cataract)? Steroid-dependent COPD? **Surgical removal of cataract may not be recommended in patients with co-existing macular degeneration, chronic or simple glaucoma, or diabetic retinopathy because of underlying blindness.**

✦ Medications: Especially note those which may contribute to cataract development—steroids, allopurinol, diuretics, tranquilizers, cholesterol-lowering medications, cancer chemotherapy.

✦ Tobacco or heavy EtOH use? **Increases risk.**

✦ **Family history of cataract increases risk.**

✦ Diet history?

✦ Reduced functional status?

✦ Social isolation?

PHYSICAL EXAMINATION

✦ General appearance. Inspect for signs of inability to perform grooming secondary to impaired vision.

✦ Eyes:

✧ Inspect with pen light. Opacity may or may not be visible depending on maturity of cataract. Yellowing of lens indicates advanced nuclear sclerosis; white opacity indicates advanced anterior cortical changes.

✧ Visual acuity examination with Snellen chart/hand-held visual card.

✧ Ophthalmoscopic examination. Red reflex may be partially or completely obscured by opacities. Black, spoke-like opacities indicate anterior or posterior cortical cataract.

✧ Most affected elderly will have bilateral cataracts. **Falls and hip fracture are more likely to occur with single cataract than if cataract in both eyes.**

✦ Neuro: observe gait. Be alert for unsteadiness caused by visual impairment rather than neurological problem.

✦ Functional assessment: note limitations secondary to decreased visual acuity.

DIAGNOSTIC TESTS

✦ **See Management.**

PREVENTION

✦ If possible, avoid prolonged use of steroids.

✦ Limit exposure to intense sunlight.

✦ Wear protective eye covering if exposed to x-rays, infrared lamps, microwaves, ultraviolet (UV) light.

✦ Antioxidant properties of vitamins (E, C) and trace minerals may be protective against development of cataract. Current data are inconclusive.

✦ Some data suggest a protective effect against cataracts with HRT; no similar protection from endogenous estrogen.

✦ **See Protocol on Prevention and Health Maintenance.**

MANAGEMENT

✦ **Refer patients with suspected cataract to ophthalmologist for slit lamp examination for confirmation of suspected cataract and to determine what part of lens is affected. Eyes will be dilated prior to examination.**

✦ For early cataract when surgery is not yet indicated, recommend:

✧ Changes in eyeglass prescription or stronger bifocals if needed.

✧ Use of low-vision aids. Stand magnifiers are useful for those with hand tremor.

✧ Large-print materials, enlarged telephone dials, books on audio tape, and closed-circuit television. Adequate lighting.

✧ Limit glare with sunglasses and hats. Use non-glare lighting.

✧ Consider application of antireflective coating to eyeglasses to reduce glare.

✧ Encourage use of reds and oranges and contrast in environment to enhance safety.

✦ Surgical removal is indicated if patient has reduced ability to work or perform ADLs/IADLs, reduced life satisfaction, increased injury risk, problems with driving, or other conditions such as phacomorphic glaucoma (need for lens extraction may be urgent) or diabetic retinopathy (lens extraction necessary to allow treatment of retinopathy).

✦ **Age is not a contraindication to surgical removal of cataract.** Most cataract extractions are done as outpatient procedures under local anesthesia.

✦ In otherwise healthy eyes, cataract removal has a 95% success rate.

✦ Because of risk, surgery will be performed on only one eye at a time. If patient is blind in one eye, ophthalmologist will counsel patient and family regarding risk prior to performing surgery.

✦ Based on patient profile, ophthalmologist will recommend one of the following procedural options for cataract extraction:

✧ Extracapsular—lens is removed and posterior capsule (outer covering of lens) is left.

✧ Phacoemulsification—lens is softened with ultrasound and removed through a needle. Posterior capsule is left.

✧ Intracapsular—both lens and capsule are removed. This option is rarely used.

✦ Topical medication is usually prescribed post-op by ophthalmologist:

✧ Genoptic (gentamicin sulfate 3 mg/ml) ophthalmic solution.

✧ Pred Forte (prednisolone acetate 1%) ophthalmic solution.

✧ Mydriacyl (tropicamide 0.5% or 1%) ophthalmic solution.

✧ Cyclogyl (cyclopentolate HCl 0.5% or 1%) ophthalmic solution.

    ✧ Diamox Sequel (acetazolamide 500 mg sustained-release capsule).
    ✧ TobraDex (tobramycin 0.3% + dexamethasone 0.1%) ophthalmic solution.
    ✧ Aquafilm/Liquid tears.

✦ Medication for pain relief will be prescribed by ophthalmologist.

✦ Following surgery, lens will be replaced with plastic disc (intraocular lens), contacts, or cataract glasses will be prescribed.

✦ Contacts may be difficult for some elderly to put in because of reduced dexterity.

✦ Patients using cataract glasses: will need 2 pairs—one for near and one for distant vision, will have restriction of visual field to area straight ahead, will have to relearn to judge distances. Peripheral fields will be distorted.

✦ Cataract glasses should only be used by patients with bilateral cataract removal or single removal but blind in other eye; otherwise, diplopia will result from use of glasses.

✦ Follow-up by ophthalmologist is required 6–12 weeks post-op to monitor for increased IOP, pain level, and efficacy of surgery.

✦ Complications of cataract surgery include: vitreous loss with anterior migration and corneal edema, intraocular hemorrhage, infection, opacification of posterior capsule, glaucoma, and retinal detachment.

✦ Consider referral to home health agency:

    ✧ Patients with physical limitations that may compromise recovery.
    ✧ Patients, especially those with second cataract remaining, who will require assistance with medication administration.
    ✧ Patients with reduced cognitive status.

KEY ISSUES

Patient/Caregiver Education

✦ Copies of the booklet "Cataract in Adults: A Patient's Guide" published by the United States Department of Health and Human Services are available by calling toll-free 1-800-358-9295.

✦ If patient undergoing surgical removal of cataract is seen in clinic by NP prior to surgery, patient/caregiver should be able to:

    ✧ Verbalize that blurring following surgery is normal.
    ✧ Verbalize that several weeks will be needed following surgery before full improvement is seen.
    ✧ Identify support person who will be able to drive patient home and remain with patient for at least 24 hr after surgery.
    ✧ List necessary home safety precautions following surgery.

✧ State understanding of topical medication regimen and importance of administering as prescribed.

✧ List potential side effects of eye drops and pain relief medications. State potential for drug interactions with medications taken for other conditions.

✧ Verbalize proper use of eye patch.

✧ Verbalize the importance of avoiding bending, lifting weight, or strenuous exercise for several weeks following surgery.

✧ List indications for notifying ophthalmologist after surgery (increased pain or change in nature of eye pain, increase in eye discharge, no improvement in vision after expected time, questions regarding medications).

Economic Considerations

✦ Limited income and limited access to transportation may prevent elderly from seeking care.

✦ Surgical removal of cataract may help patients to assume previous household duties, thus allowing care givers to return to work.

✦ In the U.S., the typical cost of cataract surgery is $2,500, making the procedure cost effective compared with the potential burden of visual impairment.

Psychosocial Considerations

✦ Visual impairment from cataract may cause loss of hobbies, recreational activities, and social isolation.

✦ Assess for anxiety/depression, social withdrawal/isolation secondary to:

✧ Low vision.

✧ Fear of further loss of vision.

✧ Change in body image.

✧ Loss of hobbies or recreational activities.

✧ Loss of independence.

Extended Care Setting

✦ Consider cataract in residents who exhibit decrease in functional status or symptoms of depression. **Incidence of blindness is increased in extended care population compared to community-dwelling elderly.**

Home Setting

✦ Home care services may be needed for administration of medications and monitoring of dietary intake in patients with cataract.

✦ Refer to OT for home safety assessment to reduce injury risk from impaired vision and for education on low-vision aids and other home adaptations.

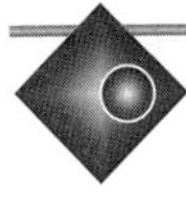

Age-Related Macular Degeneration

HISTORY

✦ Visual changes/decline? **Macular area is responsible for distinct vision and color discrimination. Leading cause of blindness in persons 65 years and older.**

✦ Loss of central vision? Intact peripheral vision? **Does not result in total blindness as an isolated disease because peripheral vision is preserved.**

✦ Onset? Sudden/gradual? Plateaus? **Normally slow, progressive decline alternating with periods of stability.**

✦ Difficulty reading? **Usually, first noted symptom.**

✦ Unilateral/bilateral? **May affect one eye initially, almost always becomes bilateral.**

✦ Visual hallucinations? **Known as Charles Bonnet syndrome: an uncommon, disturbing physiological, not psychological phenomenon in patients with bilateral loss of central vision.**

✦ History of farsightedness? Smoker? Chronic prolonged sun exposure or chronic exposure to chemicals? **All are risk factors.**

✦ History of other eye conditions such as cataracts or glaucoma?

✦ Last eye examination?

✦ Family history?

✦ Effect on ADLs and IADLs?

PHYSICAL EXAMINATION

✦ Assess iris, pupil. **Light-colored iris is a risk factor. Pupil is normal.**

✦ Ophthalmoscopic examination reveals drusen bodies in macular area of retina. **These small, lighter pink spots in the midperiphery enlarge over time, become yellow and confluent with symmetrical locations bilaterally.**

✦ Assess visual acuity using Snellen or Early Treatment Diabetic Retinopathy Sudy (ETDRS) chart and Rosenbaum or Jaeger near vision card. **Snellen chart has disadvantages, ETDRS chart is more reliable in those with low vision.**

✦ Assess vision using Amsler grid: note vertical and horizontal distortion of lines (metamorphosia) or areas of visual loss of lines (paracentral scotoma). **May detect initial abnormality in otherwise asymptomatic elder. Refer to PDR for Ophthalmology to find Amsler grid.**

✦ Perform functional evaluation asking patient to read newspaper, read medication label, tell time, count change, and read from large-print book.

DIAGNOSTIC TESTS

✦ Definitive testing is performed by ophthalmologist to diagnose and classify as:

✧ **Nonexudative (dry)**—responsible for 90% of cases, less severe visual loss. No treatment.

✧ **Exudative (wet)**—responsible for 10% of cases, accounts for most cases of legal blindness from age-related macular degeneration. Noted for hemorrhages in macula. Some elders respond to laser procedure. Amsler grid self-monitoring is important in this group.

PREVENTION

✦ No known prevention.

✦ Encourage yearly visual screening and examination to detect signs/symptoms of macular degeneration.

✦ Consider broad-spectrum antioxidant/multivitamin such as Ocuvite, although efficacy has not been substantiated.

✦ **See Protocol on Prevention and Health Maintenance.**

MANAGEMENT

✦ Positive history/physical findings require referral to ophthalmologist for definitive diagnosis.

✦ Encourage education strategies for self-assessment:

✧ Stress daily self-monitoring using Amsler grid and a near vision card.

✧ Set a routine time for daily self-monitoring.

✧ Store Amsler grid and near vision card in a highly visible place.

✧ Testing cards should be held 12–14 inches from eye with glasses in place, if prescribed.

✧ Test each eye separately, covering the opposite eye.

✧ Focus on center dot on the Amsler grid.

✧ Test for wavy lines or blank areas on the grid.

  - Mark abnormalities on grid for future reference.
  - Notify ophthalmologist of new changes.

KEY ISSUES

Patient/Caregiver Education

Patient/caregiver should be able to:

- Describe proper use of Amsler grid and near vision card.
- Describe action plan for changes noted when using Amsler grid.
- Identify and discuss functional limitations secondary to low vision.
- Demonstrate proper use of adaptive equipment.
- Demonstrate safe, adapted functions.
- Discuss anxieties and fears surrounding visual loss.
- Identify impact of low vision on social activities.

Economic Considerations

- Consider expense of low-vision adaptive aids. Some state/federal agencies provide free or reduced rate services.
- Consider costs of various modes of transportation.
- Consider costs of assistance with ADLs and IADLs.

Psychosocial Considerations

- Assess for anxiety/depression, social withdrawal/isolation secondary to:
  - Low vision.
  - Fear of progressive visual loss.
  - Change in body image.
  - Visual hallucinations.
  - Loss of independence.
  - Inability to drive.

Acute/Inpatient Setting

- Implement fall prevention program.
- Consider referral to low-vision program to assess for low-vision aids.
- Refer to PT to assess gait and safety issues to prevent functional decline.

✦ Refer to OT to assess and make recommendations for needed adaptations secondary to low vision.

✦ Implement patient education program with consideration of low-vision patient (large print, audio-presentations).

Extended Care Setting

✦ Implement a program of routine eye screening, refer patients with positive findings.

✦ Implement fall prevention program.

✦ Consider PT referral to prevent functional decline.

✦ Consider implementing self-help groups.

✦ Recommend needed adaptations secondary to low vision.

✦ Consider contacting community/state/federal agencies regarding services available for low-vision resident (i.e., audiotapes of books, music, reading of newspaper, adaptive aids, blind rehabilitation programs).

Home Setting

✦ Perform functional assessment of ADLs and IADLs (include ability to read and take medications properly).

✦ Assess for adequacy of needed social supports based on functional assessments.

✦ Consider referral to available agencies for transportation/needed social assistance secondary to low vision.

✦ Perform home safety assessment to identify and correct potential safety hazards.

✦ Consider PT and/or OT evaluations for adaptive equipment.

✦ Consider referral to blind rehabilitation services available in each state.

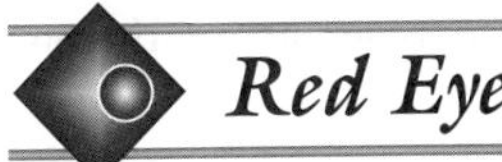

Red Eye

HISTORY

✦ Eye redness? Dryness? Increased tearing? One or both eyes? **Prevalence of dry eye is increased in the elderly. Symptoms are worse in the evening than the morning. Paradoxical reflex tearing is secondary to decreased basal tear secretion.**

✦ Burning, irritation, scratchy, gritty, or sandy sensation? Foreign body sensation? Itching?

✦ Discharge? Characteristics such as color, consistency, and amount. **Purulent discharge is usually seen in bacterial conjunctivitis, serous discharge in viral conjunctivitis, and stringy, mucoid discharge suggests allergic conjunctivitis.**

✦ Heaviness of eyelids? Swelling? Tenderness?

✦ Distorted vision? Light sensitivity?

✦ Eye pain? **Anesthetic drop relieves the pain of outer but not inner eye pathology.**

✦ Onset, duration of symptoms? Aggravating/alleviating factors? Previous episodes? Seasonal occurrence?

✦ Trauma? Fever? Sneezing or cough? Recent upper respiratory/sinus infection/fever blisters?

✦ Tobacco use? Chemical exposure? Use of or change in eye make-up or shampoo?

✦ Exposure to low humidity in cold climate, high altitudes, or airline travel?

✦ Contact lenses? Allergies?

✦ History of other eye disorders such as glaucoma or retinal hemorrhages?

✦ History of rheumatoid arthritis, Sjogren's, diabetes mellitus, lupus, sarcoidosis, psoriasis, gout, or seborrhea?

✦ Prescription/OTC medications? **Many medications taken by the elderly reduce tear secretion. Use of vasoconstrictive eye drops over time can lead to rebound vasodilation. Limit vasoconstrictive drops to 3 days at a time.**

✦ Do other family members or close contacts have similar symptoms? **Viral conjunctivitis is contagious 2 weeks after onset.**

PHYSICAL EXAMINATION

✦ Temperature, blood pressure (BP).

✦ Inspect for foreign body.

✦ Assess conjunctiva/sclera for hyperemia. **Diffuse hyperemia with conjunctivitis.**

✦ Assess extraocular movements and pupil. **Normal in conjunctivitis.**

✦ Access eyelids for color, swelling, tenderness, lash folliculitis, ectropion/entropion, masses, ptosis.

✦ Assess lid margins and conjunctiva for crusting, injection, mucus, and purulent discharge. **Purulent discharge, crusting/matting of lids and lashes is seen in bacterial conjunctivitis; serous discharge, erythema, edema of lids is seen in viral conjunctivitis.**

✦ Assess for loss of eye lashes and flaking along the lash lines.

✦ Palpate for preauricular lymphadenopathy. **Present in viral conjunctivitis.**

✦ Use Snellen and hand-held visual card to assess visual compromise.

✦ Assess ears, throat, nose, and auscultate chest to rule out infection.

✦ Assess functional status as it relates to ability to read prescription and dexterity to instill ocular medications.

DIAGNOSTIC TESTS

✦ No specific diagnostic tests.

✦ Fluorescein dye stains ulcerations; easily seen with a blue light if available.

✦ Consider gram stain, culture and sensitivity of purulent discharge or when purulent discharge persists after topical antibiotic. **External ocular infections generally respond to variety of topical antibiotics.**

✦ Schirmer test evaluates tearing. Special paper filter strips are inserted over the lower eyelid margin. The wetting is measured after 5 min. A moistened area of less than 5 mm is abnormal.

PREVENTION

✦ Teach good hand washing technique.

✦ Avoid using the same washcloth and towel to cleanse the infected and unaffected eye.

✦ Avoid rubbing infected eye, then unaffected eye.

✦ Avoidance of allergens as appropriate.

✦ **See Protocol on Prevention and Health Maintenance.**

MANAGEMENT

See Table 2-3 for differential diagnosis of the red eye.

TABLE 2-3. Differential Diagnosis of the Red Eye

	Vision	Pupil size	Conjunctival injection	Corneal clarity	Discharge	Pain	Photo-phobia	Other
Conjunctivitis								
Viral	Unchanged	Normal	Generalized	Clear	Clear, watery	Foreign body sensation	None	Itching, pre-auricular nodes, contagious
Allergic	Unchanged	Normal	Generalized	Clear	Stringy, mucoid	Foreign body sensation	None	Itching may be seasonal
Bacterial	Unchanged	Normal	Generalized	Clear	Copious, purulent	Mild	None	No preauricular nodes
Subconjunctival hemorrhage	Unchanged	Normal	Hemorrhage	Clear	None	None	None	Rule out trauma and clotting abnormality
Keratitis (inflammation of the cornea)	Decreased	Varies: normal to small	Circumcorneal (ciliary-flush) and generalized	Loss of clarity	Excess tearing	Very painful	Yes	Ocular emergency

(continued)

TABLE 2-3. Continued

	Vision	Pupil size	Conjunctival injection	Corneal clarity	Discharge	Pain	Photo-phobia	Other
Uveitis (inflammation of iris, ciliary) body, and choroid	Decreased	Small; light directed in affected eye causes pain in unaffected eye	Ciliary flush	Clear	None	Very painful	Yes	Ocular emergency
Scleritis (inflammation of the sclera)	Unchanged	Normal	Sclera may have a violet/blue hue; conjunctiva is not involved	Clear	None	Yes, severe boring type with radiation to forehead and/or jaw; may intensify with movement of eye	—	Requires referral to ophthalmologist.
Acute angle closure glaucoma	Decreased	Dilated, fixed	Ciliary flush and generalized	Cloudy	None to watery	Severe pain	Yes	Ocular emergency

Entropion

✦ Due to lid laxity and decreased muscle tone of aging. Inward turning of upper or lower eyelid margins. Excess tearing can distort vision. Lashes irritate cornea and/or conjunctiva and increase risk of secondary infection and scarring.

✦ Some find temporary relief with adhesive strips to outwardly turn the lid.

✦ Refer to ocular plastic surgeon. Consult physician.

Ectropion

✦ Outward rotation of lower lid, secondary to lid laxity and decreased muscle tone of aging. Increased exposure of eye leads to excessive drying and increased risk of secondary infection. Paradoxical tearing can occur.

✦ Frequent use of lubricating agents is helpful (see Display 2-5).

✦ Some prefer upward taping of the lid to compensate for the laxity.

✦ Refer to ocular plastic surgeon. Consult physician.

Blepharoptosis

✦ Due to structural changes, lid laxity, and decreased muscle tone. Upper lid falls over cornea.

✦ Vision can be impaired.

✦ Night-time ectropion of the upper lid can occur with its consequences. **See Ectropion.**

✦ Refer to ocular plastic surgeon. Consult physician.

Blepharitis

✦ Present with scratchy sensation and red, irritated eyelid. **Common in the elderly; may be chronic.**

✦ Inflammation of eyelid margin is due to bacteria at base of lashes. Can occur secondary to seborrheic dermatitis. **See Protocol on Seborrheic Dermatitis.**

✦ Controllable, usually not cured.

✦ Suggest 1–2 min warm water compresses using clean wash cloth for each eye bid–tid. Rewet cloth as it cools; repeat process over 5-min period. This process loosens debris; helps liquefy oily secretions to avoid chalazion formation.

✦ Gently wash the lids for 15–20 sec using washcloth and mixture of approximately 2 drops no-tear shampoo in 8 oz glass of water.

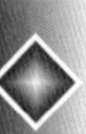

DISPLAY 2-5. *Lubricating Agent Considerations*

✦ Nonallergic reactions to preservatives and topical antibiotics are common.
✦ All preservatives have epithelial toxicity with prolonged use.
✦ Choose preservative-free agents when possible.
✦ Refrigerated drops often provide more comfort.
✦ Neomycin carries high incidence of hypersensitivity reactions.
✦ The thicker the drop, the longer it lasts.
✦ Thicker agents are likely to cause transient blurring and lash residue. Consider as safety concern.
✦ Ointments increase night-time and early morning dryness and can decrease frequency of day time drops. Consider as safety concern.
✦ **When uncertain of worsening condition, tolerance to drops, or hypersensitivity: increase frequency of drops.**
  ✧ **if hypersensitive—condition worsens.**
  ✧ **if dry—condition improves.**

✦ If severe, antibiotic ointment (erythromycin or bacitracin) can be applied to lid margins at bed time for 5–7 days.

✦ Refer to ophthalmologist if symptoms are resistant to conservative treatment. Consult physician.

Viral Conjunctivitis

✦ "Pink eye." **Caused by adenoviruses.**

✦ May be contagious for up to 2 weeks, symptoms may persist 3–4 weeks.

✦ Cool compresses for comfort.

✦ Lubricating drops.

✦ If pruritic, consider use of Naphcon-A (naphazoline HCl/pheniramine maleate) 1–2 gtts qid.

✦ Consider referral to ophthalmologist if symptoms worsen. Consult physician.

Allergic Conjunctivitis

✦ Itching and watery discharge are characteristic symptoms.

✦ Limit or eliminate allergens if possible.

✦ Cool compresses for comfort.

✦ Lubricating drops.

✦ If severe pruritus is present, consider Naphcon-A (naphazoline HCl/pheniramine maleate) 1–2 gtts qid.

✦ Use oral antihistamines with caution in the elderly secondary to sedating and anticholinergic side effects.

Bacterial Conjunctivitis

✦ Copious purulent discharge.

✦ Antibiotic as indicated by culture/sensitivity results. **Common organisms: staphylococcal species, streptococcal pneumoniae, and hemophilus species.**

✦ Topical agents such as ciprofloxacin, bacitracin, gentamicin, or erythromycin are generally used 2–3 days. **There is a high incidence of allergic reaction to neomycin-containing agents.**

✦ Refer to ophthalmologist when diagnosis is unclear, corneal involvement is suspected, or symptoms worsen. Consult physician.

Keratoconjunctivitis/Sicca

✦ Commonly known as "dry eye syndrome."

✦ Characteristic symptoms include constant foreign body sensation or gritty/sandy feeling, dryness, or paradoxical tearing. May also complain of "dry mouth."

✦ Suspect if red eye fails to respond to therapy.

✦ Especially seen in older females and patients with Sjogren's or rheumatoid arthritis.

✦ Frequent use of lubricating drops during the day and lubricating ointment at night.

Subconjunctival Hemorrhage

✦ Asymptomatic bleeding under conjunctiva.

✦ May be spontaneous but usually caused by intravascular pressure associated with coughing, sneezing, and straining.

✦ May occur with excessive rubbing of the eye.

✦ Negative history for trauma/bleeding disorders.

✦ Physical examination negative for retinal hemorrhage.

✦ No treatment required.

Corneal Abrasions/Ulcerations

✦ Incidence is high with contact lens use.

✦ Usually presents with severe pain, photophobia, and excess tearing.

✦ Refer to ophthalmologist. Consult physician.

✦ Usually resolves within 48 hr of treatment.

Keratitis

✦ Corneal inflammation.

✦ Presents with pain, photophobia, excess tearing, and decreased vision.

✦ Usually caused by adenovirus; can be caused by herpes simplex and zoster. **See Protocol on Herpes Zoster.**

✦ **Ophthalmologic emergency. Refer to ophthalmologist immediately. Consult physician.**

Uveitis

✦ Inflammation of iris, ciliary body, and choroid, the vascular supply to the outer layer of the retina.

✦ Presents with painful eye, photophobia, and decreased vision. Light directed in the uninvolved eye produces pain in the involved eye.

✦ There is inflammation of the iris and miotic pupil.

✦ Be suspect in patient who has positive history for sarcoidosis, tuberculosis, psoriasis, herpes simplex, or herpes zoster.

✦ Refer to ophthalmologist. Consult physician.

Scleritis

✦ Often presents with pain radiating to the forehead and or jaw.

✦ Sclera may have a blue hue.

✦ May become chronic.

✦ Be suspect in patients with positive history for rheumatoid arthritis, lupus, arthritis secondary to psoriasis, gout, thyrotoxicosis, pseudomonas, aspergillus, herpes simplex/zoster, and immunocompromised states.

✦ Refer to ophthalmologist. Consult physician.

Primary Angle Closure Glaucoma

✦ Common in elderly.

✦ Presents with severe pain/loss of vision. **See Protocol on Glaucoma.**

KEY ISSUES

Patient/Caregiver Education

Patient/caregiver should be able to:

✦ Verbalize understanding of etiology of red eye as it relates to their situation.

✦ Demonstrate proper instillation techniques for ocular medications.

✦ Verbalize importance of good hand washing.

✦ Demonstrate good hand washing technique.

✦ Demonstrate proper technique of contact lens cleaning/storing when appropriate.

✦ Demonstrate compliance with treatment interventions.

Economic Considerations

✦ Conditions may be chronic, requiring ongoing or recurrent treatment with frequent follow-up.

✦ Lubricating drops/ointments can be expensive, not covered by Medicare/supplement.

✦ Ask patient if he or she can afford prescribed medications before prescribing.

✦ Transportation to office setting can be costly.

Psychosocial Considerations

✦ Be alert to sleep deprivation, anxiety related to treatment requirements.

✦ Screen for depression.

Acute/Inpatient Setting

✦ Isolate contagious conditions per policy.

✦ Emphasize good hand washing technique.

✦ Be alert to latex allergies in patients receiving ocular instillations by personnel wearing latex gloves.

Extended Care Setting

✦ Be alert for red eye conditions and behavioral changes especially in the patient with dementia. Hygiene may be problematic.

✦ Teach staff to wash patients' hands frequently to prevent spread. Wash residents' hands well before allowing into congregate areas.

✦ Isolate contagious conditions per policy.

✦ Become familiar with available resources, because ophthalmology services are difficult to access at some facilities.

✦ Transportation to and from ophthalmologist may be financially difficult. Collaboration between NP and consultant is important.

Home Setting

✦ Consider OT evaluation for adaptive devices to aid ocular instillations.

✦ Assess for possible environmental allergens as indicated.

✦ Encourage patient to discard eye preparations every 3–6 months.

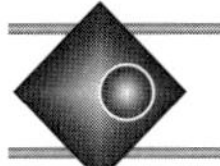

Mouth Lesions

HISTORY

✦ Onset, location, duration of lesions?

✦ Associated pain, burning, drainage?

✦ History of chronic conditions, i.e., diabetes mellitus, dementia, cancer, immunocompromised states?

✦ Recent acute infections, fever, serious illness?

✦ History of radiation therapy or chemotherapy?

✦ Presence of prodromal or systemic symptoms?

✦ Change in weight?

✦ Last dental examination? Use/fit of dentures?

✦ Oral hygiene routine?

✦ Recent stressors?

✦ Tobacco use in any form? EtOH use?

✦ Medications? **Patients on inhaled or oral steroids, oral hypoglycemics, insulin, or recent antibiotic treatment may be at risk for oral candidiasis.**

PHYSICAL EXAMINATION

✦ Temperature, hydration status.

✦ Examine oropharyngeal cavity. **Oral lesions are often asymptomatic and found during routine examination. Inspect after removing dentures. Examine area underneath tongue.**

✦ Palpate mucosal surfaces.

✦ Note location, appearance of lesion(s), condition of teeth/gums.

✦ Perform a general examination of the skin, especially in skin folds, under breasts, groin, perineal area for associated lesions.

✦ Palpate for lymph node involvement.

DIAGNOSTIC TESTS

✦ A KOH microscopic prep will demonstrate Candida; staining may reveal multinucleated epithelial (giant) cells of herpetic lesions.

✦ Consider electrolytes, BUN if suspected dehydration.

✦ Consider glucose, hemoglobin A1C if patient has diabetes.

✦ Refer for biopsy if lesions are ulcerated, raised, or firm.

PREVENTION

✦ Regular mouth care. **Especially important for patients who are at risk for mouth lesions, i.e., patients with feeding tubes, dementia, diabetes, tobacco use, immunocompromised, or those using inhaled steroids.**

✦ Encourage regular dental/periodontal care and examinations.

✦ Consider adding yogurt, buttermilk to diet during antibiotic therapy.

✦ Consider adding Lactinex one packet mixed with water tid–qid during antibiotic therapy (may be given enterally).

✦ Avoid tobacco use.

✦ Rinse mouth thoroughly after use of inhaled steroids; clean inhaler mouthpiece after each use.

✦ Maintain adequate nutrition and hydration.

✦ Maintain good control of diabetes mellitus.

✦ **See Protocol on Prevention and Health Maintenance.**

MANAGEMENT

Oral Candidiasis

Appears as painful white plaque on an erythematous base; usually involves tongue but may occur on any oral mucosa surface.

✦ Mycostatin (nystatin) oral suspension, 100,000 U/ml, 5 ml swish and swallow tid for 5 days. May be swabbed onto tongue if patient is unable to cooperate.

✦ Mycostatin pastilles (nystatin trochees), 200,000 U/ml, 1–2 dissolved slowly in mouth four to five times daily for 7–10 days.

✦ Consider Lactinex one packet in water tid–qid for 5 days.

✦ Consider adding yogurt or buttermilk to diet; avoid high sucrose foods.

✦ Xylocaine (lidocaine HCl 2%) viscous solution may help reduce discomfort early in the course of treatment.

✦ Treat topical candidiasis lesions with Mycostatin (nystatin) cream tid.

✦ Soak dentures and toothbrush in bleach (sodium hypochlorite) for 5 min daily to prevent reinfection and recurrence.

✦ Consult physician if systemic candidiasis suspected; consider oral Nizoral (ketoconazole) 200–400 mg daily, Diflucan (fluconazole) 50–200 mg daily, or Sporanox (itraconazole) 200–400 mg daily.

Herpetic Stomatitis

Vesicle or group of vesicles that evolve into ulcers; usually at vermillion border of lips; contagious; short-lived, often with 24–48 hr prodromal burning sensation.

✦ Symptomatic treatment. **Lesions usually crust in 4–10 days.**

✦ Maintain adequate nutrition and hydration during acute phase.

✦ Consider antiseptic mouth rinse.

✦ Consider oral Zovirax (acyclovir) 800 mg 5 times daily for 7 days in immunocompromised patients. Reduce dose with renal impairment.

Aphthous Ulcers

Indurated papules that progress to painful ulcers covered by yellow fibrinous membranes and surrounded with erythematous halos.

✦ Symptomatic treatment with liquid antacids, mouth rinse, or 3% hydrogen peroxide/water solution 1:1 as gargle or topical preparation of Gly-oxide (carbamide peroxide 10%) for mild episodes.

✦ Consider Xylocaine (lidocaine HCl 2%) viscous solution as a mouth wash or applied topically every 3–4 hr.

✦ Consider topical Kenalog (triamcinolone acetonide) in orabase applied after meals and at bed time.

✦ Consult physician regarding possible use of oral steroids.

✦ Consider topical antibiotic: Achromycin-V (tetracycline HCl) oral suspension 125 mg/5 ml, rinse with 2 tsp for 2 min, then swallow. Use every 6 hr for 7 days.

Angular Cheilitis

✦ Examine for erythema, scaling, fissures at corners of the mouth.

✦ Treat with topical Mycostatin (nystatin) cream bid until resolved.

✦ Soak dentures in Mycostatin (nystatin) suspension during daily cleaning.

Oral Cancer

Painless lump in the mouth, tongue, under the tongue or neck often associated with a history of tobacco or EtOH use. May present with associated symptoms of weight loss, dysphagia, ageusia, or hoarseness.

✦ **Be alert to any lesion that is increasing in size, painless, ulcerated, indurated, or in a patient with risk factors for oral cancer.**

✦ Refer any suspicious lesion to an otolaryngologist immediately.

Lesions Associated with Radiation Therapy

Patients receiving radiation therapy are at risk for oral mucosal inflammation, loss of dentition, malnutrition, and salivary gland dysfunction.

✦ Arrange for dental consultation prior to initiation of radiation therapy.

✦ Be alert to dysphagia; alter dietary consistency to maintain patient comfort and promote good nutrition. Cool foods, foods that require little chewing and dietary supplements may be helpful.

✦ A mouthwash combining Xylocaine (lidocaine HCl 2%) viscous solution, hydrogen peroxide, or Benadryl (diphenhydramine) and nystatin suspension may be soothing.

✦ Artificial saliva may be useful for xerostomia. Salagen (pilocarpine HCl) 5 mg tid–qid may be helpful with severe xerostomia associated with head and neck cancer.

KEY ISSUES

Patient/Caregiver Education

Patient/caregiver should be able to:

✦ Explain the importance of maintaining adequate nutrition/hydration during acute phases.

✦ Describe risk factors for oral lesions.

✦ Verbalize the treatment regimen prescribed.

✦ Discuss appropriate oral hygiene including denture care and need to remove dentures at night. For care of natural teeth, use soft toothbrush and toothpaste with fluoride.

✦ Discuss contact precautions when lesions are contagious.

Economic Considerations

✦ Good oral hygiene is inexpensive; prevention of oral lesions is an important treatment goal.

✦ No Medicare reimbursement for dental care/dentures; expense of even preventive dental care may be a limiting factor for many patients.

✦ Systemic antifungal agents are expensive; approval may be limited by insurance plans.

Psychosocial Considerations

✦ Poor oral conditions may limit social activity and contribute to poor nutrition, depression, isolation, and decreased functional status.

✦ Provide emotional support for patients undergoing radiation therapy.

Acute/Inpatient Setting

✦ Contact isolation for possible contagious lesions.

✦ Increase frequency of oral hygiene during acute illnesses and with patients who are mouth breathers.

✦ Be alert to increased risk of oral candidiasis in acutely ill hospitalized patient on antibiotics.

Extended Care Setting

✦ Contact isolation for possible contagious lesions.

✦ Annual and prn oral assessment by dental consultant.

✦ Stress importance of complete and regular oral care to all staff.

✦ Routine oral assessment for all patients.

Home Setting

✦ Stress important of oral hygiene especially in high-risk, homebound patients.

✦ Reinforce preventive care.

Chapter 3

Skin

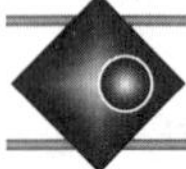

Pruritus

HISTORY

✦ Location?

✦ Burning? Pain, characteristics?

✦ Rash? Cracking? Blisters? Oozing/characteristics, amount? Crusting?

✦ Onset? Duration? Previous episodes/cyclical or seasonal? **Pruritus is most common dermatologic symptom in the elderly. Chronic pruritus may indicate systemic illness.**

✦ Contact, food, or drug allergies?

✦ Recent surgical procedures/illnesses requiring antibiotics? **Delayed drug rash can occur 2 weeks after treatment.** Recent use of contrast dyes?

✦ Recent change in bathing products, laundry detergents/softeners, or environmental exposures such as chemicals, sun, wind?

✦ What products are used for hygiene, shampoo, grooming, moisturizing? (include soaps, shampoos, conditioners, perfumes, body powder/talc, cornstarch, lotions, douching agents, and latex products as appropriate). Are lanolin products used? **Many older adults are sensitive to lanolin.**

✦ Relationship to sudden changes in environmental temperatures?

✦ What interventions have been tried? Aggravating factors? Relieving factors?

✦ Bathing habits, including water temperature preferences, frequency; use of basin, tub, or shower?

✦ Fatigue? Weight loss? Night sweats? Fever?

✦ Contact with others with similar symptoms?

✦ Pets? **Maintain high level suspicion for flea bites.**

✦ Recent travel?

✦ Recent stressors, such as relocation, financial concerns, or death of friend/relative?

✦ History of chronic renal failure, hepatitis, biliary obstruction, polycythemia vera, iron deficiency, HIV, cancer, hypothyroidism, hyperthyroidism, lymphoma, leukemia, diabetes mellitus, peripheral neuropathy, connective tissue disease, psychiatric illness?

✦ Renal dialysis? **There is a high incidence of pruritus during and after dialysis, questionably due to increased phosphorus and magnesium levels or hyperparathyroidism.**

✦ Medications, prescription/OTC? Recreational drugs? **Pruritus commonly occurs with aspirin, nonsteroidals, thiazides, opiates, estrogens, and Vitamin B complex. Be suspect of the dye, tartrazine, which provides color to medication tablets.**

✦ Residence? Type of heating/cooling, wood burning stoves, running water?

✦ How does pruritus affect sleep/activities of daily living (ADLs)?

✦ Anxiety? Depressed mood? **May cause or exacerbate pruritus.**

✦ Social support for care assistance/transportation?

PHYSICAL EXAMINATION

✦ Vital signs, weight.

✦ **Perform assessment under good lighting. Assess entire body for dermatologic abnormalities; elderly often have more than one dermatologic problem.**

✦ Inspect areas of scratching for rash, dryness, fissures, scaling, vesicles, bullae, exudate, crusting, excoriations, thickening of the tissue, hyperpigmentation, erythema, and evidence of secondary infections such as purulent exudate and foul odor.

✦ Inspect scalp for excoriations and brown mites (unhatched), gray or white mites (hatched) that cannot be easily removed along the hair shaft (suggests pediculosis capitis or head lice). Use magnifying glass or Wood's lamp if available.

✦ Assess for jaundice.

✦ Assess thyroid for palpable abnormality.

✦ Assess for lymphadenopathy.

✦ Assess for hepatomegaly and splenomegaly.

✦ Perform external genital examination/vaginal examination as appropriate.

✦ Functional assessment. **Functional decline and lack of social support can lead to poor hygiene and inability to comply with certain interventions, especially prescribed topical applications.**

✦ **See Protocol on Management of the Post-Menopausal Woman.**

DIAGNOSTIC TESTS

✦ **Diagnosis based on history, clinical findings, and response to interventions. Proceed with laboratory testing if suspicious for systemic disease or unresponsiveness to treatment intervention.**

✦ CBC with differential.

✦ Creatinine, fasting blood glucose, blood urea nitrogen (BUN), electrolytes, calcium, serum iron, bilirubin, magnesium.

✦ Urinalysis.

✦ Liver profile.

✦ Thyroid profile.

✦ Consider serum protein electrophoresis, antinuclear antibodies (ANA), rheumatoid arthitis (RA) latex fixation.

✦ Consider chest x-ray, stool hemacult.

✦ Consider stool for ova/parasites as appropriate.

✦ Consider potassium hydroxide (KOH) prep of lesions for yeast/fungus.

✦ Consider gram stain of lesions to rule out bacteria.

✦ Consult physician regarding further work-up such as prostate-specific antigen (PSA), sigmoidoscopy/colonoscopy to rule out occult malignancy as appropriate.

✦ Consider HIV testing as appropriate. Consult physician.

PREVENTION

✦ Skin hydration with emollients and superfatted, dye- and fragrance-free soaps.

✦ Fluid intake 1½–2 L daily unless otherwise contraindicated.

✦ Avoid known precipitating factors.

✦ Compliance to interventions.

✦ Timely diagnosis/treatment to prevent outbreak of scabies in adult day health, residential, and extended care setting.

✦ Avoid sharing hairbrushes, combs, and clothing.

✦ Environmental humidification as appropriate and feasible.

✦ **See Protocol on Seborrheic Dermatitis.**

✦ **See Protocol on Prevention and Health Maintenance.**

MANAGEMENT

Xerosis

✦ **Most common cause of pruritus in the elderly, secondary to decreased sebaceous and sweat gland secretions.**

✦ Incidence increases in cold environmental temperatures and decreased humidity (<60%).

✦ Characterized by fissures, scaling. May be with or without rash. Typically seen on lateral aspects of lower extremities, feet, arms, and at times, lateral trunk.

✦ Aggravated by frequent bathing, especially with hot water and defatted or alkaline soaps. Suggest generalized bathing two to three times weekly using tepid water and daily bathing of axillae and genitalia. Avoid rubbing to dry; try patting skin dry.

✦ Apply bath oils after bathing. Consider additives to be potential sensitizing agents.

✦ Apply emollients after bathing and two to three times daily. **Emollients are best absorbed through damp skin.** Petroleum is effective and inexpensive; vegetable shortening can also be used, caution of potential to stain furniture/clothing.

✦ Suggest superfatted, dye- and fragrance-free soaps.

✦ In severe cases, Lac-Hydrin 12% bid. **On open lesions, can be irritative and burn.**

✦ Cool compresses to areas of intense pruritus.

✦ Consider Atarax or Vistaril (hydroxyzine) 10–25 mg every 4–6 hr as needed. Periactin (cyproheptadine) is sometimes helpful in resistive cases but must be dosed according to body weight (maximum dose 0.5 mg/kg daily). Antihistamines are sedating, begin low dosing, titrate upward as symptoms/side effects permit.

Psoriasis

PSORIASIS VULGARIS

✦ Can occur at any age; usually of chronic nature in the elderly.

✦ Affects both genders.

✦ Stress can precipitate flares. Flares are unpredictable but seem to last longer with each occurrence. Sunlight and warm weather may help.

✦ Characteristically has chronic, scaling papules with well-demarcated borders and thick silver scales. Characteristic bleeding occurs at site of scale removal (**Auspitz sign**). Distribution is symmetrical; typically seen on scalp, elbows, knees, lower back/hips, and anogenital areas, but may become generalized.

✦ Lesions can arise at sites of trauma (**Koebner's phenomenon**).

✦ Nails may pit with separation of the nail from the nail bed. Brown discoloration and hyperkeratosis is seen frequently under the nail.

✦ Arthralgia can precede or follow eruptions of skin lesions. Distal interphalangeal joints are often involved. RA latex fixation will be negative.

✦ First line treatment involves tar shampoos, tar/salicylic acid preparations, and short-term topical steroids (approximately 2 weeks). **Select less potent steroids initially.** Ointments are generally more potent than creams; lotions are easier to apply to larger areas. Hydrocortisone 2.5% lotion, cream, ointment. Triamcinolone acetonide 0.1% lotion, cream or ointment and fluocinonide 0.05% cream or ointment. **Avoid face and genitalia—can cause skin atrophy.**

✦ Anthralin (Drithocreme) 0.1%, 0.25%, 0.5%, and 1% cream or Dritho-scalp 0.25% or 0.5% can be used in chronic psoriasis. Must be applied, then thoroughly washed off within 60 min. May stain skin, hair, fabrics, and furniture. Must be used with caution in the presence of renal disease.

✦ Referral to dermatologist for follow-up, diagnostic biopsy, and potential ultraviolet B (UVB) light or psoralens/psoralen-ultraviolet light (PUVA) treatments in resistant cases. **Psoralens may increase pruritus. An increase in the incidence of malignant skin lesion has been reported with PUVA treatments.**

✦ Dermatologist may also order systemic therapy such as Rheumatrex (methotrexate sodium), Tegison (etretinate), Sandimmune (cyclosporine), or Hydrea (hydroxyurea). All preparations carry significant side effects

✦ Soriatane (acitretin), a recently released oral retinoid agent, has shown promise in effective treatment of severe psoriasis (both plaque type erythrodermic and pustular types). **Requires close monitoring of lipids and liver function. Must be discontinued if visual changes occur and referred to ophthalmologist. Patient must be warned of increased skin sensitivity to light.**

✦ Moisturize with emollient creams/ointments.

✦ Adding oil to tub/shower bath may be hazardous.

✦ Refer to occupational therapy (OT) or physical therapy (PT) for adaptive equipment if joints have become involved.

PUSTULAR PSORIASIS

✦ Potentially life-threatening, especially in frail elderly.

✦ Begins with burning erythema, quickly spreads with pustules becoming confluent.

✦ Fever, fatigue, leukocytosis with negative blood cultures.

✦ Hospitalize, isolate, and hydrate.

Scabies

✦ Caused by *Sarcoptes scabiei* mite. Transmitted by skin-to-skin contact.

✦ Intense nocturnal itching.

✦ Look for linear or wavy burrows with a vesicle/papule at one end. Can present atypically as eczema or exfoliative dermatitis accompanied by thick crusted lesions. Erythema and generalized lymphadenopathy may be present. Located on back/buttocks in bedridden patients, inner aspect of wrists, waist, between fingers and toes, axillae, groin, gluteal fold, nipples, vulva, and penile shaft.

✦ Involves hands and feet, unlike pediculosis corporis/body lice.

✦ Treatment choices:

✧ Elimite (permethrin) 5%: drug of choice, safe/effective, requires one treatment. Apply to skin from neck to soles of feet with attention between gluteal fold, between fingers/toes, and under fingernails for 8–12 hr. Comes in 60-g tube; 30-g (1 oz) is usually adequate.

✧ Kwell (lindane) 1%: from neck down, let dry. Remove in 8–12 hr and launder clothing/bed linens using hot water. Second application required 7 days later, again allowing to dry 8–12 hr before removal. **Compliance may be problematic. Follow-up in 2 weeks.**

✦ Pruritus may continue 1–2 weeks after treatment. For more resistant cases, trial topical corticosteroids, oral antihistamines.

✦ Consider antibiotic therapy when areas are crusted and erythemic. **Suggests secondary bacterial infection.** Consider Vibramycin (doxycycline hyclate) 200 mg day 1, then 100 mg daily or Keflex (cephalexin) 250 mg qid.

✦ Treat close contacts.

Pediculosis Capitis

✦ Head lice.

✦ Treatment choices:

✧ Nix (permethrin) 1%: saturate washed/towel-dried hair and scalp. Rinse after 10 min. Use fine toothed comb to remove nits.

✧ Kwell (lindane) 1%: saturate washed/towel-dried hair and scalp. Rinse after 6 min. Comb with fine tooth comb to remove lice. Repeat in 10 days. **Compliance may be problematic.**

✦ Soak hair brushes/combs in shampoo at least 1 hr. Launder clothing, towels/wash clothes/bed linen in hot water.

✦ Refer to **Prevention.**

Metabolic Pruritus

- Systemic etiology.
- Maintain high level suspicion for systemic illness in the elderly since presentation is commonly atypical. Usually not the first sign of significant systemic illness.
- Work-up specific to suspected illness:
  - Hypersensitivity to drug or drugs.
  - Malignancy (stomach/pancreas).
  - Lymphoma (Hodgkin/non-Hodgkin).
  - Leukemia.
  - Multiple myeloma.
  - Microcytic iron deficiency anemia.
  - Polycythemia vera.
  - Carcinoid.
  - Hyperthyroidism.
  - Hypothyroidism (pruritus secondary to dry skin).
  - Diabetes mellitus.
  - Obstructive biliary disease.
  - Uremia.
  - End-stage renal disease/on dialysis.
  - Connective tissue disease.
  - Parasites.
  - Brain tumors.
- Goal: pruritic control through effective management of underlying metabolic disease.

Psychogenic Pruritus

- May accompany anxiety, depression, and dementia.
- Goal of treatment: treat psychological illness.
- Protect skin by covering with long sleeves, gauze wraps, or mittens as appropriate. Keep fingernails trimmed.
- Refer to psychiatrist; treat for xerosis in interim (dry skin can enhance itching). Consult physician.

NEURODERMATITIS

- The "nervous scratcher." May have initiated with mild contact dermatitis or insect bite. Patient continues to scratch, develops dry, scaly area.

✦ Laboratory tests are not helpful.

✦ May have signs of secondary infection.

✦ Corticosteroid ointments are effective.

✦ Cover area when possible to prevent scratching.

DELUSIONS OF PARASITE INFESTATION

✦ May present with concerns or collection of debris believed by patient to be parasites.

✦ Excoriations may be present, otherwise normal skin assessment.

✦ Refer to psychiatrist; treat for xerosis during interim. Consult physician.

KEY ISSUES

Patient/Caregiver Education

Patient/caregiver should be able to:

✦ Verbalize etiology of pruritus.

✦ Identify causative agent in hypersensitivity reactions.

✦ Verbalize treatment program and its importance. **Management is often complex; written instructions help compliance.**

✦ Identify functional restrictions preventing compliance and assist with alternative plans.

✦ Verbalize activity/interventions to prevent recurrent episodes.

Economic Considerations

✦ Treatment modalities are often costly, especially in recurrent conditions. Consider the least expensive emollients when used chronically.

✦ Treatment compliance may require paid care giver in presence of functional limitations and lack of social support.

Psychosocial Considerations

✦ Assess for development of depressive symptoms, especially in resistive, recurrent episodes.

✦ Assess for sleep deprivation.

✦ Assess for social withdrawal/isolation secondary to unresolved symptoms/time-consuming treatment protocol.

Acute/Inpatient Setting

✦ Thorough skin assessment on admission to detect pruritus secondary to infestation. Isolate per facility protocol, pending validation.

✦ Initiate patient participation in treatment program prior to discharge.

✦ Consult OT for adaptive equipment needs for shampooing, bathing, and topical applications.

Extended Care Setting

✦ Thorough skin assessment on admission for suspected infestations; isolate per facility protocol. Timely treatment.

✦ Limit generalized bathing to two to three times weekly unless otherwise contraindicated.

✦ Advocate for emollients, soaps, and shampoos that decrease potential of sensitizing/drying.

✦ Consider moisturizing skin following application of towels saturated with tepid water. **Avoid hypothermia by treating small areas at a time.**

✦ Attention to nail care to prevent excoriations/secondary infections.

✦ Avoid bath oils in shower area to prevent falls.

✦ Educate staff/patient to apply thin coat topical agents; a little goes a long way. Generally, if you can see the topical agent, you have used too much.

Home Setting

✦ Attention to safety: avoid bath oils in tub/shower; put socks and shoes on after application of emollients to feet; apply topical agents to legs by sitting with legs outstretched on the bed to prevent loss of balance.

✦ Vegetable shortening is an effective/available emollient. Caution, may stain furniture/clothing.

✦ OT consult for adaptive equipment/interventions for topical agent applications.

✦ Suggest pet evaluation if fleas are suspected.

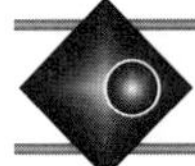

Seborrheic Dermatitis

HISTORY

✦ Onset? Duration? **Condition affects both genders but is more common among men; has a gradual onset, is chronic with periods of exacerbation; and may involve a chronic yeast (*Pityrosporum ovale*) infection.**

✦ Pruritic? **Common, especially in warm environment or during perspiration, but may be asymptomatic.**

✦ Location?

✦ Cyclical? **Usually worse in late fall and winter.**

✦ What interventions have been tried? What has been successful?

✦ Impact on daily life?

✦ Other medical conditions? **Prevalent in the elderly particularly in the presence of diabetes, facial paralysis, Parkinson's disease, HIV, alcohol (EtOH) abuse, and stress.**

✦ Social situation? Residential setting, social supports?

PHYSICAL EXAMINATION

✦ Inspect scalp and hair line, forehead, eyebrows, beard and mustache, nasolabial folds, the ear and postauricular folds, eyelids, and sternal area for white, yellow, or gray dry or greasy scales and/or crusts on an erythemic macular-papular base. Scales vary in size and thickness. Erythema without scales but the presence of fissures may be seen in the folds beneath the breasts, axillae, umbilicus, groin, and gluteal crease. **Differs from dandruff, in which scaling has no erythemic base and affects only the scalp.**

✦ Inspect for hair loss.

✦ Surrounding excoriations may indicate pruritus.

✦ Functional assessment. **Self-management requires ability to bathe, shampoo.**

DIAGNOSTIC TESTS

✦ Diagnosis is based on clinical features.

PREVENTION

- Compliance with interventions decrease risk of exacerbation.
- **See Protocol on Prevention and Health Maintenance.**

MANAGEMENT

- **Goal of treatment is decreasing the number and severity of exacerbations.**
- **Topical shampoos:** Initially, shampoo with antiseborrheic shampoo daily for 5–7 days, then a minimum of two times a week. Allow shampoo to remain on affected areas 3–5 min, then rinse well. Foam of the shampoo is effective on eyebrows and facial lesions. Shampoos containing selenium sulfide 1% or 2.5% (Selsun) or pyrithione zinc (Head and Shoulders) are usually effective used alone or on alternate days. Tar, salicylic acid, and sulfur shampoos have also been used with some effectiveness. Nizoral (ketoconazole) 2% shampoo can be added in resistant cases, alternating shampoo days. If effective, try discontinuing the selenium or pyrithione zinc agents—using ketoconazole as the primary agent.
- **Topical creams and lotions:** Apply 1–3 times a day if shampooing alone is ineffective. Hydrocortisone 1% cream or solution for areas of increased hair. Nizoral (ketoconazole) 2% cream can be applied two times a day to affected areas.
- Topical antibiotic therapy with erythromycin solution is occasionally added to shampoos, topical steroids, and antifungal agents in resistant cases or suspected secondary infection.
- Consider cutting hair to improve topical treatments.
- Initially, evaluate treatment effectiveness after 3–4 weeks.
- Consider dermatology referral in resistant or severe cases.

KEY ISSUES

Patient/Caregiver Education

Patient/caregiver should be able to:

- Verbalize understanding of the disease regarding chronicity, exacerbations, and remissions.
- Demonstrate the ability to safely and effectively apply shampoos and/or creams, lotions, solutions; verbalize need to avoid steroids in the eye.
- Verbalize the need to allow shampoos to remain on the body (in contact with scalp or skin) 3–5 min, then rinse.

✦ Determine symptomatic effectiveness of treatment regimen.

Economic Considerations

✦ Expense is increased with each additional treatment agent.

✦ Consider quantity of shampoo, creams, lotions, and solutions required for affected areas.

✦ Is there a need to hire caregiver for shampooing and bathing? This service is considered nonskilled and is not covered by Medicare/Medicare supplements.

Psychosocial Considerations

✦ Assess for concerns regarding change in body image.

✦ Assess for social withdrawal/isolation secondary to facial lesions.

Acute/Inpatient Setting

✦ Exacerbation may accompany stress of acute illness.

✦ Continue shampoos in the shower when feasible. If shampooing is not possible, continue steroid cream/lotion with/without antifungal agent.

Extended Care Setting

✦ Treatment regimen may be difficult to accomplish for bedridden person.

✦ Be alert for scratching in the elderly resident with mental status changes; inspect for clinical features of disease.

✦ Shaving men will improve effectiveness of topical treatment.

Home Setting

✦ Encourage women to avoid cosmetic application during exacerbations.

✦ Assess for adaptive needs for safe shampooing.

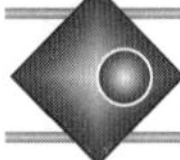

Neoplasms

HISTORY

✦ Location? Area(s) of sun exposure? Is area easily and repeatedly traumatized?

✦ Onset?

✦ Change in lesion color or size?

✦ Bleeding, oozing, crusting?

✦ Pain or tenderness? Itching?

✦ History of sun exposure? **Include prolonged/excessive exposure as a child and young adult, as well as occupational history related to outdoor activities such as fisherman, farmer, construction worker, or car/truck driver who exposes one arm to the sun through the vehicle window. Also include recreational sun exposure such as gardening/lawn care and outdoor sports such as hiking, swimming, boating, bike riding, tennis, golf, and fishing. Resulting lesions are secondary to cumulative sun exposure.**

✦ History of radiation exposure? Conditions causing impaired immune system?

✦ History of burns with scarring?

✦ History of sunscreen usage and product sensitivities/allergies?

✦ Previous history of dermatologic lesions? **Previous history of basal cell or squamous cell carcinoma carries increased risk for melanoma.**

✦ History of melanoma in first-degree relative?

✦ Smoker?

PHYSICAL EXAMINATION

✦ Fair complexion? Light-colored eyes? Blond or red hair? **All carry increased risk for skin cancer.**

✦ Systematically assess skin from scalp to soles of feet. **Sun-exposed skin that is rough, leathery textured, wrinkled, or with blotchy hyperpigmentation is predisposed to the development of premalignant/malignant neoplasms.**

✦ Assess pigmented lesions using the A, B, C, D method: A = asymmetry; B = borders; C = color; D = diameter.

✧ **Benign lesions are more likely to be symmetrical (round/oval) with even borders, can be variegated brown/pink, and are less than 6 mm in diameter.**

✧ **Melanomas should be suspected if lesions have asymmetrical shape, irregular borders, are variegated in color (more than one shade of brown/black/blue-black/white/red), and are larger than 6 mm in diameter.**

✧ **Whites are at highest risk for melanoma, but Asians and African Americans are at higher risk for melanomas on mucous membranes, the palms of the hands and soles of the feet, and under the finger and toenails, locations that are associated with a poorer prognosis.**

✦ Consider following progress of lesions with photographs, especially when multiple lesions are present.

DIAGNOSTIC TESTS

✦ Biopsy provides differential diagnosis. **Refer to dermatologist. Punch biopsies should be performed in the center of the lesion at the thickest and most irregular site.**

PREVENTION

✦ Limit sun exposure. Apply "broad spectrum" sunscreen daily prior to sun exposure.

✦ Whites should apply sunscreen with a sun protective factor (SPF) of at least 15; dark-skinned individuals can use agents with a lower SPF.

✦ Products with dibenzoyl methanes provide best protection against UVA, the long wavelength radiation promoting skin cancer and causing wrinkling and photoaging.

✦ Products with benzophenones absorb UVB, the short wavelength radiation causing redness and skin cancer, and 60% of UVA radiation.

✦ Para-aminobenzoic acid (PABA) absorbs only UVB radiation, washes off easily, and is a source of allergic reactions. Patients allergic to PABA can use sunscreens with cinnamates, which absorb UVB but only minimal UVA radiation. **PABA-containing sunscreens should be avoided by patients taking diuretics and oral hypoglycemic agents since these combinations can cause photosensitivity reactions or dermatitis.**

✦ Zinc oxide melts in the sun, providing no protection to the skin.

✦ Apply a water-resistant, high SPF sunscreen 30–60 min prior to planned, extended sun exposure, and reapply after 45–60 min of sweating or swimming. **Sweat-resistant sunscreens provide protection for approximately 30 min of perspiration. Water-resistant sunscreens provide approximately 40 min of coverage during swimming. Waterproof sunscreens provide 80 min of protection in the water.**

✦ Avoid sunbathing and tanning spas.

✦ Avoid the highest intensity of sun exposure during the hours of 10 a.m. to 3 p.m. Clouds block only 20% of ultraviolet radiation.

✦ Choose sunglasses blocking 99–100% of UVA and UVB. **Sun exposure increases risk of cataracts.**

✦ Wear at least a 3-inch brimmed hat, protecting scalp, head, eyes, ears, and neck. Cover up with protective clothing.

✦ Routine, monthly self-examination for suspicious or changing lesions. **Early detection/treatment provides greatest mortality prevention.**

✦ **See Protocol on Prevention and Health Maintenance.**

MANAGEMENT

Benign Neoplasms

SEBORRHEIC KERATOSES

✦ Common after the age of 65. More common among men.

✦ Location: face, neck, trunk, upper extremities, under breasts, groin.

✦ Characteristics: round or ovoid; flat or convex; scale covering gray or brown/black. Scale can have a waxy, granular, or papular surface and have "stuck on" appearance. Lesions under breasts and in groin have mushroom appearance.

✦ Not sun related.

✦ Treatment: cryosurgery or electrocautery.

CHERRY ANGIOMA

✦ Common after the age of 65, expected after age 80. Occurs in men and women.

✦ Location: trunk, proximal extremities.

✦ Characteristics: domed vascular papule with dull-to-shiny surface, bright red/purple. Soft, blanches with firm palpation. Up to 8 mm in diameter.

✦ May become tender if infected.

✦ If traumatized, may bleed and crust.

✦ Not sun related.

✦ Treatment is not required.

NEVI

✦ Affects men and women.

✦ Location: as single lesions on backs of hands and feet and scattered on extremities and trunk.

✦ Characteristics: firm, flat, round, or papular. Blue to black. Less than 10 mm in diameter.

✦ No treatment is required unless there is a change in patient's usual lesion. If there is a change, refer to dermatologist or plastic surgeon for surgical removal. Consult physician.

ACTINIC LENTIGINES ("LIVER SPOTS")

✦ Common among Whites but also seen in Asians and less commonly in African Americans. Occurs in men and women.

✦ Location: sun exposed areas—hands, arms, face, neck, and backs of hands/wrists.

✦ Characteristics: light yellow, light or dark brown, coarse blotches. There may be variegated browns.

✦ Treatment: bleaching agents remove blotches but leave white scarring. Sunscreens.

ACROCHORDONS ("SKIN TAGS")

✦ Common in elderly. More common among women.

✦ Location: eyelids, base of neck, axillae, groin, and beneath the breasts in women.

✦ Characteristics: color of skin, polypoid. Vary in size: < 1.0–10 mm in diameter. May become tender with trauma. Known to turn on its pedicle at which time the blood supply is obstructed and the lesion turns black and painful. The lesion dries up and falls off.

✦ Treatment is not required, but lesions may be a cosmetic concern. Lesion can be snipped with scissors.

Premalignant Neoplasms

ACTINIC KERATOSES

✦ Due to sun exposure.

✦ More common in men.

✦ Location: sun exposed surfaces—forehead, nose, cheeks, temples, lower lip, ears, neck, distal upper extremities, and backs of hands.

✦ Characteristics: round or ovoid macules and papules. Less than 1.0 cm in diameter, usually 2–5 mm. Skin colored, yellow/red to brown. Rough, dry, white scaly lesions that are adherent and have appearance of sandpaper. May be single lesions or scattered.

✦ May be pruritic or tender.

✦ May progress to squamous cell carcinoma.

✦ Treatment: 1% or 2% Efudex (5-fluorouracil) lotion applied topically bid repeated over 3–6 weeks. Cryotherapy using liquid nitrogen application followed by 5-fluorouracil applications is another option. Surgical excision. May resolve spontaneously.

Nonmelanoma Malignant Neoplasms

BASAL CELL CARCINOMA

✦ Most common skin cancer in Whites; most common in men.

✦ Secondary to sun exposure and irradiation.

✦ Location: forehead, head, neck, and upper back.

✦ Characteristics: waxy/translucent nodule, papule, plaque; may be black to violet, shiny or scaly. Irregular, smooth, rolled border with telangiectatic vessels. May have ulcerated center with crusting or scar-like plaque. May appear to be a nonhealing wound. Can spread to surrounding tissues if not excised to negative borders. Has ability to produce disfigurement if not eradicated early.

✦ Treatment: referral to dermatologist or plastic surgeon for electrodesiccation and curettage, cryosurgery, radiation therapy, chemotherapy, surgical excision, or microscopically controlled surgery (Mohs procedure). Consult physician. **Curable with early diagnosis and intervention.**

SQUAMOUS CELL CARCINOMA

✦ Commonly develops in late life; more common in men.

✦ Second most common form of skin cancer.

✦ Fair complected at greatest risk.

✦ Location: sun-exposed areas such as lips, nose, scalp, ear, dorsum of hand. Often found with a scar. Inner thigh is a common site in women; found on the glans penis in men.

✦ Characteristics: firm, red nodule or papule. May have crusted or hemorrhagic surface. Generally > 2 cm. Grows faster than basal cell carcinoma. Can metastasize and cause death.

✦ Lesions on ears and lips carry a higher risk of metastasis.

✦ Treatment: electrodesiccation and curettage, cryotherapy, surgical excision, or Mohs procedure. Radiation is an option for a patient who will not accept surgery or is considered a poor risk.

Melanoma

✦ Responsible for the most number of deaths related to skin cancer.

✦ Location: around the mouth, anus, vulva, scalp, back; more common on the legs between knees and ankles in women and toes and soles of feet in dark-skinned patients.

LENTIGO MALIGNA MELANOMA ("HUTCHINSON'S FRECKLE")

✦ A type of melanoma common among the elderly.

✦ Location: sun-exposed areas, especially the neck and head.

✦ Characteristics: tan/brown macule with irregular borders. Papules/nodules within macula can develop. May take years before changes occur in growth and/or irregular pigmentation.

✦ Curable if treated early.

KEY ISSUES

Patient/Caregiver Education

Patient/caregiver should be able to:

✦ Identify their individualized risk factors

✦ Verbalize understanding of prevention strategies and demonstrate knowledge in selection of the appropriate sunscreen based on individualized needs. **See Prevention.**

✦ Demonstrate ability to complete thorough self-examination using needed adaptive equipment to visualize back and soles of feet.

Economic Considerations

✦ Treatment of premalignant and malignant lesions is medically necessary and covered by health insurance policies.

✦ Cosmetic treatments may have limited coverage.

Psychosocial Considerations

✦ Be alert for cosmetic concerns especially related to facial lesions. **Consider advantages of plastic surgery referral vs. dermatology referral.**

Acute/Inpatient Setting

✦ Take advantage of admission history/physical to identify possible dermatology issues.

✦ Most surgical procedures are done as outpatient.

Extended Care Setting

✦ Provide sunscreens to residents spending time out of doors.

✦ Yearly routine screening for skin lesions.

Home Setting

✦ Emphasis on preventive strategies, especially daily application of sunscreens when working outdoors—even if overcast.

✦ Assess environment for mirrors and other adaptive equipment to assist with routine monthly self-assessments of skin.

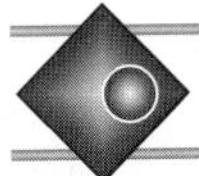

Contact Dermatitis

HISTORY

✦ General condition of skin: location of eruption?

✦ Presence of papules, vesicles, bullae, scaling, weeping, lichenification, hyperpigmentation, pruritus, heat, swelling, tenderness?

✦ Duration: acute occurrence or chronic condition?

✦ Possible stimuli? Elicit history of contact with possible stimuli, duration of contact, and latency period between contact and symptoms. **Consider pets, hobbies when eliciting history.** Change in soap, deodorant, lotion, shampoo, make-up?

✦ History of venous or other lower extremity ulcers?

✦ Medications? Note especially OTC medications used to treat other underlying condition such as venous ulcer (neomycin), topical hydrocortisone, topical lidocaine, benzocaine, lanolin, or topical preparations containing PABA.

✦ Occupational history? Note possible stimuli in workplace and especially "wet work" occupations such as hairdressers, custodians, agricultural workers, cooks.

PHYSICAL EXAMINATION

✦ Vital signs, temperature.

✦ Inspect skin at site of occurrence. Distinguish widespread erythema from sharply demarcated area. Note presence of heat, edema, scaling. Inspect for papules, vesicles, bullae. Note configuration (e.g., linear vs. annular).

DIAGNOSTIC TESTS

✦ Consider KOH stain of scraping to differentiate fungal infection if resistant to treatment.

✦ Patch test—useful only for allergic contact dermatitis. Strip of hypoallergenic tape implanted with allergens is applied to skin (usually on back); removed after 48 hr. Evaluated on removal and again 4–7 days later. Consult dermatologist or allergist.

PREVENTION

✦ Maintain good skin hygiene, including lubrication. **See Chapter on Special Hygiene Needs.**

✦ Daily, brief bathing in warm, not hot, water.

✦ Avoid harsh soaps.

✦ Use wet compresses with tepid tap water to ease itching.

✦ Once identified, avoid causative agents by wearing gloves or other measures.

✦ **See Protocol on Prevention and Health Maintenance.**

MANAGEMENT

✦ Contact dermatitis is an eczematous condition rarely accompanied by urticaria.

✦ **Incidence increases with aging, secondary to increased use of topical medications and seniors spending more time during retirement in direct contact with environmental stimuli.**

✦ Is differentiated between two types, allergic or irritant. Irritant contact dermatitis is more prevalent.

Irritant Contact Dermatitis

✦ Direct tissue damage occurs after contact with irritating stimulus.

✦ Reaction usually occurs within 48 hr of contact and is diminished by 96 hr.

✦ Frequently caused by contact with water, detergents, solvents, soaps, greases. Patients who perform "wet work" may react to otherwise innocuous substances.

✦ Hands and face are common sites. Reaction at eye area usually caused by dusts, fumes, or cosmetics on hands (nail polish) rather than eye make-up. If occurs in nonexposed area, probably due to a substance that is applied (e.g., cosmetic lotion).

✦ Reaction does not spread but is more limited to site of contact (look for "branding sign" distribution).

✦ Vesicles may be accompanied by heat, swelling, tenderness. Erythema usually demarcated sharply and may be intense.

✦ Generally less pruritic than allergic contact dermatitis.

✦ No diagnostic test. History is confirmatory.

TABLE 3-1. Topical Corticosteroids Commonly Prescribed for Contact Dermatitis

Agent	Vehicle/potency	Instructions for use
Low potency		
Hydrocortisone	Cream 0.5%, 1%, 2.5% Lotion 0.25%, 0.5%, 1%, 2.5% Ointment 0.5%, 1%, 2.5%	Apply to affected area tid–qid
Aristocort, Kenalog (triamcinolone acetonide)	Ointment 0.025%, 0.1%, 0.5% Cream 0.025%, 0.1%, 0.5% Lotion 0.025%, 0.1%	Apply to affected area tid–qid
Moderate potency		
Valisone (betamethasone valerate)	Cream 0.1% Ointment 0.1% Lotion 0.1%	Apply to affected area qd–bid
Synalar (fluocinolone acetonide)	Cream 0.01%, 0.025% Ointment 0.025% Solution 0.01%	Apply to affected area bid–qid
High potency		
Cyclocort (amcinonide)	Cream 0.1% Ointment 0.1%	Apply to affected area bid–tid
Halog (halcinonide)	Cream 0.025%, 0.1% Ointment 0.1% Solution 0.1%	Apply to affected area bid–tid

- Management goals:
  - Identification of offending agent and prevention of future contact.
  - Symptom control.
  - Prevention of secondary infection.
  - Prevention of scarring.
- Topical steroid therapy (see Table 3-1). Potential for side effects increases with potency. Begin with lowest potency. Avoid high potency steroids on face and near eyes.
- Topical steroid therapy may be difficult for elderly to apply. Possible side effects include atrophy, hypopigmentation, telangiectasia, striae, burning, purpura, and, less frequently, cataracts and glaucoma.
- Oral steroids used only for severe cases. Consider a tapered dose such as a Medrol dose pack.
- Dependent on patient's condition, consider antibiotic prophylaxis against staph/strep secondary infection:

- ✧ Keflex (cephalexin) 250–500 mg PO qid.
- ✧ Dynapen, Pathocil (dicloxacillin) 250–500 mg PO qid.
- ✧ Erythromycin 250–500 mg PO bid–tid with meals.

✦ Antihistamines may be of some value for pruritus.

Allergic Contact Dermatitis

✦ Reaction occurs hours to several days following contact; may require many days to resolve.

✦ Common causative agents: cosmetics, plants, germicides, nickel, chromium, topical medications, latex.

✦ Sites with thinner skin (eyelids, ear lobes, genital area) are most susceptible.

✦ **Xerosis that commonly accompanies aging increases vulnerability.**

✦ Initial reaction may present with large vesicles and bullae overlying erythema and pruritus.

✦ Later presentation is with erythema and pruritus, smaller vesicles, peeling, and possible hyperpigmentation.

✦ Management goals:

- ✧ Identification and avoidance of offending agent.
- ✧ Symptom control.
- ✧ Prevention of secondary infection.
- ✧ Prevention of scarring.

✦ Treat with topical steroids and/or oral steroids, antibiotic prophylaxis **See Protocol on Irritant Contact Dermatitis.**

✦ Refer to allergist or dermatologist for patch test if chronic recurrence, unresolving eczema, or lichenification.

KEY ISSUES

Patient/Caregiver Education

Patient/caregiver should be able to:

✦ List preventive measures.

✦ Verbalize medications prescribed, how to apply/take and frequency.

Economic Considerations

✦ Necessary avoidance of causative agents in the workplace may pose economic burden in working elders.

Psychosocial Considerations

✦ Patient may be unwilling to avoid contact with pets or causative agents related to leisure-time activities.

Acute/Inpatient Setting

✦ Be alert to reactions to new environmental agents (detergents, sheets, creams, and lotions).

Extended Care Setting

✦ Educate staff to be aware of signs/symptoms of contact dermatitis and to seek to identify possible causative agents.

✦ Screen cosmetics, toiletries provided to residents by visitors for possible irritants.

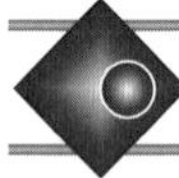

Dermal Candidiasis

HISTORY

- ✦ Description of skin condition: color, nature of vesicles, odor?
- ✦ Location, onset, duration of lesions?
- ✦ Associated symptoms: pruritus, erythema, burning, excoriation?
- ✦ Alleviating treatment?
- ✦ Comorbid conditions: diabetes mellitus, incontinence, poor hygiene?
- ✦ Medications? Recent course of antibiotic therapy?

PHYSICAL EXAMINATION

✦ Skin: inspect for erythema, satellite lesions, excoriation, secondary bacterial infection—especially in perineal/groin and within skin folds (inframammary and abdominal).

✦ Mouth: inspect oral cavity for signs/symptoms of oral candidiasis—white patches or plaques.

DIAGNOSTIC TESTS

- ✦ Consider KOH stain of scraping.

PREVENTION

- ✦ Avoid moisture on skin.
- ✦ If antibiotic course is necessary, consider adding yogurt to diet.
- ✦ Optimal blood glucose control in diabetes.
- ✦ **See Protocol on Urinary Incontinence.**
- ✦ **See Chapter on Special Hygiene Needs.**
- ✦ **See Protocol on Prevention and Health Maintenance.**

MANAGEMENT

✦ Optimal management of diabetes mellitus. **See Protocol on Diabetes Mellitus.**

TABLE 3-2. Antifungal Agents Commonly Prescribed for Dermal Candidiasis

Agent	Potency/vehicle	Instructions for use
Micatin (miconazole nitrate)	2% cream	Apply to affected area bid
Lotrimin (clotrimazole)	1% cream 1% lotion	Apply to affected area bid
Spectazole (econazole nitrate)	1% cream	Apply to affected area once daily
Mycostatin (nystatin)	100,000 U/g cream 100,000 U/g ointment	Apply to affected area

- ✦ Manage with application of antifungal agent. See Table 3-2.
- ✦ Consider nystatin powder in patient with increased diaphoresis as causative agent.
- ✦ Consider oral antifungal agents if problem persists following trial of topical products.
- ✦ Use of amphotericin B (Fungizone) and itraconazole (Sporanox) is usually not necessary except for treatment of resistant Candida in immunocompromised hosts.
- ✦ May co-exist with intertrigo, a common condition in elderly with diabetes mellitus, obesity, incontinence, bedridden state, or poor hygiene. Intertrigo is an inflammation caused by moisture and friction that can be successfully managed by:
  - ✧ Wearing of nonbinding, cotton undergarments.
  - ✧ Application of talc to reduce friction. Cornstarch increases risk of fungal/yeast infection.
  - ✧ Applying barrier such as zinc oxide in incontinence.

KEY ISSUES

Patient/Caregiver Education

Patient/caregiver should be able to:

- ✦ List preventive measures.
- ✦ Verbalize medication regimen.
- ✦ Identify increased risk if accompanying diabetes mellitus.

Economic Considerations

✦ Newer antifungal agents may be expensive, not available in all formularies.

Acute/Inpatient Setting

✦ Common occurrence in persons with diabetes and patients receiving antibiotics for bacterial infection.

Extended Care Setting

✦ Consider applying cotton mitts to hands of patients with dementia to prevent excoriation secondary to pruritus.

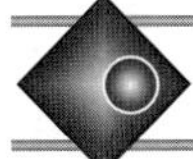

Lower Extremity Ulcers

HISTORY

✦ Pain? Quality, location, onset, duration, aggravating and alleviating treatments/factors/positions?

✦ History of trauma to lower extremity?

✦ Comorbid conditions: diabetes mellitus, history of peripheral vascular disease(PVD)/deep vein thrombosis, previous ulcers, congestive heart failure (CHF), tobacco or EtOH use?

✦ Medications, prescribed and OTC? Note especially steroids (use may impair healing) and vasoconstrictors.

✦ Diet history—deficiency of Vitamins A, C, and zinc may retard healing.

✦ Reduced functional status?

✦ Social support/caregiver?

PHYSICAL EXAMINATION

See Table 3-3.

✦ Assess temperature (possible sign of infection).

✦ Inspect skin of lower extremities. Eczematous and hemosiderin deposits suggest venous insufficiency.

✦ Assess shape of lower extremities. **Chronic venous stasis gives the leg a bowling pin or champagne bottle shape.**

✦ Assess muscles of lower extremities. **Muscle atrophy suggests chronic ischemia of arterial insufficiency.** Palpate calves for tenderness.

✦ Assess for dependent rubor. If there is pallor of the leg with elevation and intense redness in dependent position, advanced arterial disease is suspected. The redness is secondary to hyperemia due to cutaneous vasodilation.

✦ Auscultate and palpate peripheral pulses from groin to feet. **Bruits are loudest in systole and extend to diastole in severe arterial disease.** Assess for varicosities.

✦ Assess presence, extent of peripheral edema.

✦ Inspect for abdominal distention which may present proximal obstruction to lower extremity blood flow.

✦ Assess temperature of lower extremities; compare right with left.

✦ Assess ulcerations. Decreased elasticity and decreased adherence to dermis associated with aging may increase risk of ulcer formation. Record size

TABLE 3-3. **Differentiation of Lower Extremity Ulcers**

Type of ulcer	Usual location	Border	Ulcer base	Drainage	Surrounding tissue	Pulses	Pain
Venous	Ankle area above medial malleolus	Irregular; may be erythematous, friable	Pale; shallow or deep	Moderate to copious	Ruddy, pigmented, edematous; rubor of venous disease does not resolve rapidly with elevation	+; may require Doppler secondary to edema	Stinging, burning, aching; increases in dependent situations; may be pruritic
Arterial	Feet and toes, distal	Regular, punched out appearance when chronic; if secondary to trauma, conforms to irregularity	Pale/yellow grey/eschared; no granulation; shallow or deep	Minimal in dry gangrene, but may drain if tissue is macerated or secondarily infected	Pale pigmentation, gray, scaly, shiny, no edema; rubor of arterial insufficiency resolves with elevation of leg	Absent	Severe—burning, stabbing; increases on elevation of extremity; relief with dependency; worst at night
Diabetic	Commonly on foot or pressure points	—	Dry, necrotic, deep	None to moderate	Dry, thin	May be present	Painless or numbness/burning; associated with neuropathy

in two dimensions; draw or trace on thin paper. Document status of wound bed and surrounding tissue as well as description of drainage/odor. **Use of photographs is helpful to evaluate treatment.**

✦ Assess for foot abnormalities. **Charcot's joint is often seen in diabetic patient with foot ulcer.** Assess for foot drop.

✦ Assess toenails. Thick and slow-growing nails are characteristic of arterial insufficiency. Assess footwear.

✦ Assess feet for blisters, corns, and calluses.

✦ Assess soles of feet for dryness and fissures and between the toes for maceration.

✦ Evaluate motor and sensory nerve function, proprioception, Achilles/patellar reflexes.

✦ Assess gait and balance for ability to avoid trauma to lower extremities, risk of falls.

DIAGNOSTIC TESTS

✦ CBC.

✦ Serum glucose, blood urea nitrogen, creatinine, sedimentation rate if infection is suspected.

✦ Serum albumin/prealbumin to detect malnutrition—**possible deterrent to healing.**

✦ Cultures of wounds can be misleading due to colonization.

✦ Consider x-ray or bone scan of extremity to rule out osteomyelitis; foreign objects in patient with sensory neuropathy; and fractures.

✦ Doppler/duplex studies of arterial and venous systems.

✦ In suspected arterial insufficiency, ankle-brachial index (ABI). Carried out by taking the blood pressure in both upper extremities and recording the highest systolic blood pressure. Apply a standard arm cuff to leg above malleoli. Use Doppler to find dorsalis pedis or posterior tibial pulse. Use the strongest signal for the screening examination. Inflate cuff until signal is inaudible. Slowly deflate and record systolic pressure at which the signal returns. ABI is calculated by dividing the ankle pressure by the higher of the two arm systolic pressures. **Results:** Normal ratio = 1.0; Moderate disease = 0.75–0.90; Severe disease = 0.5–0.75. If <0.45, the wound has poor prognosis of healing and patient is at risk of amputation. Pressures may be falsely elevated in diabetic. Refer patient for transmetatarsal and/or toe pressures.

PREVENTION

✦ Avoid trauma to lower extremity.

✦ Foot care including proper shoes especially in patient with diabetes or arterial vascular disease. Consider referral to orthotist or pedorthist.

✦ Recommendations for venous disease patients:

✧ Regular walking or other exercise.

✧ Wear compression stockings with 20–30 mm Hg pressure.

✦ **See Protocol on Prevention and Health Maintenance.**

MANAGEMENT

✦ Begin with differentiation of ulcer etiology. See Table 3-3.

✦ If signs of infection (fever, lymphangitis), **see Protocol on Cellulitis.**

✦ **See Chapter on Special Hygiene Needs** for basic care recommendations.

✦ Consider Vitamin C (ascorbic acid) 500 mg qd, zinc sulfate 220 mg qd, and a multiple vitamin with minerals to enhance wound healing. **Vitamin A 25,000 IU qd should also be considered but short term (5–7 days).**

✦ Adequate nutrition is imperative to wound healing. Consult nutritionist.

Arterial/Ischemic Ulcers

✦ Characterized by claudication that requires exertion. **Disease in the femoral-popliteal artery causes pain or fatigue in the calf muscles that resolves by stopping the exertional activity. If the stenosis is in the iliac artery, the pain is felt in the affected buttock. Arterial ischemic pain at rest is usually felt in the distal forefoot and is usually described as a severe burning pain. The pain is worse at night and with elevation of the extremity. Relief is usually obtained when the extremity is in a dependent position such as dangling off the bedside. Claudication is usually present before the onset of pain at rest.**

✦ **There are no pigment changes over the shin and the tissue has a shiny, scaly, atrophic appearance with little or no hair growth. There may be fissures noted on the shins and heels. Signs of inflammation can develop rapidly with compromised circulation.**

✦ **Wound bed is yellow/gray/eschared with no granulating tissue. There is usually no bleeding following ulcer bed manipulation. Surrounding tissues may appear pale or mottled. Wet or dry gangrene may be present. Wet gangrene indicates probable secondary infection. Gangrene warrants immediate referral.**

✦ Management goals:

✧ Increased blood flow to leg. **Best accomplished by revascularization surgery or balloon angioplasty. Maximize medical management if patient is not a surgical candidate.**

✧ Comfort, pain relief.

✧ Prevention of further deterioration of wound by local care.

✦ Consider enzymatic debriding agent (Elactase, Debrisan).

✦ If antibiotics are required to treat secondary infection, oral antibiotic treatment is often less effective than IV route due to poor circulation to the area.

✦ Consult physician for referrals as appropriate to vascular/plastic surgeons, infectious disease specialist, wound/ostomy/continence nurse, OT, and PT.

✦ Use occlusive dressings with caution because wound cannot be viewed.

✦ Consider allowing wound to dry naturally, or painting with betadine bid to avoid tissue maceration and secondary infection.

Venous Ulcer Disease

✦ Caused by retrograde blood flow from incompetent, absent, or malfunctioning veins.

✦ May co-exist with arterial insufficiency, neuropathy, or lymphatic obstruction.

✦ May be characterized by edema that is often unilateral, chronic lymphedema, pruritic, or burning skin, brown or red skin discoloration (secondary to hemosiderin deposits), co-existing varicosities, purpura, telangiectasias, scaly skin, weeping dermatitis. Woody induration and fibrosis of skin may be present in chronic, late-stage disease.

✦ Ulcers may begin with slight trauma.

✦ Most are colonized with bacteria. **Antibiotics are not necessary in the absence of signs of local or systemic infection.**

✦ Treatment consists of three modalities:

✧ Elevation to correct venous hypertension and relieve pain. Recommend bed rest 2 hr bid with legs elevated above level of heart. Avoid sitting with legs in dependent position. Encourage walking.

✧ Compression to improve venous return and decrease superficial pressure. **Compression is contraindicated if venous stasis co-exists with arterial insufficiency.** Elastic wraps provide compression but are hard to apply and pressure varies. **Fitted elastic support garments can be custom fit with specific pressure (30–40 mm Hg). Often difficult to apply. Consider stocking with zipper or refer to OT for adaptive equipment such as stocking holder frame. Cannot be used if ulcers are present secondary**

to risk of trauma and leakage. Unna boot (gauze wrap with calamine, zinc oxide, gelatin, and glycerine topped with elastic dressing)—applied weekly. Good choice for elderly who cannot change dressings or apply compression stockings. Must be applied properly to prevent irritation. **Pressure may vary with different persons applying dressing. Contraindicated if cellulitis is present.**

✧ Occlusion/debridement provides for removal of necrotic tissue. Wet-to-dry saline dressings will debride but must be used with caution when granulation tissue is present. Occlusive dressings provide optimum debridement. Use cautiously with infected ulcer or cellulitis because these dressings prevent wound viewing. Steady improvement should be seen every week. If no improvement within 2–4 weeks, reassess treatment modality.

✦ Consult physician for ulcers recalcitrant to treatment, for surgical debridement, or growth factor therapy.

✦ Pain medication as indicated. Consult physician if pain is severe.

✦ If no improvement for 3 months, consider referral for biopsy for squamous cell or basal cell carcinoma.

Diabetic Ulcers

✦ Occur over pressure points.

✦ Motor, sensory, and autonomic neuropathies as well as vascular diseases are underlying problems.

✦ Usually painless, therefore unnoticed.

✦ Patient education is the key to prevention and treatment.

✦ High risk for amputation.

✦ Elevated blood glucose may be first clue to infection.

✦ Provide moist wound environment:

✧ Saline damp to dry q 12 hr if debridement is required.

✧ Saline damp to damp ever 6–8 hr to provide moist environment.

✧ Calcium alginates can be used with infected wound.

✧ Avoid occlusive agents and use caution with hydrogels. **Excess moisture can lead to maceration and wound deterioration.**

✦ Avoid cytotoxic cleansing agents such as Dakin's solution (diluted sodium hypochlorite), acetic acid, hydrogen peroxide, and betadine.

✦ Blood glucose control is necessary for wound healing.

✦ Pressure relief, non-weight bearing status (NWBS). Refer to PT/OT for adaptive equipment and assistive devices for ambulation. Consider referral to orthotist or pedorthist for secondary options for patient unable to maintain NWBS.

✦ Osteomyelitis (common when bone is exposed) requires prolonged IV antibiotics (5–6 weeks). Consult physician for referral to infectious disease specialist for antibiotic choices.

✦ Consider sharp debridement. Consult physician for referral to surgeon.

KEY ISSUES

Patient/Caregiver Education

Patient/caregiver should be able to:

✦ Verbalize importance of checking shoes for foreign objects/frayed seams prior to wearing, especially if patient with diabetes. Consider referral to diabetes educator.

✦ Verbalize principles of good skin care, foot hygiene.

✦ Perform dressing changes if possible.

✦ Verbalize proper use of medications.

✦ Identify signs/symptoms that mandate contacting nurse practitioner (NP) or physician.

✦ Explain importance of avoiding application of tape directly to skin.

Patients (caregivers) with venous disease should be able to:

✦ State importance of avoiding OTC topical ointments that could cause contact dermatitis.

✦ Verbalize importance of avoiding scratching of skin in the presence of pruritus.

✦ If indicated, demonstrate application of compression dressing with prescribed pressure.

Economic Considerations

✦ Ulcerations/claudication/pain can be disabling and lead to lost days of work or decreased function.

✦ Treatment modalities are costly and chronically recurrent.

✦ Osteomyelitis requires prolonged IV antibiotic therapy often not reimbursed by insurance.

Psychosocial Considerations

✦ Wound care can be overwhelming to patients and caregivers.

✦ Be aware that loss of body image and social isolation may result from presence of ulcers. **Wounds have a negative emotional impact.**

✦ Be alert for depression secondary to chronic illness requiring multiple treatment modalities.

✦ Odor associated with severe ulcers/infection can lead to social isolation.

Acute/Inpatient Setting

✦ More frequent dressing changes, IV antibiotics/diuretics may hasten healing. Consider if failed home treatment.

Extended Care Setting

✦ Refer to PT to promote ability to exercise.

Home Setting

✦ Patients with diminished functional status should be referred to home health agency for dressing application. Must meet homebound criteria under Medicare.

✦ Diabetic ulcers require close follow-up (every 7–10 days). Consider transportation issues.

✦ Consider functional alteration if NWBS is required.

✦ Monitor medication compliance.

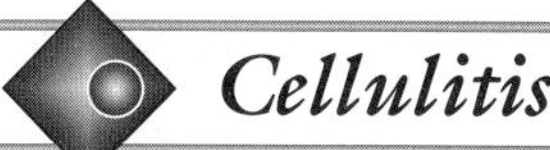

Cellulitis

HISTORY

✦ **Cellulitis is infection of skin and subcutaneous tissue characterized by nondistinct margins, accompanying erythema, tenderness, or pain.**

✦ Condition at site: location (usually occurs in lower extremity but possible in any part of body), discharge, odor, erythema, edema, pruritus, tenderness, or pain?

✦ Associated symptoms: fever, chills, rigor, malaise, lymphadenopathy, tinea infection, mental status changes?

✦ Comorbid conditions?

✦ **History of PVD, diabetes mellitus, immunosuppressed status, or extremity edema (CHF) increases risk of complications.**

✦ History of IV drug use?

✦ History of coronary artery bypass graft or femoropopliteal bypass surgery (occurs more frequently at vein graft sites)?

✦ Medications? Note steroids and other drugs that suppress immunity.

✦ Functional status?

✦ Social situation and supports?

PHYSICAL EXAMINATION

✦ Vital signs, temperature.

✦ Cardiovascular: auscultate for heart murmur (may occur as a result of bacteremia).

✦ Respiratory: note signs of CHF.

✦ Lymph: palpate nodes for tenderness and enlargement, especially those proximal to site.

✦ Skin: inspect condition of skin at suspected site. Inspect for signs of tinea at other areas. Note degree of edema and erythema. Streaking extending proximally from site with tender lymph nodes suggests lymphangitis. Assess for drainage and odor. Palpate for fluctuance and crepitus.

✦ Neuro: assess mental status.

DIAGNOSTIC TESTS

✦ CBC with differential.

✦ Culture of discharge or tissue does not usually identify causative agent, only surface contamination.

✦ Serum glucose (fasting, if possible). Cellulitis may be initial presentation of diabetes mellitus in elderly.

✦ Consider blood cultures if patient is immunocompromised or severely ill.

✦ Consider ultrasound or x-ray to rule out foreign body if suspected.

✦ Consider x-ray or bone scan of affected part to rule out osteomyelitis if diabetic, immunocompromised, or history of previous injury/surgery.

✦ Consider x-ray or CT/MRI if crepitus, fluctuance, or devitalization of tissue and to rule out underlying abscess.

PREVENTION

✦ Control edema in underlying CHF and vascular insufficiency.

✦ Optimize blood glucose control in diabetes mellitus.

✦ Administer tetanus immunization if open wound is present and not previously inoculated or no booster within past 5 years.

✦ **See Protocol on Prevention and Health Maintenance.**

MANAGEMENT

✦ **Increased risk for complications in the elderly.**

✦ Commonly caused by group A *Streptococcus* or *Staphylococcus aureus.*

✦ Gram-negative organisms are more prevalent in diabetics.

✦ Differentiate from thrombophlebitis by noting presence of palpable, tender vein.

✦ Usually managed outpatient if serious soft-tissue infections are excluded. **See Indications for Acute Hospital Admission** (below).

Indications for Acute Hospital Admission (Consult Physician)

✦ Cellulitis of orbit, face, or perineum.

✦ Animal or human bites.

✦ Accompanying fever and lymphangitis.

✦ Inability to care for self at home.

✦ Immunocompromised.

✦ Failed outpatient management.

Outpatient Management

✦ **Consult physician when cellulitis is suspected on basis of history and physical examination.** If abscess is present, consult physician or surgery clinic for incision and drainage.

✦ **Empiric treatment is usually effective.** Limit attempts to culture to those who have failed antibiotic therapy or for complex infections.

✦ Suspect pathogen of anaerobic origin when crepitus and/or discharge with foul odor are present.

✦ Empiric oral antibiotic agents:

✧ Dynapen, Pathocil (dicloxacillin) 125–250 mg PO qid for 10–14 days.

✧ Keflex (cephalexin) 250–500 mg PO qid for 10–14 days.

✧ Erythromycin 250–500 mg PO qid for 10–14 days.

✧ Duricef (cefadroxil) 500 mg PO bid for 10–14 days. Adjust dose if renal impairment.

✦ For patients with diabetes mellitus, cutaneous ulcers are usually polymicrobial in origin:

✧ Keflex (cephalexin) 250 mg PO qid and Cipro (ciprofloxacin HCl) 250–500 mg PO bid provide broad-spectrum coverage. Adjust dose of Cipro if renal impairment.

✦ Outpatient parenteral antibiotic therapy may be tried to avoid inpatient admission. Suspicion of deep infection or serious illness should prompt referral for hospitalization and parenteral antibiotic administration.

KEY ISSUES

Patient/Caregiver Education

Patient/caregiver should be able to:

✦ Demonstrate ability to perform wound care.

✦ State accurate antibiotic dosing.

✦ State signs/symptoms of nonhealing and complications that require contact of NP/physician.

✦ Verbalize importance of resting (elevating) affected area.

Economic Considerations

✦ Parenteral antibiotics are extremely costly and may not be covered by third party carriers. Medicare rules are changing on coverage of home care provision of IV therapy. Daily office administration may be required.

✦ Parenteral antibiotics justify skilled and acute care classification.

Psychosocial Considerations

✦ Chronic infection can debilitate and depress patients and strain caregivers. A multidisciplinary approach is a crucial management strategy.

Acute/Inpatient Setting

✦ Required for extensive debridement and parenteral antibiotic management of serious or resistant infections.

Extended Care Setting

✦ Consult physician to initiate parenteral antibiotics when appropriate to avoid inpatient admission.

Home Setting

✦ Assess social/caregiver support and patient's ability to follow treatment regimen at home. Refer to home health agency as appropriate.

✦ Chronic infection is a serious risk for further disability, malnutrition, functional decline.

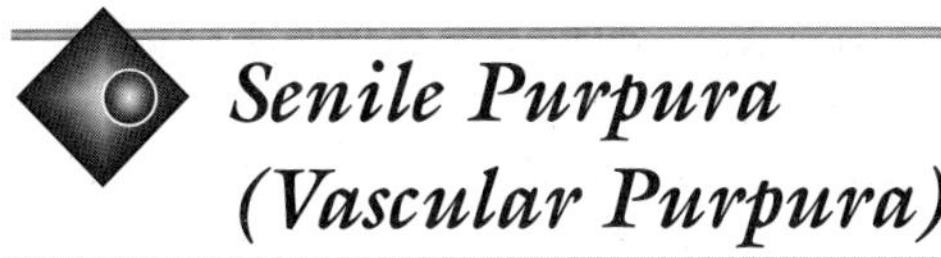

Senile Purpura (Vascular Purpura)

HISTORY

- ✦ Unexplained superficial bruising? Location?
- ✦ Onset? Trauma? Recent fall? History of falls?
- ✦ **If history is positive for prolonged bleeding with cuts and scratches; onset with infections or use of steroids, nonsteroidal antiinflammatory drugs (NSAIDS) or aspirin; EtOH intake; or malnutrition, rule out causes other than senile purpura, which is a benign condition.**
- ✦ Social situation, supports? **Be alert for possibility of physical abuse in the elderly patient.**

PHYSICAL EXAMINATION

- ✦ Assess for nonpalpable ecchymotic areas on forearms, especially radial/extensor surfaces.
- ✦ Assess for blanching. **Blanching is not expected with senile purpura.**
- ✦ Assess for hemosiderin (rust) deposits suggestive of recurrent, chronic condition.

DIAGNOSTIC TESTS

- ✦ Platelet count and coagulation studies. **Will be normal with senile purpura.**
- ✦ CBC and differential. **Will be normal with senile purpura.**

PREVENTION

- ✦ Implement interventions to decrease risk of trauma specific to elder.
- ✦ **See Protocol on Prevention and Health Maintenance.**

MANAGEMENT

- ✦ There is no specific treatment.

✦ Ascorbic acid 500 mg/day has been trialed, but if decreases bruising, is still not diagnostic of senile purpura.

✦ Consider clothing that protects the extremities.

KEY ISSUES

Patient/Caregiver Education

Patient/caregiver should be able to:

✦ Verbalize this is a recurrent, chronic condition.

✦ Verbalize condition is benign.

Psychosocial Considerations

✦ Assess for social withdrawal/isolation secondary to change in body image.

Acute/Inpatient and Extended Care Settings

✦ Consider padded side rails, especially in patient with cognitive changes.

✦ Consider clothing with long sleeves for protection.

✦ Implement fall prevention program. **See Protocol on Falls.**

✦ Avoid restraints.

Home Setting

✦ Environmental safety evaluation.

✦ Attention to fall prevention.

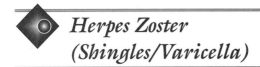

Herpes Zoster (Shingles/Varicella)

HISTORY

✦ Dermatomal pain, itching, or burning, pre-eruptive hyperesthesia along dermatome(s)? **Pain may precede eruption by days to weeks.**

✦ Prodromal symptoms of chills, fever, malaise?

✦ Blurring of vision? Periorbital edema?

✦ Severity of pain/discomfort? Use of a pain scale can help quantify pain.

✦ Onset? Duration of symptoms? Location of symptoms? **Most commonly affected areas are thoracic, cervical, and ophthalmic regions.**

✦ Characteristic lesions? Erythematous plaques initially; developing into papulovesicular lesions in clusters arising from erythematous bases following unilateral dermatomal pattern; pustulate and crust in 7–10 days. Successive eruptions possible over next 5–7 days; total resolution in 1 month.

✦ Postherpetic neuralgia: presence of pain more than 1 month after onset of zoster eruption? **Pain is neuropathic. Incidence is greatly increased with each decade over age 60; incidence increased in ophthalmic zoster.**

✦ Effect on daily life: altered sleep, mood, appetite, ability to perform ADLs?

✦ Recent acute illness or stressors?

✦ Comorbid conditions?

PHYSICAL EXAMINATION

✦ Examine affected areas for characteristic lesions, pre-eruption hyperesthesia, paresthesia, pruritus, or secondary infection.

✦ Examine face, eyes for possible ophthalmic involvement.

✦ Palpate for lymph node enlargement in regional distribution.

DIAGNOSTIC TESTS

✦ Usually unnecessary due to characteristic appearance of lesions.

✦ Vesicle scraping: presence of giant cells, stained multi-nuclear epithelial cells characteristic of this viral infection (Tzanck preparation).

PREVENTION

✦ Contact isolation of infected individuals, especially from pregnant or immunosuppressed individuals without varicella immunity, until vesicles have resolved.

✦ Strict hand washing, wound and contact precautions when examining or treating affected patients.

✦ **See Protocol on Prevention and Health Maintenance.**

MANAGEMENT

Acute Phase

✦ Avoid dressings and topical agents which may exacerbate pain or macerate tissues. Consider premedication with analgesics 45–60 min prior to dressing change.

✦ Apply wet compresses of Burrow's solution or tepid water several times daily for 30 min, then pat dry; may be helpful as lesions begin to crust.

✦ Trial of scheduled Tylenol (acetaminophen) or NSAIDs for pain management

✦ For severe pain, consider a trial of low dose narcotics. Consult with physician.

✦ If lesions become secondarily infected, give systemic oral antibiotics such as Keflex (cephalexin) 250–500 mg every 6 hr; available in suspension 125–250 mg/5 ml; E.E.S. 400 (erythromycin ethylsuccinate) 400 mg every 6 hr; available in suspension 200–400 mg/5 ml; or Pathocil (dicloxacillin) 125–250 mg every 6 hr, available in suspension 62.5 mg/5 ml. **Be alert to administration guidelines and common side effects, especially GI symptoms.**

✦ Refer any patient with eye or facial involvement to an ophthalmologist for identification and treatment of possible herpes corneal involvement.

✦ Antiviral therapy **if patient presents within the first 72 hr of rash** (speeds healing of the rash, decreases pain and ocular complications). Adjust dose if renal impairment is present.

- ✧ Zovirax (acyclovir) 800 mg five times daily for 7 days; or
- ✧ Valtrex (valacyclovir) 1,000 mg tid for 7 days; or
- ✧ Famvir (famcyclovir) 500 mg tid for 7 days.

✦ If no contraindications (i.e., diabetes mellitus, hypertension, or glaucoma) to corticosteroids: consider prednisone 40–60 mg/day, tapered over a period of 21 days. **Initiate within first week. Corticosteroids may hasten recovery from severe infections, but do not prevent postherpetic neuralgia.**

✦ Follow-up in 5–7 days or sooner if patient is frail.

✦ Consider hospitalization if frail patient, if more than 3 dermatomes are affected, or for severe infection with systemic symptoms. Consult with physician.

Postherpetic Neuralgia

✦ Topical therapy with lidocaine 5% gel or lidocaine-prilocaine cream or Zostrix (capsaicin). Apply five to six times daily; may initially cause some burning.

✦ Trial of analgesic or low dose narcotic medications (assess benefit in 1–2 days) and taper over time.

✦ If pain is constant: consider adding a tricyclic antidepressant, Norpramin (desipramine) 12.5–25 mg at bed time. Use cautiously in older patients; increased incidence of adverse side effects: increased confusion, dry mouth, constipation, urinary retention, and falls.

✦ If pain is lancinating: consider Tegretol (carbamazepine) 100–200 mg/daily, increase as needed; available as suspension 100 mg/5 ml. Can cause blood dyscrasias; monitor CBC.

✦ If pain persists: consider alternative antidepressant or anticonvulsant medications or combination therapy.

✦ Consider nonpharmacologic approaches, i.e., transcutaneous electrical nerve stimulation (TENS) unit, behavioral management, or referral to a neurologist or Pain Management Clinic.

KEY ISSUES

Patient/Caregiver Education

Patient/caregiver should be able to:

✦ Verbalize the cause of herpes zoster and prolonged condition of postherpetic neuralgia.

✦ Demonstrate understanding of treatment modalities.

✦ Identify signs and symptoms of secondary infection.

✦ Demonstrate correct techniques for contact isolation to protect family/care givers with no varicella immunity.

✦ Assess and manage pain appropriately.

Economic Considerations

✦ Antivirals are costly and may require prior approval on some health plan formularies.

Psychosocial Considerations

✦ Patient may have altered mood/depression, especially if pain course is prolonged.

✦ Patient may have altered sleep patterns secondary to pain.

✦ Inform patient that lesions rarely leave permanent scarring.

Acute/Inpatient Setting

✦ Maintain contact isolation until all lesions are crusted.

✦ Assess pain level and provide adequate pain management. Adjust regimen as needed. Pain may be exacerbated by an acute illness.

✦ Observe for secondary infections.

✦ Consider IV antiviral therapy if within 3 days of onset.

✦ Monitor for electrolyte imbalance and nutritional needs.

Extended Care Setting

✦ Maintain contact isolation until all lesions are crusted.

✦ Be especially alert to pain in the patient with dementia who may be unable to express pain verbally.

Home Setting

✦ Maintain contact isolation until all lesions are crusted.

✦ Provide for increased need for assistance with ADLs during acute phase or with postherpetic neuralgia.

Chapter 4

Cardiovascular System

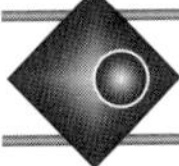

Chest Pain

HISTORY

✦ Thoracic pain may be difficult to evaluate as many organs in this region supply pain pathways to the spine, with many crossed synapses between T1 and T6, making pain localization a challenge.

✦ Description of pain? Sharp, stabbing, burning, tearing, dull, aching, squeezing, pressure, or fullness? The elderly may have atypical presentation due to altered pain sensation. Angina may present as shortness of breath without chest pain.

✦ Description of pain on a scale of 0 to 10? Mild, moderate, severe? Is the pain constant or intermittent when present?

✦ Onset? Sudden or gradual? Is pain new, if not when did it last occur?

✦ How often does it occur? How long does it last?

✦ Location? Radiation?

✦ Associated symptoms: dyspnea, cough, hemoptysis, diaphoresis, eructations, nausea, vomiting, diarrhea, dizziness/syncope, headache, palpitations, fever, anxiety, fatigue, or swelling in the extremities?

✦ If pain is recurrent, does it occur with exertion or a particular activity; rest; change in environmental temperature or oral intake of icy foods/drink; excitement/emotion, either positive or negative; stress; respiration; body position; certain foods or on an empty stomach? What activity was going on with this occurrence?

✦ Does chest pain occur at a particular time of the day or night?

✦ Is the pain frightening?

✦ Baseline functional status? Effect of pain on baseline functional status? Quality of life secondary to pain?

✦ Recent cognitive changes? Falls?

✦ What relieves or alleviates the pain? Rest, medication (nitroglycerin/antacids/other), change in position, eating, or warmth? How quickly is it relieved?

✦ Can symptoms be reproduced by applying pressure to the area of pain?

✦ How does this episode of pain differ from previous episodes?

✦ Tobacco use? Alcohol (EtOH) use? Caffeine use?

✦ History of diabetes mellitus, hypertension (HTN), coronary artery disease (CAD), hyperlipidemia, valvular heart disease, chronic obstructive pulmonary disease (COPD), gastrointestinal or musculoskeletal disorders?

✦ Recent surgery or infection? **Risk of myocardial infarction (MI)/pneumonia is increased.**

✦ Family history of CAD, HTN, diabetes mellitus, or hyperlipidemia?

PHYSICAL EXAMINATION

✦ Vital signs with blood pressures (BPs) lying, sitting, and standing; weight. Oxygen saturation using pulse oximeter.

✦ Assess gait/posture. Note guarding/expressions of pain.

✦ Observe for signs of anxiety.

✦ Assess skin for pallor, cyanosis, and moisture.

✦ Assess for rash or scarring of the thorax. **May suggest herpes zoster.**

✦ Palpate cervical spine for trigger points, pain, or limitation in movement with flexion, extension, and rotation. **Suggestive of osteoarthritis.**

✦ Observe respirations for rate, rhythm, ease or distress of breathing Assess for cough; assess sputum for color, quantity as appropriate.

✦ Assess lungs for crackles, wheezes, absent breath sounds, increased tactile fremitus, egophony ("eee" sounds like "ay"), and rubs. **All suggest pulmonary pathology.**

✦ Auscultate for arrhythmia, tachy- and brady- rates; murmurs and rubs. Auscultate for aortic, renal, iliac, and femoral bruits.

✦ Palpate costochondral area bilaterally. **Costochondritis typically involves second through the fourth costochondral junctions and xiphoid.**

✦ Assess for guarded respiration and pain with change of position. **May suggest fractured rib(s), especially with history of falls or EtOH usage.**

✦ Assess abdomen for distention, bowel sounds and bruits, tenderness, and organomegaly.

✦ Assess for peripheral pulsations and peripheral edema.

DIAGNOSTIC TESTS

✦ 12-Lead electrocardiogram (ECG).

✦ Creatine phosphokinase (CPK), isoenzyme CPK-MB fractions, CBC and differential, glucose, blood urea nitrogen (BUN), creatinine, electrolytes, Free T4, and thyroid-stimulating hormone (TSH).

✦ Posterior/anterior and lateral chest x-ray.

✦ Consider barium swallow to rule out esophageal strictures/gastroesophageal reflux disease (GERD). **Rule out cardiac etiology first.**

✦ Consider referral to cardiologist for further work-up (Holter monitoring/exercise tolerance testing/thallium stress test/arteriogram/heart catheterization) if findings are suggestive of coronary or valvular heart disease. Consult with physician.

✦ CT scanning/MRI are considered to document cervical osteoarthritis with nerve root compression.

PREVENTION

✦ **See Protocols on Prevention and Health Maintenance; Chronic Obstructive Pulmonary Disease; Pneumonia; Gastroesophageal Reflux Disease; Abdominal Pain; Falls; and Anxiety.**

✦ Avoid precipitating factors.

✦ Modify ischemic heart disease risk factors. **Emphasis is on smoking cessation, exercise, and HTN. Lipid control in the younger elder.**

✦ Aspirin 81 mg daily.

MANAGEMENT

Differential diagnosis and management is often difficult in the elderly due to atypical presentation, co-existing chronic diseases, and presence of dementia and/or delirium. Treatment of chest pain is an emergent condition until proven otherwise. Differential diagnoses of chest pain may include:

✦ **Cardiac:** angina, MI, aortic dissection.

✦ **Pulmonary:** pneumonia/pleurisy.

✦ **Gastrointestinal:** GERD, peptic ulcer, cholecystitis.

✦ **Musculoskeletal:** costochondritis (Tietze's syndrome), hypertrophic osteoarthritis of cervical spine with radiculopathy, rib fractures.

✦ **Neurologic:** herpes zoster.

✦ **Other:** anxiety disorders.

Refer to Display 4-1.

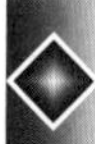

DISPLAY 4-1. *Differential Diagnosis of Chest Pain by Site of Origin*

Myocardial Ischemia

Retrosternal
Interscapular
Epigastric
Shoulder
Arms, especially left
Jaw

Aortic Dissection

Retrosternal
Back

Pneumonia/Pleurisy

Right lower anterior chest
Left lower anterior chest
Shoulder
Epigastric
Back

Gastric/Duodenal Pathology

Epigastric
Right lower anterior chest
Back

Cholecystitis

Interscapular
Epigastric
Shoulder, especially right

Costochondritis (Tietze's Syndrome)

Second to fourth costochondral junction
Shoulder

Hypertrophic Osteoarthritis of Cervical Spine (Cervical Spondylosis)

Arms
Shoulder

Gastroesophageal

Retrosternal
Epigastric

Angina

✦ Typical presentation is pressure/squeezing/heaviness substernally with radiation to neck and left arm. Nitroglycerin sublingually usually relieves pain. If unrelieved by nitroglycerin, and accompanied by dyspnea, nausea, and vomiting, suspect unstable angina/MI. **Emergent, consult physician.**

✦ Management requires understanding of baseline function and activity typically prompting anginal episode.

✦ Untreated HTN, COPD, hyperthyroidism, arrhythmias, and infection require appropriate work-up and management to decrease frequency and severity of angina.

✦ In patient with known angina, change in pattern, such as: pain at rest, increase in frequency, or unrelieved by nitroglycerin, may represent unstable angina.

✦ Use of tobacco causes vasoconstriction. Smoking cessation decreases the susceptibility to angina by eliminating carbon monoxide/vasoconstriction.

✦ Medications include: sublingual, transdermal, or oral nitrates; beta blockers such as Inderal (propranolol HCl), Tenormin (atenolol), Lopressor or Toprol-XL (metoprolol), Cogard (nadalol). **Use cautiously in congestive failure.** Calcium channel blockers such as Procardia or Adalat (nifedipine), Isoptin or Calan (verapamil HCl), Cardizem (diltiazem HCl), or Norvasc (amlodipine).

✦ Patient may be instructed to use sublingual nitrates prior to activities known to precipitate angina.

Myocardial Infarction (MI)

✦ **Emergent condition. Refer immediately to the nearest emergency department. Consult physician.**

✦ Most older than 85 years of age do not complain of chest pain during MI. **Dyspnea, mental status changes, agitation, weakness, syncope, and/or anorexia may be the only manifestations of MI.** History is basis for hospitalization.

✦ Initial treatment includes: nitroglycerin (0.4 mg) sublingually; aspirin 325 mg orally (or chewed); IV morphine for pain unresolved with nitroglycerin sublingually; and oxygen therapy.

✦ Thrombolytic therapy and beta blockers are used in elderly if not contraindicated. **Adverse drug effects are more common among the elderly.**

✦ Hospitalization for close monitoring and supportive care. **Arrhythmias are a common complication.**

Aortic Dissection

✦ Presents with sudden onset of severe, tearing chest pain with radiation into both extremities and into back. **Suspect in patient with history of HTN. May also occur as a result of late stage syphilis. Emergent. Refer immediately to nearest emergency department. Consult physician.**

✦ Emergent goal is BP control.

✦ May find unequal pulses/BPs. May rapidly develop MI, arrhythmia, congestive heart failure (CHF).

✦ Chest x-ray demonstrates widening of mediastinum.

Pneumonia/Pleurisy

✦ **See Protocol on Pneumonia.**

✦ Pain is described as aching (in pneumonia) and sharp or breath catching in pleurisy. Pain is usually located in the lower chest.

✦ Upper respiratory track infection may have preceded the pain.

✦ Associated symptoms may include fever, dyspnea, cough.

Gastrointestinal

✦ **See Protocols on Gastroesophageal Reflux Disease and GI Bleeding.**

Cholecystitis

✦ **See Protocol on Abdominal Pain.**

Costochondritis (Tietze's Syndrome)

✦ Pain is described as constant, aching, and stabbing pain. Pain is worse on palpation and with coughing, deep respirations, or any movement of the involved joints. It is constant for days at a time.

✦ Usually involves the second to fourth costochondral junction, the xiphoid, and may radiate into the shoulders and arms and across the precordium.

✦ May be recurrent.

✦ Patients having experienced a viral illness, cancer, or rheumatologic illnesses are at greatest risk.

✦ Activities such a gardening/pruning may aggravate the condition.

✦ Heat often helps relieve the pain.

✦ Treat with nonsteroidal antiinflammatory agents or scheduled acetaminophen.

Hypertrophic Osteoarthritis of Cervical Spine (Cervical Spondylosis)

✦ A radiculopathy due to irritation of sensory nerve roots.

✦ Onset is gradual and may follow exertional activities involving the upper chest wall, such as bending, lifting, painting, or gardening, and prolonged periods of lying or sitting.

✦ Pain is recurrent and described as a heavy, pressure, or vice-like constriction (similar to angina). Pain is unrelieved by nitroglycerin or rest.

✦ Pain is moderate to severe and may radiate bilaterally to the neck, jaw, and back (depending on the dermatome involved). Substernal or precordial pain may be present and radiate into the left arm, neck, or jaw.

✦ Pain can be reproduced by palpation of posterior cervical trigger points and may be associated with lightheadedness or syncope, as vertebral arteries may be compressed.

✦ Treat with nonsteroidal antiinflammatory agents. If ineffective, consider steroid taper, physical therapy, cervical collar, or traction. Refer to orthopedics or neurosurgery for resistant cases.

✦ MRI and CT/myelogram may be the indicated diagnostic tests.

Rib Fracture

✦ Pain is of sudden onset at time of trauma and may worsen after the first few days of injury. Movement of thorax as well as deep breathing aggravates the pain.

✦ Pain is sharp, moderate to severe.

✦ Posturing toward the affected side, or splinting the area is common.

✦ Rule out lung trauma in presence of 12–24-hr delay in dyspnea, cough, hemoptysis, or fever.

✦ EtOH, benzodiazipine, or tricyclic usage increases the incidence of falls, which increase the risk of rib fractures. Osteopenic patients are particularly vulnerable. **See Protocol on Falls.**

✦ Treat with nonsteroidal antiinflammatory agents, scheduled acetaminophen; narcotics should be considered acutely.

✦ Consider Zostrix (capsaicin) applications to site of pain qid.

✦ Ice/heat should be considered. **Use cautiously if using Zostrix, because either can potentiate treatment.**

Herpes Zoster

✦ **Elderly are at increased risk.**

✦ Gradual, progressive onset or may be postherpetic and chronic.

- ✦ Sharp, stinging, burning pain. Aggravated by any contact of the skin.
- ✦ Moderate to severe pain. Rash may not appear until days after onset of pain.
- ✦ **See Protocol on Herpes Zoster.**

Anxiety Disorder

✦ May be sudden or gradual onset and lasts at least 30 min and may be continuous for days.

✦ Pain is often vague and diffuse; patient may feel disabled by the pain.

✦ Patient may have associated hyperventilation. **May cause T-wave inversion and ST segment depression, as well as low pCO_2 on blood gas testing.**

✦ Patient often reports multiple treatments with variable results.

✦ Be alert to multiple somatic complaints; history of anxiety/depression.

✦ Rule out organic causes.

✦ Refer to psychologist for psychometric testing/psychotherapy; refer to psychiatrist for potential pharmacologic intervention. **Consult physician.**

✦ Treat underlying emotional state (psychotherapy and/or antidepressant/anxiolytic agents). **Consult physician.**

KEY ISSUES

Patient/Caregiver Education

Patient/caregiver should be able to:

✦ Identify and verbalize precipitating activities and risk factors associated with underlying illness.

✦ Describe how to personally control/eliminate precipitating activities and risk factors.

✦ Verbalize understanding of medications to treat underlying cause and demonstrate compliance with treatment regime.

✦ Verbalize signs and symptoms that should prompt emergent treatment from professional care provider.

Economic Considerations

✦ Unnecessary hospitalization of patients with chest pain costs $1.5–3.5 billion annually. Emergency room protocols have been developed based on clinical history, ECG, and baseline laboratory values to predict likelihood of ischemic disease and recommendations for hospitalization.

✦ Coronary arteriogram/heart catheterization should be reserved for the patient who is a surgical candidate and desires surgical correction if indicated.

✦ Due to the chronicity of most chest pain etiologies, treatment plans/medications can become very expensive.

Psychosocial Considerations

✦ Be alert to signs and symptoms of depression and anxiety related to altered sense of well being.

✦ Assess functional/cognitive status to determine changes associated with chest pain.

✦ Refer to social services to coordinate community resources to assist the patient in remaining within the community despite functional loss.

✦ Consult physician/cardiologist and occupational therapist (OT)/physical therapist (PT) for exercise program specific for patient.

Acute/Inpatient Setting

✦ All chest pain must be considered emergent until proven otherwise.

✦ Cardiovascular work-up can be done as an outpatient.

✦ Presentation may be acute onset delirium—proceed with work-up as indicated for emergent conditions.

Extended Care Setting

✦ Dementia complicates differential diagnosis—staff must be educated to be alert to any change in baseline behaviors.

✦ Due to limited resources, the nurse practitioner (NP) often performs the ECG and makes appropriate referrals.

✦ An interdisciplinary approach often prevents unnecessary hospitalization.

Home Setting

✦ Emphasis on preventive strategies.

✦ Assess routinely for compliance with medication and management interventions, which are often complex.

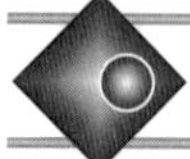

Hypertension

HISTORY

✦ Prior diagnosis of elevated BP?

✦ Previous treatments for HTN?

✦ Headaches? Location? Onset? Duration? Treatment?

✦ Dizziness? Vertigo? Syncope? Altered balance? History of falls?

✦ Vision changes? Last eye examination?

✦ Chest pain? Location? Onset? Duration? History of angina or heart disease?

✦ Shortness of breath? **Angina often presents atypically in the elderly; dyspnea is often presenting symptom.**

✦ Recent weight gain or loss?

✦ Edema? Location?

✦ Comorbid conditions: history of MI, cerebrovascular accident (CVA), transient ischemic attacks (TIA), peripheral vascular disease (PVD), CHF, renal disease, diabetes mellitus, hyperlipidemia, COPD?

✦ History of prostate problems, urinary retention, or incontinence?

✦ History of dementia or depression?

✦ Family history of HTN, heart disease, diabetes mellitus, hyperlipidemia?

✦ Medications: prescription/OTC? **Be alert to medications which may increase BP, e.g., NSAIDs, antihistamines, decongestants, tricyclic antidepressants.**

✦ Tobacco use? EtOH use?

✦ Allergies?

✦ Diet history? Sodium/fat intake?

✦ Activity level? Exercise history?

✦ Stressors?

✦ Mood? Sexual function? Sleep habits?

✦ Presence of major risk factors places patient into a high risk category. Risk factors include: smoking, dyslipidemia, diabetes mellitus, age > 60 years, male gender, postmenopausal status, family history of CV disease.

✦ Risk categories are: Group A—no risk factors, no target organ disease (TOD)/CV disease; Group B—at least one risk factor excluding diabetes mellitus, no TOD/CV disease; Group C—TOD/CV disease and/or diabetes mellitus with or without risk factors.

PHYSICAL EXAMINATION

✦ Vital signs; BP in both arms in three positions on initial visit. On follow-up visits, take BP in arm in which BP was highest. Include Osler maneuver each visit.

✦ Weight on each visit.

✦ Fundoscopic: **Observe for arteriolar narrowing, focal spasm of arterioles. Papilledema, hemorrhages, and/or exudates indicate malignant HTN.**

✦ Cardiovascular examination: assess heart, auscultate for bruits, palpate peripheral pulses, observe for signs of PVD.

✦ Respiratory examination: assess for signs of CHF.

✦ Abdominal examination: assess for aneurysm, bruits, hepatomegaly.

✦ Consider neurological examination if suspected TIAs.

DIAGNOSTIC TESTS

✦ Initial visit:

✧ Fasting lipid profile.

✧ Serum electrolytes, BUN, creatinine, CBC.

✧ Hemoglobin A1C (if patient is a diabetic or if fasting blood sugar [FBS] is in borderline range).

✧ Urinalysis.

✧ 12-Lead ECG.

✧ Consider a chest x-ray if target organ disease present (see Display 4-2).

✧ Consider carotid Doppler study if carotid bruits present.

✧ Consider an echocardiogram if symptoms of CHF.

✦ Follow-up visits:

✧ Diagnostic testing should be customized to the individual based on risk factors, comorbid conditions, and treatment regimen. Minimum of annual electrolytes, BUN, and creatinine.

PREVENTION

✦ Weight reduction and referral for nutritional counseling if appropriate.

✦ Diet instruction. **Major dietary restrictions should be avoided. A no-added-salt diet is usually sufficient; a reduction to less than 4 g of sodium is rarely necessary. Reduction of caffeine recommended. Consult with nutritionist.**

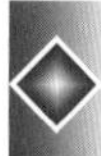

DISPLAY 4-2. *Manifestations of Target Organ Disease*

Cardiac:	CAD, left ventricular hypertrophy, CHF
Cerebrovascular:	TIA, CVA
Peripheral vascular:	Aneurysm, reduced pulses with or without claudication
Retinopathy:	Hemorrhages, exudate, papilledema
Renal:	Elevated creatinine (> 1.5 mg/dL), proteinuria

- ✦ Regular exercise as tolerated; aerobic exercise is of greatest benefit.
- ✦ Annual eye examinations.
- ✦ Smoking cessation.
- ✦ Reduction or cessation of EtOH.
- ✦ Stress management/relaxation techniques.
- ✦ **See Protocol on Prevention and Health Maintenance.**

MANAGEMENT

- ✦ If possible, discontinue medications that may increase BP.
- ✦ Optimal management of comorbid conditions.
- ✦ Consult with physician if newly diagnosed, refractory to treatment, hypertensive emergency, or evidence of target organ damage.
- ✦ Consider referral for specialty evaluation for secondary HTN (see Display 4-3), if refractory to treatment or with target organ damage.
- ✦ Refer immediately to emergency department if hypertensive emergency.
- ✦ Definition/classification:

Optimal BP	≤ 120/80 mm Hg
Normal BP	≤ 130/85
High normal	130/85 to 139/89
Stage I (mild)	140/90 to 159/99
Stage II	160/100 to 179/109
Stage III	≥ 180 to ≥ 110

- ✦ Goal is to maintain average diastolic BP (DBP) at < 90 mm Hg with at least a 10-mm Hg decrease below pretreatment pressure over a prolonged period with avoidance of significant medication side effects.

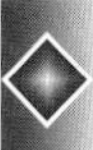

DISPLAY 4-3. *Manifestations of Secondary Hypertension (HTN)*

Pheochromocytoma:	Headache, palpitations, labile or refractory HTN, weight loss, endocrine disorder
Renovascular:	Malignant or refractory HTN, abdominal bruits, renal insufficiency
Primary aldosteronism:	Refractory HTN, hypokalemia
Cushing's syndrome:	Characteristic body habitus, skin changes

✦ Isolated systolic HTN is more common in the older population; goal is a 15–20-mm Hg decrease in systolic BP (SBP) or an SBP of < 160 mm Hg. **Systolic HTN is more highly associated with cardiovascular morbidity/mortality than diastolic HTN.**

✦ Consider antihyperlipidemic agent. **See Protocol on Hyperlipidemia.**

✦ Tailor medication regimen to the older patient. Keep regimen as simple as possible. **Goals of BP reduction should be modified if medication side effects are significant. See Chapter on Medication Issues.**

✦ Initial antihypertensive choice and dose is determined by patient's age, risk factors, presence or absence of cardiac, renal, neurological, or vascular disease, allergies or other comorbid conditions, essential versus secondary HTN, and cost to patient. Consider "two for one" concept, i.e., beta blockers for patient with glaucoma/HTN or arteriosclerotic cardiovascular disease (ASCVD)/HTN; calcium antagonists for angina/HTN or atrial fibrillation/HTN.

✦ If little or no response to the initial agent: increase dose, add a second agent, or change to a different class of drugs.

✦ Frequency of follow-up varies depending on the stability of BP control and other comorbid conditions. Follow-up within 1–2 weeks when changing medication regimen.

✦ Medication choices: **Dosages given are usual adult starting dose; start low/go slow with the elderly patient. Examples are given in each class. See Chapter on Medication Issues.**

✧ **Diuretics:** Inexpensive, effective; may increase cholesterol and low-density lipoprotein (LDL); may affect glucose control in diabetics. Useful with associated dependent edema.

✧ **Thiazides:** HCTZ (hydrochlorothiazide) 12.5–25 mg daily.

✧ **Loop diuretics:** Lasix (furosemide) 20–40 mg daily. Patients with impaired renal function and/or CHF may require much higher doses. May be used IV in acute setting.

✧ **Potassium-sparing:** Aldactone (spironolactone) 25–50 mg daily/bid.

✧ **Combination:** Dyazide (hydrochlorothiazide 25 mg and triameterene 37.5 mg) 1–2 tablets daily, Maxzide (hydrochlorothiazide 50 mg and triameterene 75 mg) 1 tablet daily.

✧ **Quinazoline:** Zaroxolyn (metolazone) 2.5–5 mg daily, maximum dose 20 mg/daily. Use cautiously in frail elders at risk for dehydration.

✧ **Central antiadrenergic agents:**

✧ Catapres (clonidine HCl) 0.1 mg bid, maximum dose 2.4 mg daily, transdermal patch weekly (start with 0.1 mg, available in 0.2 mg and 0.3 mg).

✧ Aldomet (methyldopa) start with 250 mg bid and titrate slowly as needed.

These agents have significant sedative effects and may be associated with increased risk of confusion and depression in the elderly. The clonidine patch may be useful in patients who are unable to take oral medications. Rebound HTN may occur if patient is noncompliant or if clonidine is discontinued abruptly or used prn in the acute setting.

✧ **Beta blockers: Not as effective as monotherapy in elderly patients.**

✧ Tenormin (atenolol) 25–50 mg daily, maximum dose 50 mg bid.

✧ Lopressor (metoprolol tartrate) 50 mg bid, maximum 450 mg/daily, available in an extended-release form.

✧ Corgard (nadolol) 20–40 mg daily, maximum 320 mg daily.

✧ **Direct vasodilators:**

✧ Apresoline (hydralazine HCl) 10 mg qid, maximum 300 mg daily. BID dosing may be adequate.

✧ Loniten (minoxidil) 2.5–5 mg daily, maximum 100 mg daily.

Potent agents; may cause edema formation.

✧ **Alpha-1 blockers:**

✧ Cardura (doxazosin mesylate) 1 mg daily, maximum 16 mg daily.

✧ Minipress (prazosin HCl) 1 mg bid/tid, maximum 40 mg daily.

✧ Hytrin (terazosin HCl) 1 mg at bed time, maximum 20 mg daily.

Indirect vasodilators; may also be used for urinary retention in patients with neurogenic bladder.

✧ **Angiotensin-converting enzyme (ACE) inhibitors:**

✧ Lotensin (benazepril HCl) 5–10 mg daily, maximum 40 mg daily.

✧ Capoten (captopril) 6.25–12.5 mg bid/tid, maximum 300 mg daily.

✧ Vasotec (enalapril maleate) 2.5–5 mg daily, maximum 40 mg daily.

✧ Monopril (fosinopril sodium) 10 mg daily, maximum 40 mg daily.

✧ Accupril (quinapril HCl) 5–10 mg daily, maximum 80 mg daily.

✧ Prinivil, Zestril (lisinopril) 2.5–10 mg daily, maximum 20 mg daily.

✧ Altace (ramipril) 1.25–2.5 mg daily, maximum 20 mg daily.

Research indicates a lower mortality with use of ACE inhibitors in patients with CHF and a renal protective component in patients with diabetes. Monitor renal function and potassium levels, which can increase with use of ACE inhibitors. When possible, stop diuretics 2–3 days before beginning ACE inhibitors. If not possible, begin with lowest dose and monitor closely. See Protocol on Heart Failure.

✧ **Calcium channel blockers: May cause constipation.**

✧ Norvasc (amlodipine) 2.5–5 mg daily, maximum 10 mg daily.

✧ Cardizem (diltiazem HCl) 30 mg qid, maximum 360 mg daily, available in once-daily sustained-release (Cardiazem CD or Dilacor XR: 120, 180, 240, 300, or 360 mg) and twice-daily sustained-release (Cardiazem SR: 60, 90, or 120 mg).

✧ Plendil (felodipine) 5 mg daily, maximum 20 mg daily.

✧ Procardia XL, Adalat CC (nifedipine) once-daily sustained-release 30, 60, or 90 mg.

✧ Calan (verapamil HCl) 80 mg tid, maximum 360 mg daily, available in once-daily sustained-release (Calan SR: 120, 180, or 240 mg).

✧ **Angiotensin II receptor antagonists: Less likely to produce cough than ACE inhibitors.**

✧ Cozaar (losarten potassium) 25–50 mg daily, maximum 100 mg daily.

✧ Diovan (valsarten) 80 mg daily, maximum 320 mg daily.

✧ Avapro (irbesartan) 150 mg daily, maximum 300 mg daily.

KEY ISSUES

Patient/Caregiver Education

Patient/caregiver should be able to:

✦ Verbalize recommended nonpharmacological techniques.

✦ Identify medications and verbalize regimen.

✦ Discuss potential target organ effects of HTN.

✦ Demonstrate correct technique for monitoring BP (when appropriate).

✦ Verbalize understanding of dietary restrictions.

Economic Considerations

✦ Consider cost of medications, and if covered by insurance.

✦ Consider cost of follow-up visits, laboratory testing, special foods with restricted diet.

Psychosocial Considerations

✦ Patients who take diuretics may avoid or limit social interactions or may not take the medication on days when they have outside activities planned.

✦ Simplify regimen to maximize compliance; consider medication reminders or pill organizers.

Acute/Inpatient Setting

✦ Reassess antihypertensive regimen during acute hospitalization; patient may not require as much medication during that time.

✦ Be alert to potential for orthostasis and falls. **See Protocol on Falls.**

✦ Avoid overly aggressive lowering of BP in acute stroke; maintain BP > 140/90. **See Protocol on Transient Ischemic Attack (TIA)/Cerebrovascular Accident (CVA).**

✦ Acute management of elevated BP: use the rapid-acting oral agent, clonidine 0.1 mg; observe for rebound.

✦ Antihypertensive agents may need to be administered IV or transdermally during acute hospitalization.

Extended Care Setting

✦ Be alert to potential for orthostasis and falls. **See Protocol on Falls.**

✦ Transfer patients from lying to sitting to standing slowly to prevent orthostasis.

✦ Consider use of supervised rocking chair for patients with orthostasis.

✦ Acute management of elevated BP: use the rapid-acting oral agent, clonidine 0.1 mg; observe for rebound.

✦ Be alert for atypical presentations of associated cardiovascular problems, i.e., silent MI, TIA, CVA.

Home Setting

✦ Have patient/caregiver maintain BP record and bring to follow-up visits.

✦ Home health referral for homebound patients with refractory BP or other risk factors.

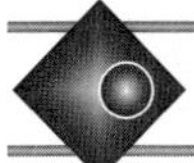

Heart Failure

HISTORY

✦ Symptoms occur due to the heart's decreased ability to adequately pump and circulate blood, resulting in overload and congestion of the circulatory system. Symptoms of salt and water retention will also be present because failure of the cardiac pump activates the renin–angiotensin–aldosterone system.

✦ Depending on which side of the heart has compromised function, presentation will include classic symptoms and physical findings. See Display 4-4. **Be aware that heart failure may present atypically in the elderly: mental status changes, lethargy, insomnia, agitation, decreased functional status, incontinence, weight loss. Symptoms may be attributed to aging rather than heart failure.**

✦ **In the elderly, symptoms may be attributed to comorbidity: edema to venous insufficiency rather than to heart failure.**

✦ Comorbid conditions: CAD, HTN, MI (note date), arrhythmia, mitral and aortic valve disease, cardiomyopathy, renal insufficiency, vascular disease, anemia, diabetes mellitus, hyperthyroidism, hypothyroidism, COPD? **HTN, ischemia, and aortic stenosis are the most common causes of heart failure in the elderly.**

✦ EtOH or tobacco use?

✦ History of rheumatic fever?

✦ Family history of cardiac disease?

✦ Medications? Especially note use of beta blockers, prednisone, estrogen, testosterone, NSAIDs (sodium retention), antiarrhythmics, antineoplastics.

✦ Diet history?

✦ Cognitive status?

✦ Change in functional status? Activity level? Reduced ability to walk, climb stairs, carry groceries without shortness of breath? Postural dyspnea?

✦ Social support/caregiver?

PHYSICAL EXAMINATION

See Display 4-4.

✦ Weight—critical for monitoring edema, adjusting medication.

✦ Vital signs: Assess for uncontrolled HTN. Note respiratory rate.

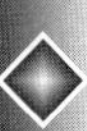

DISPLAY 4-4. *Signs/Symptoms/Physical Findings in Heart Failure*

Failure rarely remains isolated to one side of the heart; left-sided failure usually ultimately results in right-sided failure.

LEFT-SIDED FAILURE

Dyspnea
Orthopnea
Paroxysmal nocturnal dyspnea
Cough
Blood-tinged sputum
Pulsus alternans
S_3 gallop

RIGHT-SIDED FAILURE

Peripheral edema (dependent edema, ascites)
Anorexia
Nausea and vomiting
Hepatomegaly + hepatojugular reflex
Jugular venous distention
Pulmonary edema
Point of maximal impulse (PMI) displaced to left

BIVENTRICULAR FAILURE

Cachexia
Cyanosis
Fatigue
Tachycardia
Cardiomegaly

✦ Lungs: Observe for signs of air hunger, use of accessory muscles, presence of dyspnea with activity. Evaluate oxygenation if indicated with pulse oximeter or arterial blood gases (ABGs). Auscultate for crackles, wheezes. **Crackles may be present in elderly with comorbid conditions (COPD, atelectasis).** Assess capillary refill, shortness of breath when supine (orthopnea).

✦ Cardiovascular: Observe for signs of fatigue with slight exertion. Palpate point of maximal impulse (PMI may be displaced to left or right). Auscultate heart sounds and rate. Note presence of S_3 (best heard at apex while in left lateral recumbent position). S_4 may be heard in patients with HTN or ischemic disease. Assess for elevated jugular venous pressure (JVP). Assess for hepatojugular reflex (reliable sign in the elderly). If positive sign, normal JVP at rest will rise with compression of right upper quadrant of abdomen. Palpate peripheral pulses; note presence of pulsus alternans.

✦ Abdomen: Inspect abdominal girth. Palpate for tenderness. Note presence of ascites. Percuss/palpate for increased liver span.

✦ Extremities: Note presence of dependent peripheral edema. Record degree of pitting.

✦ Skin: Inspect for cyanosis. Note hyperpigmentation or induration of skin over extremities.

✦ Neuro: Observe for mental status changes, anxiety, restlessness, or lethargy.

DIAGNOSTIC TESTS

✦ Screening tool to assess ability to perform activities of daily living (ADLs).

✦ CBC to assess for anemia, which may precipitate or aggravate heart failure.

✦ Serum electrolytes. If on diuretic therapy, note especially potassium, sodium, magnesium. Sodium is often low in heart failure due to activation of renin–angiotensin–aldosterone system.

✦ Creatinine. **Be aware that creatinine level may be normal despite abnormal kidney function due to decreased muscle mass in the elderly.**

✦ Blood urea nitrogen (BUN may be increased by diuretic therapy).

✦ Serum albumin level: increased risk for hypoalbuminenia resulting from volume overload.

✦ Liver function tests.

✦ Oxygenation assessed by pulse oximeter or ABGs.

✦ Urinalysis: proteinuria suggests nephrotic syndrome; presence of cast or red blood cells (RBCs) suggests glomerulonephritis.

✦ Free T_4, TSH levels, especially in presence of atrial fibrillation.

✦ Chest x-ray to assess for cardiac enlargement, prominence of superior pulmonary veins (early sign of pulmonary venous congestion), interstitial edema, pleural fluid, effusion.

✦ ECG will reveal no diagnostic changes in heart failure but may identify underlying causes, left ventricular hypertrophy (LVH), tachycardia or arrhythmia, MI.

✦ Echocardiogram for evaluation of systolic function, diastolic function, and coronary arteries. Assesses for enlarged chambers and thickened walls (LVH), and valvular disease.

PREVENTION

✦ Control of HTN.

✦ Dietary modification.

✦ Medication compliance.

✦ Patients with asymptomatic LVH should consider ACE inhibitor therapy to prevent development of clinical heart failure. Persons with diabetes especially benefit due to protective effect on renal function.

✦ **See Protocol on Prevention and Health Maintenance.**

MANAGEMENT

Acute Failure

✦ Elderly who present with heart failure accompanied by the following should be hospitalized: Consult physician. **See Acute/Inpatient Setting.**

- ✧ Acute ischemia.
- ✧ Pulmonary edema.
- ✧ Respiratory distress/O_2 sat < 90%.
- ✧ Severe illness.
- ✧ Uncontrolled HTN.
- ✧ Hypotension/syncope.
- ✧ Inadequate social support system.
- ✧ Heart failure unresponsive to outpatient treatment.

✦ **Determine etiology (systolic vs. diastolic dysfunction) based on echocardiogram.** If ejection fraction (EF) < 35–45%, systolic dysfunction. If EF is normal, consider diastolic dysfunction.

✦ Correct precipitating causes. See Display 4-5.

Chronic Failure

✦ Most elderly patients with chronic heart failure will present for management by NP, followed collaboratively with physician. (See Table 4-1).

✦ Systolic dysfunction occurs when the ventricles are unable to eject a normal volume of blood (EF < 45%).

✦ Diastolic dysfunction is a result of the ventricles' inability to accept a normal volume of blood (abnormal LV relaxation and compliance; reduced LV filling volume with increased LV end-diastolic pressure). Seen in myocardial ischemia, aging, HTN. LVH treatment includes judicious use of diuretics, nitrates, possibly calcium antagonists; control of HTN.

✦ **For the elderly, improved quality of life rather than prolonged survival may be biggest goal.** Counsel patients/caregivers regarding prognosis, medications, importance of compliance, diet, and activity levels. **See Patient/Caregiver Education.**

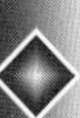

DISPLAY 4-5. ***Possible Precipitating Causes of Heart Failure***

Ischemia/MI
Arrhythmia
Uncontrolled HTN
Medications that retain sodium (hormones, NSAIDs)
EtOH use
Poor compliance with medications
Infection, sepsis
Anemia, especially acute
COPD exacerbation/pneumonia
Renal dysfunction
Pulmonary emboli
Anascara
Rapid IV fluid replacement, blood transfusion

✦ Consult nutritionist for counseling concerning sodium and fluid restrictions, adequate protein and calorie intake, maintenance of potassium. **Strict sodium restriction is not advisable in elderly unless hyponatremic or failure to respond to diuretics.** Caution that some salt substitutes contain excess potassium.

SYSTOLIC DYSFUNCTION

✦ If signs/symptoms are mild (fatigue or mild dyspnea), therapy may begin with an ACE inhibitor. ACE inhibitors improve survival for patients in New York Heart Association classes II through IV, improve exercise capacity and functional level in all heart failure patients, and have been shown to increase survival in post-MI patients with heart failure.

✦ ACE inhibitors can worsen renal failure in patients with pre-existing renal disease, may cause hyperkalemia especially when used in conjunction with potassium-sparing diuretics, and are contraindicated in patients with renal artery stenosis. Monitor potassium, BUN, and serum creatinine. Creatinine clearance is better indicator of renal function in the elderly. **See Chapter on Medication Issues.**

✦ The most common side effects of ACE inhibitor therapy are persistent cough (10%), hypotension, and rash.

✦ For symptoms of volume overload (orthopnea, paroxysmal nocturnal dyspnea, crackles, elevated JVP, dyspnea on exertion), add a diuretic agent. Begin therapy with the lowest effective dose of a thiazide diuretic.

✦ Complications of rapid diuresis include hypotension, syncope, falls, CVA, and MI. Diuretic doses should be adjusted based on presence of

TABLE 4-1. Medications Used in Heart Failure

Medication	Usual initial adult dose	Usual initial geriatric dose	Maximum dose
ACE inhibitors			
Vasotec (enalapril maleate)	2.5 mg PO bid	2.5 mg PO bid	40 mg PO bid
Capoten (captopril)	25 mg PO tid	6.25–12.5 mg PO tid	100 mg PO tid
Prinivil, Zestril (lisinopril)	5 mg PO daily dose	2.5 mg PO daily dose	20 mg PO daily dose
Altace (ramipril)	5 mg PO bid	2.5 mg PO bid	10 mg PO bid
Thiazide diuretics			
Hydrochlorothiazide	25 mg PO qd	25 mg PO qd	50 mg PO qd
Loop diuretics			
Lasix (furosemide)	20 mg PO qd	10 mg PO qd	600 mg PO qd
Digitalis glycosides			
Lanoxin (digoxin)*	0.125 mg PO qd	0.125 mg PO one to three times/week: creatinine clearance < 10 mL/min; 0.125 mg PO qd: creatinine clearance < 30 mL/min; 0.25 mg PO qd: creatinine clearance > 30 mL/min	0.25 mg qd
Vasodilators			
Apresoline (hydralazine HCl)	10 mg PO qid	10 mg PO tid	300 mg PO qd
Isordil titradose (isosorbide dinitrate)	5–20 mg PO tid	5 mg PO tid	40 mg PO tid

*Follow blood levels.

orthostasis or BUN:creatinine ratio; ratio > 20:1 indicates need for reduction in dosage.

✦ Monitor closely for hypotension or renal insufficiency with concomitant ACE inhibitor and diuretic therapy.

✦ When patient becomes resistant to thiazides or when renal function is decreased significantly, loop diuretic therapy is indicated. **Loop diuretics often precipitate urinary incontinence in the elderly.** Advise patients not to take before social event or too late in the day.

✦ If large doses (160–240 mg/qd furosemide) are required, a potassium-sparing diuretic may be added to the loop diuretic. Careful monitoring of potassium levels is necessary with multiple diuretic therapy.

✦ For severe symptoms of systolic dysfunction, digoxin (digitalis) may be added to the diuretic and ACE inhibitor combination. Digoxin increases ventricular performance in patients with left-ventricular systolic dysfunction and controls heart rate in atrial fibrillation.

✦ **Digoxin must be used with caution in the elderly because they often have impaired renal excretion and a smaller body mass, which can lead to digitalis toxicity. Elderly may experience toxicity at serum levels within usual therapeutic range. Signs and symptoms of digitalis toxicity include nausea, vomiting, anorexia, visual disturbances, and arrhythmias. Be aware of atypical presentation of toxicity in the elderly: confusion, fatigue, irritability. See Chapter on Medication Issues.**

✦ Monitor digoxin level when there is change in renal function, suspected toxicity, concomitant hypothyroidism, hyperthyroidism, or other conditions that can modify digoxin pharmacokinetics.

✦ Risk of interactions between digoxin and other medications taken by the elderly is high. Monitor medications carefully. See Display 4-6.

✦ Consult physician for referral to cardiologist for:

✧ Persistent symptoms despite treatment with ACE inhibitor/diuretic/digoxin.

✧ Patient with contraindications to ACE inhibitor or digoxin.

✧ Patient with concomitant angina or pulmonary edema.

✦ Adjunct therapy for heart failure includes oral anticoagulation in setting of embolic events, chronic/paroxysmal atrial fibrillation, documented LV thrombus.

DIASTOLIC DYSFUNCTION

✦ 40% of patients with heart failure have diastolic dysfunction with normal systolic function manifested by pulmonary congestion and low cardiac output. **Especially common in elderly as a result of HTN, LVH, ischemic heart disease, and aortic valve disease.**

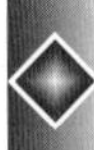

DISPLAY 4-6. ***Medications with Potential for Interaction with Digoxin***

Verapamil	Antacids	Indomethacin
Nifedipine	Kaolin	Ibuprofen
Amiodarone	Pectin	Diclofenac
Quinidine	Cholestyramine	Antineoplastics

✦ ACE inhibitors, diuretics, and vasodilators are used for treatment. See Table 4-1. **Consult physician for persistent symptoms.**

✦ Digoxin is not of value in diastolic dysfunction if there is normal left ventricular EF and sinus rhythm.

KEY ISSUES

Patient/Caregiver Education

Patient/caregiver should be able to verbalize:

✦ Understanding of prognosis of disease. **A 5-year mortality rate near 50% has been found in several studies of heart failure. 40% of patients with heart failure will die suddenly. Establishment of advance directives and future planning is crucial for families. See Chapter on Legal and Ethical Issues.** Cardiopulmonary resuscitation (CPR) training for family members may be indicated based on patient's preference.

✦ Reasons for taking medications, correct dosing requirements, and potential side effects. Use of a daily medication record is helpful. For those on digoxin therapy, importance of checking heart rate before dose is given.

✦ Need to consult NP before taking OTC medications. Many OTCs for headache and heartburn contain sodium carbonate or sodium bicarbonate.

✦ Recommendations for dietary sodium and fluid restrictions; need to record daily fluid intake if indicated.

✦ Importance of keeping a record of daily weights, weighing in the morning after urinating but before breakfast.

✦ Understanding of when to contact NP:

✧ Sudden weight change or when weight increases 3–5 pounds or greater in 1 week.

✧ Fever.

✧ Increase of symptoms.

✦ Need to limit EtOH intake to no more than 1 drink per day.

✦ Significance of remaining active to maintain exercise tolerance. Aerobic exercise (after baseline stress test) should be encouraged in stable patients. Weight lifting should be avoided. Patients with more severe disease should be advised to pace activities to avoid shortness of breath.

Economic Considerations

✦ **It is estimated that more than $10 billion is spent in direct costs for patients with heart failure.**

Psychosocial Considerations

✦ Provide counseling related to end-of-life issues for patients and family members. **See Chapter on Palliative Care.**

✦ Refer to support groups for heart failure patients/family members.

Acute/Inpatient Setting

✦ **Heart failure is most common reason for hospitalization of adults older than 65 years of age. Elderly are at increased risk for readmission.**

✦ **Be aware that IV fluid replacement is the most common precipitator of acute heart failure in the elderly.**

✦ Patients with pulmonary edema may need hospitalization for rapid diuresis with IV loop diuretics, oxygen therapy, nitrates.

✦ Patients with untreatable symptoms may be admitted for coronary artery bypass graft (CABG), valve replacement/repair, placement of left ventricular assistive device, or heart transplant (rare).

Extended Care Setting

✦ Educate staff to monitor for worsening of symptoms to avoid rehospitalization.

Home Setting

✦ Most common precipitator of worsening failure in outpatient population is medication/dietary noncompliance.

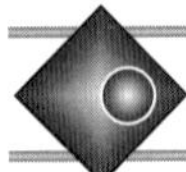

Atrial Fibrillation

HISTORY

✦ **Atrial fibrillation in the elderly is often asymptomatic on initial presentation.**

✦ Associated symptoms: palpitations, fatigue, angina, lightheadedness, cough, dyspnea with accompanying CHF? *May be first sign of hyperthyroidism.*

✦ History of angina, arrhythmia, HTN, MI, CAD, CVA, CHF, mitral valve prolapse, mitral stenosis and regurgitation, atrial septal defect, COPD, trauma to chest, pulmonary embolus, pneumonia, anemia, hyperthyroidism? **In 65–70 year olds, the stroke rate is 4–5% higher with atrial fibrillation.**

✦ History of EtOH or tobacco abuse? Consider possibility of "holiday heart." Caffeine use?

✦ Family history of HTN, CAD, CVA, diabetes mellitus, hyperlipidemia?

✦ Medications? Note especially use of theophylline, tricyclic antidepressants, Aricept, stimulants.

✦ Functional status?

✦ Cognitive status?

✦ Social situation, supports?

PHYSICAL EXAMINATION

✦ Vital signs: If heart rate is irregular, auscultate apical rate for full minute. Assess for orthostasis.

✦ Head/neck: perform range of motion to assess for dizziness.

✦ Eyes: fundoscopic examination for papilledema, hemorrhages, and/or exudates indicative of malignant HTN.

✦ Lungs: auscultate for wheezing (may be indicative of CHF or pulmonary embolus). Note presence of crackles especially in bases.

✦ Cardiovascular: inspect for jugular vein distention; palpate peripheral pulses; assess capillary refill. Auscultate heart sounds with bell and diaphragm of stethoscope in sitting, standing, and left lateral recumbent positions. S_3 may be present in CHF. S_4 is absent in atrial fibrillation. Auscultate for carotid bruits. Palpate for thrills, heaves, and apical impulse. Assess for dependent edema.

✦ Neuro: assess for focal neurologic findings because peripheral emboli accompanying atrial fibrillation may present as TIA/CVA.

DIAGNOSTIC TESTS

- ✦ Serum electrolytes.
- ✦ Serum drug levels as indicated (digoxin, quinidine, amiodarone).
- ✦ CBC.
- ✦ Thyroid function tests. T_3 and free T_4. New sensitive TSH test values are below normal in atrial fibrillation.
- ✦ Chest x-ray.
- ✦ 12-Lead ECG. Common findings in atrial fibrillation include normal QRS, ventricular rate 80–180, atrial rate ⩾400, and loss of distinct p waves. If atrial fibrillation is found on ECG or suspected based on symptomatology, consult physician and consider 24-hr Holter monitor to evaluate if arrhythmia is paroxysmal or sustained.
- ✦ Proceed to echocardiogram to assess left ventricular function, valvular function, atrial size, and presence of cardiac thrombi. **If transthoracic echo is negative, consider transesophageal echo (TEE) for detecting left atrial thrombi; TEE not available at all facilities and carries a risk of aspiration and patient discomfort.**
- ✦ If pulmonary embolus is suspected, consult physician for consideration of ventilation-perfusion (VP) scan, arterial blood gases, or oxygen saturation determination.
- ✦ International normalized ratio (INR)—standard of care for monitoring effectiveness of anticoagulation therapy. Standardizes prothrombin time by correcting for variability in reagent sensitivity. **See Outpatient Management of Anticoagulation**.

PREVENTION

- ✦ Control HTN.
- ✦ Strive for normalization of lipids.
- ✦ Encourage regular aerobic exercise.
- ✦ Encourage weight management.
- ✦ Encourage stress management.
- ✦ **See Protocol on Prevention and Health Maintenance.**

MANAGEMENT

- ✦ May have rapid or slow ventricular response.
- ✦ May be chronic or paroxysmal. In the elderly, both types require anticoagulation therapy unless multiple 24-hr monitors have shown infrequent

TABLE 4-2. Therapeutic Recommendations for Atrial Fibrillation

Patient profile	Recommended therapy
Elderly with high risk of bleed	Aspirin 81 or 325 mg PO qd
Elderly > 75 years, with low risk of bleed	Warfarin: INR goal 1.5–2.5
Patient < 75 years, with other risk factors (HTN, diabetes mellitus, previous CVA/TIA)	Warfarin: INR goal 2.0–3.0
Patient < 60 years, with lone atrial fibrillation, no other risk	Aspirin 325 mg PO qd

fibrillation episodes or patient has contraindication to anticoagulation. Antiplatelet therapy indicated in such cases.

✦ See Table 4-2.

✦ Risk of CVA as complication of atrial fibrillation increases with aging and with comorbidity: CHF, HTN, diabetes mellitus, history of CVA/TIA, previous arterial thromboemboli, abnormal left ventricular function, enlarged left atrium.

✦ Patients with history of past head trauma, dizziness, EtOH use must be excluded from anticoagulation therapy. Assess risk of falls in determining risk/benefit ratio of anticoagulation.

✦ Peripheral emboli as complication of atrial fibrillation may present as ischemic limb or bowel.

Initial Therapy

✦ Consult physician for in-patient admission for rate control and anticoagulation with heparin in patients with accompanying CHF or ischemia, symptomatic hypotension, or ventricular rate > 170.

✦ Management goals:

✧ Improvement of cardiac performance by controlling ventricular rate.

✧ May be achieved by pharmacological or electrical cardioversion. Electrical cardioversion is good option for those with recent or acute onset and who have normal echocardiograms. Candidates must be acutely anticoagulated with heparin before cardioversion and have no cardiac or embolic risk. If duration of fibrillation > 48 hr, will require anticoagulation for 3–4 weeks prior to cardioversion, and 2–4 weeks afterward.

✧ Antiarrhythmic therapy for rate control with digoxin, verapamil, propanolol, atenolol, metroprolol, amiodarone, or quinidine may be instituted. Monitor closely for toxic side effects. Follow serum drug levels if indicated (digoxin, quinidine, amiodarone). **See Chapter on Medication Issues.**

TABLE 4-3. Therapeutic Goals Recommended for Oral Anticoagulation

	INR
Prevention of systemic embolism Valvular heart disease Atrial fibrillation	2.0–3.0*
Pulmonary embolism and venous thrombosis	2.0–3.0*
Prevention of venous thrombosis	2.0–3.0*
Mechanical heart valves	2.5–3.5

*For elderly > 75 years, INR 1.5–2.5. Rate of intracranial hemorrhage in one trial increased two-fold for those > 75 years compared with overall population.

✧ ECG should be obtained periodically to evaluate if normal sinus rhythm is maintained or should have patient on continuous monitoring.

✧ Symptom relief (control of rate, heart failure).

✧ Prevention of embolism with anticoagulant or antiplatelet therapy.

✧ In symptomatic atrial fibrillation refractory to pharmacological management and electrical cardioversion, consider referral for AV node ablation and pacemaker implantation.

Outpatient Management of Anticoagulation

✦ See Table 4-3.

✦ Oral anticoagulation is instituted with dose of Coumadin (warfarin sodium) 2.5–5.0 mg PO in one daily dose and may be started while patient is hospitalized and receiving heparin. Response is dependent on dose, Vitamin K intake, presence of liver disease, GI dysfunction, nutritional status, and concomitant medications. See Display 4-7.

✦ Steady state is established in 5–7 days. Maximal effect is seen in 14 days. Have patient return to clinic (RTC) q 4–7 days for dosage adjustments until therapeutic level is maintained.

✦ Dosage adjustment recommendations:

✧ INR < 1.5: increase dose by 20%.

✧ INR 3.1–3.5: decrease dose by 20%.

✧ INR 3.6–4.0: consider holding one dose and decrease dose by 20%.

✧ INR > 4.0: consider holding two doses and decrease dose by 20%.

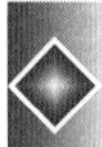

DISPLAY 4-7. *Medications That May Affect Anticoagulant Effect of Warfarin*

DECREASE INR

Rifampin	Barbiturates
Griseofulvin	Antihistamines
Pencillin	Carbamazepine
EtOH	

INCREASE INR

NSAIDs	Propanolol
Isoniazid	Quinidine
Tamoxifen	Anabolic steroids
Levothyroxine	Ciprofloxacin
Phenytoin	Erythromycin
Vitamin E (large doses)	Bactrim
Acetaminophen	Metronidazole
Selective serotonin reuptake inhibitors (SSRIs)	Miconazole
	Simvastatin
	Omeprazole
Cimetidine	Antibiotics (current/recent)

✦ RTC monthly for evaluation of INR and dosage adjustment as indicated.

✦ Avoid multiple prescriptions of different dose strengths. Advise to break 5-mg tablet in half for 2.5-mg dose.

✦ Provide table of days of week with dose to be taken each day.

✦ Major complication of anticoagulation is bleeding (risk increases when INR $>$ 3.0). Assess for signs of bleeding with urinalysis, CBC, and fecal occult blood test q 4 months and as needed.

KEY ISSUES

Patient/Caregiver Education

✦ Patient/caregiver should be able to:

✧ Verbalize correct regimen for anticoagulation therapy, including how and when to take medication, when to take a missed dose.

✧ List OTC medications, foods, and beverages that can affect warfarin levels.

✧ State signs and symptoms of bleeding and bruising.

✧ State importance for anticoagulated patients to restrict EtOH use to avoid traumatic injury.

✧ Acknowledge necessary restrictions of dietary stimulants (caffeine).

✧ Identify when anticoagulated patient should seek emergency treatment.

✦ Inform patient/caregivers that medical identification bracelets/necklaces are available to identify anticoagulation patients.

✦ Advise patients that foods high in vitamin K may be eaten, but drastic dietary changes should be avoided.

Acute/Inpatient Setting

✦ Acute rate control may be achieved by IV infusion of beta blockers (metoprolol), digoxin, or calcium-channel blockers (verapamil).

✦ Institute fall risk protocol for all anticoagulated patients.

✦ Patients on Coumadin (warfarin sodium) prior to admission require discontinuation of the drug 1 week prior to elective surgical procedures. Check prothrombin time and INR on day of procedure and consult physician regarding management and consideration of heparin. INR should be 1.5 or less before surgery.

Extended Care Setting

✦ Educate staff on key issues for anticoagulated patients. **See Patient/Caregiver Education.**

✦ Institute fall risk protocol for all anticoagulated patients.

✦ Consult OT/PT for safety assessment and precautions.

✦ Ensure that anticoagulated patients do not receive razor blades for shaving.

✦ Consult with dietary services regarding necessary food/beverage restrictions for anticoagulated patients.

Home Setting

✦ Assist patients in outlying areas to establish plan for monitoring of INR. Network with community providers to facilitate lab access. Portable finger stick INR monitors are available but results may vary from laboratory measurements depending on reagent used. Portable monitors may be useful for those who are homebound, live long distances from a laboratory, or have poor venous access.

- Refer to home health as appropriate for monitoring.
- Consult OT for home safety assessment.

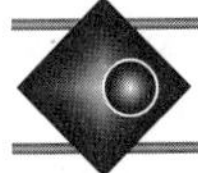

Abnormal Heart Sounds

HISTORY

✦ **If an abnormal heart sound is auscultated on physical examination, goal is to screen for evidence of underlying cardiovascular disease and/or the impact on cardiovascular function.**

✦ Associated symptoms: dizziness/syncope, chest pain, shortness of breath, dyspnea on exertion, orthopnea, nausea, palpitations, altered mental status, anxiety, nervousness, nonproductive cough, change in weight, or increased fatigue?

✦ History of CAD, angina, MI (note date/location), arrhythmia, valvular disease, CHF, heart block, murmur, CVA, TIAs, PVD, chronic renal insufficiency (CRI)?

✦ Cardiovascular procedures (note date): percutaneous transluminal coronary angioplasty (PTCA) with or without stenting, CABG, valve replacement (note which valve, type of prosthesis, anticoagulation), pacemaker implantation (note type of pacemaker), carotid endarectomy, peripheral artery bypass surgery?

✦ Pertinent past medical history/risk factors: rheumatic fever, congenital heart disease, anemia, hyper/hypothyroidism, HTN, diabetes mellitus, hyperlipidemia, obesity? **Rheumatic fever can be underlying etiology for aortic stenosis (AS), mitral regurgitation (MR), tricuspid regurgitation (TR), mitral stenosis, or aortic insufficiency (AI).**

✦ History of EtOH or tobacco use?

✦ Family history of HTN, heart disease, CVA, diabetes mellitus, hyperlipidemia?

✦ Medications? Note use of antihypertensives, antiarrhythmics, anticoagulants, other cardiac drugs, lipid-lowering agents.

✦ Diet? Note diet high in fat or salt. Restrictions of fat, salt, fluids, carbohydrates?

✦ Functional status? Note sedentary lifestyle.

✦ Cognitive status?

✦ Social situation, supports?

PHYSICAL EXAMINATION

✦ Weight. Vital signs. Check for orthostasis. Note heart rate and rhythm.

✦ Fundoscopic: assess for papilledema, hemorrhages, and/or exudates, which are indicative of malignant HTN.

✦ Cardiovascular examination: assess for jugular vein distention, auscultate for carotid bruits, palpate for thrills, heaves, and apical impulse. Auscultate for heart rate and rhythm and for heart sounds with bell and diaphragm of stethoscope in sitting, lying, and left lateral recumbent positions. Have patient sit up and lean forward to accentuate heart sounds. **Note intensity of heart sounds, presence of splitting, or of S_3, S_4, murmurs, clicks, or opening snap. Note location on chest wall, timing in heart cycle (systole or diastole). With murmurs, also note shape or configuration, pitch (frequency), location of maximal loudness, radiation, intensity, and changes with respirations or maneuvers.** See Display 4-8.

✦ Normal changes of aging can result in diminished arterial compliance, turbulent blood flow, and benign systolic murmurs. These murmurs may be mistaken for a pathologic murmur or mask the murmur of AS. Changes in ventricular diastolic function associated with aging or HTN can produce an S_4 that may be a common physical finding in the elderly.

✦ Palpate peripheral pulses. Auscultate for bruits in abdomen and groin.

✦ Respiratory examination: note presence of crackles especially in bases.

✦ Note presence, location, degree of dependent edema.

✦ Consider neurological examination for focal neurological findings.

DIAGNOSTIC TESTS

✦ 12-Lead ECG, especially if new patient or new finding on physical examination.

✦ Check drug levels when appropriate, i.e., digoxin, theophylline, antiarrhythmics.

✦ Baseline CBC, electrolytes, BUN, creatinine, albumin, liver function tests, thyroid stimulating hormone, free T4, and lipid profile.

✦ Monitor prothrombin time and INR if on Coumadin (warfarin sodium). **See Protocol on Atrial Fibrillation.**

✦ Consider P/A and lateral chest x-ray if signs of CHF. **See Protocol on Heart Failure.**

✦ Consider echocardiogram if findings suggestive of CHF or to evaluate possible valvular disease.

✦ Consider TEE if question of prosthetic valve dysfunction or of valvular vegetation with suspected endocarditis.

✦ Consider carotid Doppler studies if bruits noted or with neurological symptoms suggestive of TIA or CVA.

✦ Consider 24-hr Holter ECG monitoring to evaluate arrhythmias. Consult with physician.

✦ Refer to cardiologist for further testing for new finding, or in patient refractory to treatment.

PREVENTION

✦ Educate patient on modification of risk factors as appropriate, i.e., smoking cessation, increased activity/exercise, dietary modifications with decreased fat and salt, limited fluid intake, no/moderate EtOH. **Avoid excessive dietary restrictions in the elderly who may be at increased risk of decreased appetite and malnutrition.**

✦ Consider enteric-coated aspirin 81 mg PO daily.

✦ Patients with history of valve replacement surgery, known valvular disease, or congenital heart defects should receive prophylactic antibiotics prior to dental and surgical procedures. Recommend ampicillin or amoxicillin 1 g PO or IV 1 hr prior to procedure, followed by 500 mg every 6 hr for four doses. Vancomycin 1 g IV or erythromycin 500 mg PO may be substituted for penicillin-allergic patients.

✦ Patients on Coumadin (warfarin sodium) require careful monitoring. Stop Coumadin 1 week prior to elective surgical procedures and administer heparin 5,000 units subcutaneously every 12 hr or Lovenox (enoxaparin sodium) 30 mg subcutaneously bid. Check prothrombin time, INR, and partial thromboplastin time (PTT) on day of procedure. Consult with physician on management. **See Protocol on Atrial Fibrillation.**

✦ Patients with history of mechanical valve replacements should remain on anticoagulation therapy throughout life. Porcine valves do not require chronic anticoagulation.

✦ Following PTCA with stent placement, patients generally are placed on Ticlid (ticlopidine HCl) for a specified period of time (usually 4 weeks, during which weekly CBC and platelet counts should be monitored).

✦ **See Protocol on Prevention and Health Maintenance.**

MANAGEMENT

✦ Recognition of pathologic versus benign sounds is important in management. Consult with physician as needed. See Display 4-8.

✦ Assess and treat comorbid conditions.

✦ Consult with physician if new finding or with acute exacerbation of known cardiac problem. Refer to cardiologist.

✦ **See Protocols on Anemia; Chest Pain; Atrial Fibrillation; Heart Failure; Transient Ischemic Attack (TIA)/Cerebrovascular Accident (CVA);**

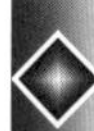

DISPLAY 4-8. *Heart Sounds and Murmurs*

Benign (Innocent) Murmurs

✦ Most are systolic, low in intensity (Grade I or II) without radiation, abnormal heart sounds, or ejection sounds, and with a normal ECG.
✦ Aortic area: aortic sclerosis associated with aging produces the most common benign murmur in the elderly.
✦ Left sternal border: murmur associated with anemia, hyperthyroidism, tachycardia.

Pathologic Murmurs

✦ Diastolic murmurs, pansystolic murmurs, and continuous murmurs are pathologic.
✦ Very loud murmurs are usually pathologic.
✦ Murmurs associated with evidence of underlying cardiac disease are pathologic, i.e., ASCVD, valvular replacement, CHF.
✦ Examples of pathologic systolic murmurs:

✧ **Aortic stenosis (AS):** most common clinically significant cardiac valvular abnormality in the elderly. Characteristics: rough, medium-pitch, diamond-shaped murmur, peaks in mid-systole; best heart in aortic area or left sternal border (LSB) with radiation to right mid-clavicular area and carotids; may be associated with diminished S_2, paradoxical split S_2, S_4, or ejection click. Associated symptoms: angina, exertional dyspnea, and syncope.

✧ **Idiopathic hypertrophic subaortic stenosis (IHSS):** Characteristics: medium-pitched murmur of long duration, best heard at LSB with radiation to apex; increased with standing, diminished with squatting; associated with loud S_2. Associated symptoms: dyspnea, angina, fatigue, syncope, sudden death during or after physical exertion.

✧ **Pulmonic stenosis:** Characteristics: murmur is similar to AS but best heard in pulmonic area; S_2 may be widely split or single. Associated symptoms: fatigue, dyspnea, right ventricular failure, syncope.

✧ **Mitral regurgitation:** Characteristics: pansystolic murmur, decreased with inspiration, radiates from lower LSB to apex and midaxillary line; S_3 may be present in advanced disease. Associated symptoms: CHF.

✧ **Tricuspid regurgitation:** Characteristics: high pitched, heard best along LSB in 4th and 5th intercostal spaces (ICS), increased with inspiration, no radiation. Associated symptoms: may be well tolerated for years before development of severe right ventricular failure.

(continued)

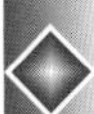

DISPLAY 4-8. *Continued*

✦ Examples of pathologic diastolic murmurs:

✧ **Mitral stenosis:** Two-thirds of patients with mitral stenosis are women; most cases result from rheumatic fever. Characteristics: low pitched, rumbling murmur, heard best in apex with the bell; S_2 may be intensified and may be associated with an opening snap (OS) after S_2. Associated symptoms: dyspnea, pulmonary edema, atrial arrhythmias, hemoptysis.

✧ **Aortic insufficiency:** Characteristics: high-pitched, blowing murmur, heard best with diaphragm in 2nd and 3rd left ICS with patient leaning forward; immediately follows S_2. Associated symptoms: palpitations, exertional dyspnea, orthopnea, chest pain.

ABNORMAL HEART SOUNDS

✦ Loud S_1: may be associated with mitral stenosis or anemia.
✦ Widely split S_2: associated with right bundle branch (RBBB), pulmonic stenosis, atrial septal defect (ASD), ventricular septal defect (VSD), or mitral regurgitation.
✦ S_3: associated with CHF.
✦ S_4: associated with HTN; absent in atrial fibrillation; may be heard with normal aging changes.

Hypertension; Hypothyroidism; Hyperthyroidism; and Hyperlipidemia.

Aortic Stenosis (AS)

✦ Recommend avoidance of strenuous activity especially with severe AS.

✦ Consider diuretic and ACE inhibitor therapy for systolic dysfunction.

✦ Assess severity of lesion with Doppler echocardiogram and consider referral for possible valve replacement surgery, which is the definitive treatment for AS.

✦ ASCVD commonly co-exists with AS.

Idiopathic Hypertrophic Subaortic Stenosis (IHSS)

✦ Diagnosed by echocardiogram.

✦ Consider careful medical management with beta blockers, calcium-channel blockers, and antiarrhythmics as indicated.

✦ Nitrates, diuretics, and ACE inhibitors may be used as adjunct treatment for CHF.

Pulmonic Stenosis

✦ Congenital heart disease.

✦ Manage right-sided heart failure with diuretics and ACE inhibitors.

✦ **See Protocol on Heart Failure.**

Mitral Regurgitation (MR)

✦ Commonly occurs due to rheumatic heart disease, LVH, or following an MI.

✦ Consider vasodilator therapy with ACE inhibitors or peripheral vasodilators; digoxin and diuretics may be added for left ventricular dysfunction.

✦ Treat atrial fibrillation which is commonly present.

✦ Cardiac function may be followed by echocardiogram; mitral valve replacement (MVR) is indicated for progressive symptoms.

✦ **See Protocol on Atrial Fibrillation.**

Tricuspid Regurgitation

✦ Uncommon; seen in congenital heart disease and with endocarditis.

✦ Often well tolerated.

✦ Manage right-sided heart failure if present.

Mitral Stenosis

✦ Commonly occurs due to rheumatic heart disease.

✦ Manage heart failure symptoms, control atrial fibrillation, which is commonly present.

✦ Beware of excessive volume depletion and vasodilator therapy, which reduces cardiac output.

✦ Consider referral for surgical intervention for progressive symptoms.

Aortic Insufficiency (AI)

✦ Commonly occurs due to rheumatic heart disease or with endocarditis.

✦ Acute AI is poorly tolerated.

✦ Symptomatic relief with diuretics, ACE inhibitors, and optimum control of HTN is important. Refer for possible surgical intervention.

KEY ISSUES

Patient/Caregiver Education

The patient/caregiver should be able to:

✦ Describe medication regimen, desired effects, and possible adverse effects of medications.

✦ Discuss nonpharmacological management strategies, i.e., dietary modifications, weight management, stress management, exercise program, smoking cessation strategies.

✦ Recognize physiological changes which should prompt contact with the health care provider, i.e., change in frequency, timing, or character of chest pain, syncope, weight gain in CHF.

Economic Considerations

✦ Cardiovascular disease is the number-one cause of mortality in the U.S., and a major factor in morbidity and health care cost.

Psychosocial Considerations

✦ Cardiovascular disease impacts functional status both in the working elder and in the frail elder. Maintaining functional health is an important goal of care.

✦ Be alert to depression, sleep disturbances, sexual disturbances in elders with cardiovascular disease.

Acute/Inpatient Setting

✦ See specific protocols for parameters necessitating acute hospitalization.

Extended Care Setting

✦ Be alert to subtle signs that may indicate acute change in cardiovascular status.

Home Setting

✦ Assist patient/caregiver in establishing a process for monitoring cardiovascular status in the home. Consider home health referral when appropriate.

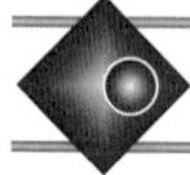

Peripheral Vascular Disease

HISTORY

✦ Pain, cramping, aching, tiredness or weakness in calf? Hip, thigh, and/or buttock pain with ambulation, resolving with rest? **Calf symptoms suggest femoral or popliteal stenosis; buttock, hip, and thigh symptoms suggest aorto-iliac stenosis. Symptoms are usually bilateral and progressive.**

✦ Distance of ambulation before onset of symptoms? **Patients who have difficulty ambulating related to other conditions may not demonstrate claudication. The first signs may be resting pain and/or leg ulceration.**

✦ Onset of symptoms? **Arterial insufficiency occurs after the age of 50, is most common after the age of 75. Men are affected with arterial insufficiency more often than women.**

✦ Aching or heaviness not particularly associated with activity? **Characteristic of venous insufficiency.**

✦ Alleviation of pain by positioning lower extremities? **Symptoms of arterial origin are typically alleviated by dangling the legs, whereas those of venous origin are alleviated by elevation.**

✦ What interventions have been tried? What has worked?

✦ History/onset of CAD? **Peak occurrence of PVD (arterial) is 10 years after the onset of symptomatic CAD. Symptomatic CAD and cerebral ischemia can co-exist with PVD.**

✦ History of CHF, HTN, TIA, CVA, hyperlipoproteinemia, polycythemia, or diabetes mellitus? **Distal vessels (popliteal, peroneal, and tibial arteries) are affected more frequently in the diabetic patient. Aorto-iliac segments are affected more frequently in the nondiabetic patient.**

✦ Male impotence?

✦ Tobacco use? EtOH?

✦ Family history of HTN, heart disease, CVA, diabetes mellitus, hyperlipidemia?

✦ Medications?

✦ Functional status? Effect of symptoms on function?

✦ Social situation, supports?

✦ **It is not uncommon to have a mix of both arterial and venous PVD.**

PHYSICAL EXAMINATION

✦ Vital signs, with BP both arms. Weight.

✦ Brachial artery index (BAI). **Systolic pressure is greater in the brachial artery than in the ankle. See Protocol on Lower Extremity Ulcers.**

✦ Cardiovascular: assess rate, rhythm, heart sounds, murmurs, and gallops.

✦ Lungs: assess for signs of CHF.

✦ Auscultate for bruits from abdomen to bilateral groin. **Heard over aorta or iliac/femoral arteries.**

✦ Observe for pulsating abdominal mass. **Detected in < 50% of patients with abdominal aortic aneurysm.**

✦ Palpate abdominal aorta by using the palmar surface of both hands with fingers extending on the midline. Press the fingers deeply inward on each side of the aorta, feeling for pulsation. Normally, the pulsation is directed anteriorly. A lateral pulsation suggests an aortic aneurysm. **The incidence of abdominal aneurysm increases with age. Expected rate of expansion: 0.2–0.4 cm yearly. Surgical intervention is indicated for aneurysms > 6 cm.**

✦ Assess lower extremity temperature and skin. **Tissue will appear thin, tight, and shiny with cool extremities in arterial PVD. Dependent rubor with blanching and pallor upon elevation.**

✦ Assess lower extremities for presence or absence of hair on toes and anterior tibial areas. **Often present in early disease and often a nonspecific finding in the elderly.**

✦ Palpate for peripheral pulses. **Distal pulses are weak or absent.**

✦ Assess for evidence of ulcerations of arterial insufficiency. **Painful, gangrenous leg ulcers are common. Arterial leg ulcers are typically seen over the first metatarsophalangeal joint, toes, dorsum of foot and heel, lateral malleolus, and distal pretibial region. See Protocol on Lower Extremity Ulcers.**

✦ Assess for peripheral edema and hemosiderin deposits. **Assess for signs of venous insufficiency, which affect women more often than men.**

✦ Assess for ulcerations suggestive of venous insufficiency. **Venous ulcerations are usually painless and located along the medial aspect of the leg, especially the medial malleolus. See Protocol on Lower Extremity Ulcers.**

✦ Assess for diffuse erythema, suggestive of cellulitis.

✦ Assess for localized erythema or tenderness, suggestive of superficial phlebitis.

✦ Stand patient to assess for varicose veins.

DIAGNOSTIC TESTS

✦ BUN, creatinine, sodium, potassium, and glucose.

✦ Fasting lipid profile.

✦ 12-Lead ECG.

✦ Consider abdominal ultrasound and abdominal CT scan in the presence of suspected abdominal aneurysm. **Consult physician. Serial ultrasounds are suggested every 6 months to 1 year in the presence of an aneurysm.**

✦ Doppler ultrasound to determine flow in the vessels. **Helpful to determine baseline and treatment outcomes.**

✦ Ankle brachial index. **Measurements of ≥ 0.9 is normal; 0.6–0.8, moderate disease; and < 0.5 or ankle pressure of ≤ 70 mm, severe obstructive disease with prediction of surgical bypass within 6.5 years.**

✦ Consider treadmill testing to determine baseline functional capacity. **The presence of arterial PVD suggests concomitant coronary and cerebrovascular disease.**

✦ If indicated, refer to vascular surgeon for angiography if patient is a willing and appropriate surgical candidate. **Consult physician. Surgical intervention involves bypass procedures, percutaneous angioplasty, debridement, skin grafting, and possibly amputation.**

PREVENTION

✦ The most important risk factors for peripheral arterial disease are cigarette smoking and diabetes mellitus. Other risk factors to be controlled are HTN, and hyperlipidemia. **See Protocols on Diabetes Mellitus; Hypertension; and Hyperlipidemia. See Chapter on Substance Abuse.**

✦ Exercise program.

✦ Consider lipid-lowering drugs to treat hyperlipidemia in young elders.

✦ Injury prevention to legs and feet.

✦ Optimal nutrition, especially in the presence of leg ulcers. **High calorie, high protein with supplementation of multiple vitamin with minerals, zinc, ascorbic acid, and short-term vitamin A. See Chapter on Pressure Ulcers.**

✦ Control of pruritus and stasis dermatitis, if present. **Skin emollients and corticosteroids are often useful. See Protocols on Lower Extremity Ulcers and Pruritus.**

✦ Low-dose heparin or Lovenox (enoxaparin sodium), low molecular weight heparin, is indicated to prevent venous thrombosis in high risk patients.

✦ **See Protocol on Prevention and Health Maintenance.**

MANAGEMENT

✦ Avoidance of tobacco in any form. **Tobacco hastens atherogenesis. Carbon monoxide causes further tissue hypoxia and nicotine causes**

vasospasm for 60 minutes following use. Counsel patients, suggest pharmacologic interventions (patches/gum/inhalants) and individual/group therapy.

✦ Aspirin 81–650 mg PO daily.

✦ For venous insufficiency: compression therapy and elevation of legs while sitting. Avoidance of long periods of standing. **Compression stockings may be customized for individual patients.**

✦ Treat secondary leg ulcers, both arterial and venous. **See Protocol on Lower Extremity Ulcers.**

✦ Coumadin (warfarin sodium) anticoagulation is used for at least 3–6 months in the presence of thrombophlebitis. **Permanent warfarin therapy should be considered for recurrent thrombi. Oral anticoagulants must be used with caution in the elderly, especially those at risk of falling.**

✦ Daily walking program. Instruct to walk to the point of pain (claudication), then stop, resume walking after pain subsides. **This process stimulates the development of collateral circulation.**

✦ Good foot hygiene. **Cleanliness along with drying well between the toes to prevent tinea pedis.**

✦ Instruct to wear warm socks in cold temperatures.

✦ Avoid heating pads and hot water.

✦ Avoid injury to lower legs and feet. Wear protective clothing and proper fitting footwear. Instruct to run hand inside shoes before each application, checking for foreign objects (such as pebbles, BBs, etc.), worn areas, and breakdown of seams.

✦ Moisturize legs and feet daily and more often if extremely dry. Dry between the toes after application of moisturizer. **Skin becomes dry, soles of feet are often excessively dry, tissue is thick and often cracked—a source of secondary infection.**

✦ Consider nutritionist referral for obesity or malnutrition. **Obesity can complicate both arterial and venous insufficiency.**

✦ Consider PT consult for balance and gait evaluation.

✦ Consider OT consult for adaptive equipment to prevent injury during ADLs.

✦ Consider elevating the head of the bed with 6–10" blocks to alleviate arterial resting pain, usually experienced at night. **Some find relief by sleeping in recliner with feet in a more dependent position.**

✦ Avoid vasodilating drugs.

✦ Trental (pentoxifylline) is controversial. It is thought to work on RBC membranes, facilitating movement through narrow, diseased vessels. Dosage is 400 mg with meals tid. If effective, results will be seen in 1 to 2 months.

✦ The use of Ticlid (ticlodipine) has improved symptoms of arterial PVD in some, but is also controversial.

✦ Consider referral to pain clinic for unsuccessful pain management. **Mexillitine and gabapentin have recently been tried with some success in the control of nocturnal neuropathic pain.**

✦ Consider referral to vascular surgeon for consideration of arteriogram, and balloon angioplasty or bypass grafting if indicated. **Surgical intervention may improve the patient's quality of life and prevent amputation in the treatment of pain and leg ulcerations. Amputation may be the ultimate decision when pain, progressive gangrene, or secondary infection of ulcerations cannot be controlled by other means.**

KEY ISSUES

Patient/Caregiver Education

Patient/caregiver should be able to:

✦ Identify their individualized risk factors.

✦ Verbalize understanding of prevention strategies as they apply. **See Prevention.**

✦ Verbalize and demonstrate proper management techniques.

Economic Considerations

✦ Management of leg ulcers and dermatologic consequences of PVD is chronic and expensive.

✦ Elders who continue to work may be required to retire or reduce their hours significantly.

✦ Compression stockings vary from relatively inexpensive (TED hose) to customized and very expensive. **Coverage under insurance is limited.**

Psychosocial Considerations

✦ Be alert to social isolation due to significant pain/leg ulcerations.

✦ Intervention may be required for symptoms of anxiety/depression associated with chronicity of illness or smoking cessation.

Acute/Inpatient Setting

✦ The acute care process most often surrounds the needs associated with the elder undergoing vascular evaluation, surgical intervention, wound care, or a complicating illness associated with PVD, such as arterial embolism, acute arterial thrombosis, acute ischemia, ruptured aortic aneurysm, ischemic bowel, or thrombophlebitis.

✦ Initiate rehabilitation program with involvement of PT and OT as early as possible to maximize functional status.

Extended Care Setting

✦ Be alert to exercise intolerance and nonverbal clues to pain, especially in the elder with dementia.

✦ Develop walking programs addressing the special needs of those with claudication. Movement of rocking chairs may be substituted for walking in the nonambulatory patient (helps stimulate development of collateral circulation).

✦ Develop or include in smoking cessation program as appropriate.

Home Setting

✦ Self-application of compression stockings may be unrealistic. Observe for difficulty and consider stockings with zipper opening/closure. Consider OT referral for adaptive equipment such as stocking holder frame. Compression stockings may be more easily applied over regular hosiery.

✦ Include in smoking cessation program.

✦ Consider referral to psychologist for smoking cessation as appropriate.

✦ Assess environment for safety.

✦ Consider pain center referral for intractable pain (claudication, rest pain, or neuropathic pain).

Chapter 5

Pulmonary System

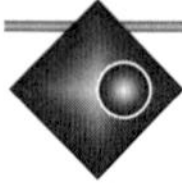

Chronic Obstructive Pulmonary Disease (COPD)

HISTORY

✦ Shortness of breath? At rest? On exertion? Recent increase? Elderly may under-report symptoms.

✦ Cough? When occurs (early a.m.)? Frequency? Sputum amount, sputum characteristics?

✦ Associated signs/symptoms: fever, edema, chills, fatigue, angina, orthopnea, change in weight?

✦ Allergies? Home environment? Home oxygen? Home nebulizers?

✦ Past medical history: Frequent upper respiratory infections (URI), bronchitis, pneumonia, exposure to environmental toxins, tuberculosis (TB) exposure, tobacco use (pack-year history), previous diagnostic testing (last chest x-ray, purified protein derivative [PPD], pulmonary function testing (PFTs)?

✦ Comorbid conditions: cardiovascular disease (CVD), peripheral vascular disease (PVD)?

✦ Medications—especially current inhaler or steroid therapy/OTC inhalers?

✦ Effects of symptoms on activities of daily living (ADLs), work, walking?

PHYSICAL EXAMINATION

✦ Vital signs/weight.

✦ General appearance: color, posture, gait, affect, change in anterior/posterior chest diameter (**increase can occur with normal aging**), extent of respiratory difficulty. Note tachypnea, use of accessory muscles, decreased diaphragm movement.

✦ Neuro: mental status. **Be aware of atypical presentation in the elderly.**

✦ Lungs: assess for rhonchi, wheezing, hyper-resonance.

✦ Cardiac: distant heart sounds common.

In Long-Term COPD Patients

✦ Look for signs of **right-sided heart failure**: peripheral edema, jugular venous distention, hepatomegaly.

✦ Look for signs of **pulmonary hypertension**: fatigue, cyanosis, lightheadedness, clubbing of digits, murmur.

✦ Look for signs of **cor pulmonale**: dyspnea, cough, fatigue, increased sputum production, S_3 gallop, peripheral edema, jugular venous distention.

DIAGNOSTIC TESTS

On New Diagnosis of COPD

✦ PPD. **See Protocol on Tuberculosis.**

✦ **Chest x-ray** for baseline (if not recently performed).

✦ **12-Lead ECG** for baseline (if not recently performed).

✦ **Arterial blood gases (ABGs)—PaO_2 declines with normal aging**; however, PaO_2 < 55 mm Hg indicates chronic hypoxemia and requires continuous oxygen therapy.

✦ **PFTs** to define nature of pulmonary dysfunction. Decreased residual volume (RV) and decreased forced expiratory volume in 1 second (FEV_1) indicates restrictive disease. Increased RV and decreased forced expiratory volume (FEV) with FEV_1/forced vital capacity (FVC) (FEV_1:FVC ratio) < 0.80 indicates obstruction. Decreased diffusion capacity of carbon monoxide (DLCO) suggests emphysema. **Because FEV_1, FEV_1/FVC, and DLCO decline with age, values should be age-adjusted by laboratory for interpretation.** PFTs should be repeated with topical beta agonist if obstructive disease is suggested to exclude asthma and determine usefulness of bronchodilator therapy. **Some elderly may have difficulty performing spirometry. Other measures, such as distance walked without symptoms, may be more reliable than PFTs.**

✦ Serum electrolytes, blood urea nitrogen (BUN), creatinine.

✦ CBC with differential (screen for polycythemia, which may accompany COPD).

✦ Alpha-globulin peak level to rule out α_1-antitrypsin deficiency is especially important for patients with no smoking history.

On Routine Visits for COPD

✦ Oxygen saturation by pulse oximeter at rest and with activity, on room air if possible. Consider ABGs if indicated by O_2 sat results or symptoms. Some patients will have chronically high $PaCO_2$ levels while metabolically compensated (elevated serum bicarbonate with normal pH). New onset of reduced sats may indicate heart failure.

✦ Theophylline level if applicable. Usual accepted level for adults is 10–20 μg/ml. Because of high frequency of toxic side effects in the elderly, level may be better maintained at 10–14 μg/ml.

✦ Blood glucose level if on steroids.

On Acute Exacerbation of COPD

✦ **P/A and lateral chest x-ray** (exclude pneumonia, pulmonary embolus).

✦ **Sputum culture and Gram stain.**

✦ **ABGs.**

✦ **Serum electrolytes, glucose, creatinine, BUN.**

✦ **Theophylline level,** if applicable.

✦ **CBC** to rule out infection, assess for anemia.

PREVENTION

✦ Avoid respiratory irritants (smoke, aerosol sprays).

✦ Avoid extreme temperatures.

✦ The importance of increasing fluid intake to mobilize secretions has not been established.

✦ Avoid wine and spicy foods that may cause bronchospasm.

✦ Maintain adequate nutrition with small, frequent (5–6 per day) meals or snacks.

✦ Employ energy-saving techniques. **See Patient/Caregiver Education.**

✦ Emphasize importance of early treatment of infection. Consider giving prescription for antibiotic to be started at first signs of infection.

✦ Administer Symmetrel (amantidine HCl) or Flumadine (rimantadine) on exposure to Influenza A. Usual adult dose: 200 mg daily for 2–7 days: geriatric dose: 100 mg daily for 2–7 days. **Can cause confusion in the elderly.**

✦ **See Protocol on Prevention and Health Maintenance.**

MANAGEMENT

Patient with New Diagnosis of COPD

✦ Mainstays of therapy for long-term maintenance in COPD are bronchodilators (beta-adrenergic agonists, anticholinergic agents) and steroids. Maximum effect is achieved by using combination of all three therapies.

✦ **There is increased risk for toxic side effects from systemic therapies in the elderly.** Metered dose inhaler (MDI) is the preferred delivery route for the elderly.

✦ MDIs may be difficult for the geriatric patient due to arthritis, tremor, dementia, or poor eyesight. Use of a spacer with MDI is recommended.

✦ Begin with **one** of the beta-adrenergic inhalers or anticholinergic inhalers listed below. If symptoms are not relieved, add second inhaler from previously unselected class.

✦ **Beta-adrenergics:** wait 1–2 min between first and second inhalation.

✧ **Proventil, Ventolin (albuterol)** 2 inhalations q 4–6 hr.

✧ **Brethaire (terbutaline sulfate)** 2 inhalations q 4–6 hr.

✧ **Serevent (salmeterol xianfoate)** 2 inhalations bid, not for acute symptoms.

✧ **Alupent (metaproterenol sulfate)** 2–3 inhalations q 4–6 hr, maximum 12 inhalations/24 hr.

✦ **Combination anticholinergic and beta-adrenergic:**

✧ **Combivent (ipratropium bromide + albuterol)** 2 inhalations qid, maximum 12 inhalations/24 hr.

✦ If combination of beta-adrenergic and anticholinergic is used, inhale beta-adrenergic first; WAIT 5 MINUTES; and then use anticholinergic.

✦ **Anticholinergics:**

✧ **Atrovent (ipratropium bromide)** 2 inhalations q 4–6 hr, maximum 12 inhalations/24 hr.

✦ If still symptomatic, add adrenocorticoid inhaler.

✦ **Adrenocorticoids:**

✧ **Azmacort (triamcinolone acetonide)** 2 inhalations tid–qid, maximum 16 inhalations/24 hr.

✧ **AeroBid (flunisolide)** 2 inhalations bid, maximum 8 inhalations/24 hr.

✧ **Beclovent, Vanceril (beclomethasone dipropionate)** 2 inhalations tid–qid, maximum 20 inhalations/24 hr.

✦ If combination of three medications is used, inhale beta-adrenergic first; wait 5 minutes and inhale anticholinergic; wait another 5 minutes and inhale adrenocorticoid.

✦ The elderly may complain of palpitations and tachycardia with beta-adrenergic inhalers; however, these side effects are usually transient.

✦ Advise patients to rinse mouth after steroid inhaler use to prevent candidiasis. Clean inhaler after use.

✦ For the elderly who are maintained on theophylline therapy, use lowest dose necessary to maintain theophylline level at 10–14 μg/ml. **See Diagnostic Tests. Consider discontinuing oral theophylline therapy because the elderly experience a high frequency of toxic side effects (nausea, tremor, headache, insomnia).**

✦ Patients whose symptoms are unabated with inhaler therapy may be treated with a trial of oral steroids:

✧ **Medrol (methylprednisolone)** usual adult dose: 32 mg daily; geriatric dose: same as adult. Taper per Medrol Dose Pack.

✧ **Deltasone (prednisone)** usual adult dose: 40 mg daily; geriatric dose: same as adult except modify in patients with altered CNS state, diabetes mellitus, congestive heart failure (CHF), wounds, infections except lung.

✦ If oxygen therapy is warranted (PaO_2 < 55 mm Hg), 1–3 liters/min is sufficient for most patients and best delivered on a 24-hr basis. Selected patients (who suffer from exercise-induced dyspnea or insomnia from nocturnal dyspnea) with PaO_2 < 55 mm Hg may benefit from intermittent therapy.

Patient with COPD

If following conditions exist, proceed to Interventions I:

✦ Stable weight.

✦ Maintaining functional ability with no increase in symptoms.

Interventions I:

✦ Review management with patient and caregiver.

✦ Return visit to nurse practitioner (NP) q 3–6 months.

If following conditions exist, proceed to Interventions II:

✦ Inadequate nutrition evidenced by weight decrease.

✦ Increase in symptoms.

✦ Decreased ability to perform ADLs.

Interventions II:

✦ Refer to nutritionist.

✦ Revise pharmacological therapy as needed. **See Management of Patient with New Diagnosis of COPD.**

✦ Consider need for home health visits and refer to social worker.

✦ Follow-up by telephone or return visit to NP.

- Refer to physician if:
  - Refractory to treatment.
  - Developing signs of cardiac failure.

Patient with Acute Exacerbation of COPD

If following conditions exist, proceed to Interventions:

- Presence of fever, edema, chills, fatigue, angina, orthopnea, colored sputum, weight change, or increase in dyspnea despite therapy.
- High $PaCO_2$ levels without metabolic compensation.

Interventions:

- Assess ABGs. Maintain $PaO_2 \geqslant 90\%$.
- Determine underlying cause of exacerbation:
  - Worsening CHF?
  - Pneumonia?
  - Acute bronchitis?
  - Pulmonary embolus?
- Refer to physician for hospital admission if:
  - Worsening CHF.
  - Pneumonia.
  - Pulmonary embolus.
  - Angina.
- Treat exacerbation secondary to bronchitis with inhaled beta-adrenergic agonist, two to four inhalations, repeat after 30–60 min; if no relief, refer to physician for admission for IV steroids (**See Acute/Inpatient Setting**). If symptoms relieved after first treatment, prescribe antibiotic therapy for at-home use.
  - **Antibiotic choices:**
    - **Bactrim DS (trimethoprim 160 mg/sulfamethoxazole 800 mg)** usual adult dose: one tablet bid for 14 days; geriatric dose: if CrCl is 15–30 ml/min, reduce dose to **Bactrim (trimethoprim 80 mg/sulfamethoxazole 400 mg)** one tablet bid; If CrCl <15 ml/min, not recommended.
    - **Amoxil (amoxicillin)** usual adult dose: 250–500 mg tid for 10 days; geriatric dose same as adult.
    - **Cipro (ciprofloxacin HCl)** usual adult dose: 250 mg bid for 10 days; geriatric dose same as adult. Avoid use with theophylline; may increase levels.
    - **E-mycin (erythromycin)** usual adult dose: 250 mg qid for 10 days; geriatric dose same as adult.

✧ **Achromycin V, Sumycin (tetracycline)** usual adult dose: 250–500 mg qid for 10 days; geriatric dose: 250 mg qid for 10 days. Take 1 hr before or 2 hr after meals.

KEY ISSUES

Patient/Caregiver Education

Patient/caregiver should be able to:

- Explain indications and potential side effects of medications.
- Identify signs of impending exacerbation.
- Demonstrate proper use of oxygen therapy equipment.
- Demonstrate proper use of MDI and/or large-volume spacer.
- Demonstrate test for empty inhaler.
- Explain disadvantages of smoking. Patient **must** be able to identify personal motivation for cessation. Once motivation is established, plan for cessation should be established with reinforcement/support from NP.
- Explain importance of monitoring weight and reporting changes.
- Explain importance of eating small, frequent meals.
- Identify appropriate dietary choices (more fats, fewer carbohydrates).
- Demonstrate energy-saving techniques such as pacing, diaphragmatic exercises, and pursed-lip breathing.

Economic Considerations

- Expense of oxygen therapy restricts use by elderly on limited incomes.
- Criteria for Medicare reimbursement for chronic oxygen therapy:
  - $PaO_2 < 55$ mm Hg.
  - With CHF, $PaO_2 < 59$ mm Hg.
  - O_2 sat < 88% after complete medical treatment.
  - With CHF, O_2 sat < 90% after complete medical treatment OR desaturation to above levels with activity.
- Consider use of demand pulsing delivery or reservoir cannula to reduce cost of oxygen.
- Inhalers and other medications may be restricted from certain HMO/PPO formularies.
- Prescribe substitute therapy or file for formulary exception if indicated.

Psychosocial Considerations

- Be aware of potential for caregiver burden..
- Evaluate for depression resulting from:
  - Decreased ability to perform ADLs.
  - Financial burden of management.
  - Dependence on oxygen therapy.
  - Long-term prognosis.
  - Changes in self-concept related to coughing and sputum production.
  - Inability to voice/vent frustration because emotional upset may impair breathing.
- Evaluate for social isolation resulting from:
  - Dependence on oxygen therapy.
  - Confinement for avoidance of environmental pollutants.
- Patient requiring constant oxygen therapy may have anxiety related to:
  - Possibility of insufficient oxygen supply.
  - Insecurities about equipment use/failure.

Acute/Inpatient Setting

- Steroid therapy greatly potentiates the elderly's risk for:
  - Glucose intolerance.
  - GI ulcer.
  - Osteoporosis.
  - Cataracts.
  - Skin breakdown.
  - Mental status changes—**Be alert for delirium.**
- Consider H_2 blocker with steroid therapy to prevent ulcer.
- Consult respiratory therapist for nebulizer therapy and instruction on home oxygen therapy.
- Oxygen therapy should be available (**at time of discharge**) for transfer to home or extended care.

Extended Care Setting

- IV antibiotic therapy may be initiated to prevent hospital admission.

Home Setting

- Initiate orders for home health that include parameters for assessment of:

  - ✧ Worsening signs/symptoms.
  - ✧ Decreasing ability to perform ADLs.
  - ✧ Depression and anxiety.
  - ✧ Weight/nutritional status.
  - ✧ Increasing caregiver stress.
  - ✧ Effectiveness of oxygen therapy (sats).
  - ✧ When to notify NP of status change.
  - ✧ Plan for reinforcement of proper use of oxygen therapy equipment.
  - ✧ Plan for continuous reinforcement of proper MDI technique.
  - ✧ Laboratory monitoring.

✦ Need for respiratory therapist visits and nebulizer treatments may accelerate level of care to extended care facility.

✦ Oxygen and nebulizer therapy will qualify most elderly COPD patients for home health visits.

✦ Assessment for presence of smokers in home is critical if oxygen therapy is to be used.

✦ Most COPD patients have concomitant disease. Accurate home health assessment is needed to differentiate from multiple chronic illnesses and treat symptomatology.

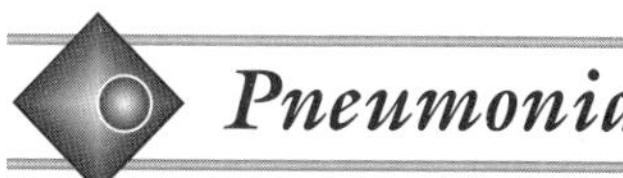

Pneumonia

HISTORY

✦ Rhinorrhea? Sore throat? Cough? Sputum production/amount/characteristics? **Commonly absent in the elderly.**

✦ Chills? Fever? **Febrile state in the elderly is defined as 2-degree elevation of temperature above the patient's baseline temperature. Absence of fever is common; hypothermia may indicate sepsis.**

✦ Pleuritic chest pain? Location? Duration?

✦ Anorexia? Fatigue, malaise, weakness?

✦ Change in mental status/depressed mood? Atypical presentations common.

✦ Headache, bradycardia, abdominal pain, diarrhea, muscle aches? **Rule out Legionella—carries increased incidence of mortality in elderly.**

✦ Onset and duration of symptoms?

✦ Smoker? History of COPD?

✦ Pneumovax?

✦ History of neurologic disease such as cerebrovascular accident (CVA), Parkinson's disease, Alzheimer's disease, or late stage multiple sclerosis with known or suspected dysphagia?

✦ Immunocompromised? Alcohol (EtOH) intake?

✦ Hypnotics? Anxiolytics? Other medications causing sedation?

✦ Difficulty swallowing, choking or coughing while eating? Enteral feeding? History of high residuals or constipation if fed enterally? **See Protocol on Management of the Enterally Fed Patient. Aspiration is common cause of pneumonia in the elderly. Impaired clearance of bacteria in the oropharynx increases risk of pneumonia secondary to decreased cough and gag reflex.**

✦ Rapid decline in function? Falls?

✦ Residential setting? Community, hospital, extended care facility?

✦ Recent environmental epidemic exposure or contact with another infected individual? **Symptoms in the elderly are more subtle, sepsis at diagnosis is not uncommon.**

PHYSICAL EXAMINATION

✦ Assess cognitive status, compare with baseline.

✦ Vital signs. **Respiratory rate > 25 breaths/min may be best and only indication of pneumonia in the elderly; hypotension may co-exist.**

✦ Observe characteristics of respiration: orthopnea, cyanosis, tachypnea, poor inspiratory effort, or use of accessory muscles and/or intercostal retraction.

✦ Percuss chest, dullness is a common finding.

✦ Auscultate lungs, typically diminished breath sounds; wheezes, crackles and rhonchi do not clear with cough. Egophony (spoken "eee" sounds like "ay") associated with consolidation.

✦ Perform oxygen saturation at rest and during activity.

✦ Perform functional assessment of ADLs; compare with baseline.

DIAGNOSTIC TESTS

✦ Posterior/anterior (P/A) and lateral chest x-ray.

✦ Sputum specimen for Gram stain, culture, and sensitivity in presence of productive cough. **Sputum must be from deep cough/not oropharyngeal secretions. Less than 10 squamous epithelial cells and more then 25 leukocytes/100 × field—indicates lower respiratory tract specimen. Gram stain is useful in initiating treatment while awaiting culture report.**

✦ CBC with differential may demonstrate low or normal white count, may have shift to the left. Leukopenia and anemia have been associated with increased mortality.

✦ Blood cultures in the presence of fever. One-third of elderly with pneumonia will have positive cultures, increasing risk of mortality secondary to sepsis.

✦ BUN, creatinine, and electrolytes to assess hydration, electrolyte imbalance, and renal function. **Assessment of renal function is critical in determining creatinine clearance and appropriate antibiotic selection/dosing.**

✦ Albumin/prealbumin to assess nutritional status. **Prealbumin is most reliable determinant of current nutritional status. Albumin level of < 2 g/dL carries poorer prognosis.**

✦ Consider three early morning sputums for acid-fast bacillus stain and culture to rule out TB. **See Protocol on Tuberculosis.**

✦ Consider urine for *Legionella pneumophia* antigen if suspicion is high. Consult physician.

PREVENTION

✦ Encourage annual influenza vaccine. Educate about risk/benefits and myths/misunderstanding regarding immunization.

✦ Encourage pneumococcal vaccine (Pneumovax) in those > 65 years and those with chronic disease (currently suggested once in life-time, every 6 years in high-risk patient). **Risk of pneumonia increases with age secondary to physiologic changes, altered immunity and increased incidence of chronic disease. It is the most common cause of infection-related deaths in the elderly.**

✦ Annual dental examination. **Caries predispose to pneumonia due to increased oral bacteria.**

✦ Adequate nutrition and hydration. Two quarts of fluid daily unless otherwise contraindicated.

✦ Educate caregiver in techniques such as positioning, feeding techniques, altered consistency of diet/fluids to prevent aspiration in at-risk patients (those with gastroesophageal reflux disease [GERD], dementia, neurologic conditions, enterally fed, substance abuse).

✦ Assess and educate regarding proper technique in use of respiratory inhalers. **See Protocol on COPD.**

✦ Frequent positional changes during periods of bed rest; avoid prolonged bed rest.

✦ Encourage smoking cessation.

✦ Instruct and encourage proper use of incentive spirometer, when appropriate.

✦ Encourage frequent, proper hand washing technique.

✦ Avoid warm, steam vaporizer. Educate in proper cleaning of cool-mist vaporizer.

✦ Clean/dry medication receptacle in nebulizer between use.

✦ Infection control: isolation of *Staphylococcus aureus* and other resistant pathogens in hospital/extended care setting. During influenza epidemics, restrict affected admissions, visitors, and/or health care providers.

✦ Use sterile water in oxygen humidification.

✦ **See Protocol on Prevention and Health Maintenance.**

MANAGEMENT

✦ Encourage appropriate hydration; oral/parenteral. If parenteral, adjust volume and rate of administration to prevent fluid volume overload.

✦ Treat malnutrition. Consult nutritionist at onset of treatment.

✦ Consult speech pathology for bedside swallow study, video fluoroscopy, if indicated.

✦ Be alert to potential for silent aspiration.

✦ Supplemental O_2 if indicated. Important in preventing CHF in patients with a history of cardiovascular disease.

✦ Respiratory therapy, if indicated. Incentive spirometry, oral inhalers, or nebulization treatments if inhaler technique is inadequate to control symptoms.

✦ Proper and frequent repositioning of bed-bound patients; encourage appropriate out-of-bed mobilization to optimize pulmonary function.

✦ Aggressive suctioning if unable to mobilize secretions.

✦ Consider oral inhalers, expectorants, antitussive agents as appropriate.

✦ Antibiotic therapy appropriate to residential setting (inquire about and account for institution's pathogen profile and resistant organisms), epidemic prevalence, diagnostic findings (sputum Gram stain and organism identification/x-rays), and creatinine clearance. Antibiotic therapy should be initiated when pneumonia is suspected.

✦ Consider hospitalization for frail, at-risk patient or those for whom sepsis is suspected.

✦ Radiologic resolve is delayed 10–12 weeks in the elderly. Clinical improvement is key in determining progress.

✦ Rule out TB/cancer in resistant cases. (See Displays 5-1 and 5-2.)

Antibiotic Therapy

✦ Treat empirically based on likely pathogen to setting. **Mortality is decreased by prompt treatment.** Combination therapy is recommended when clinical status poor.

✦ Correct antibiotic therapy once pathogen is identified by diagnostic studies.

✦ Calculate creatinine clearance; alter dosages accordingly. Closely monitor appropriate peak and troughs and subsequent renal function.

✦ Consult pharmacokinetic services if available.

✦ Is organism beta lactamase positive? (If so, do not use Amoxil [amoxicillin trihydrate], consider Augmentin [amoxicillin/clavulanate potassium] 250–500 mg PO q8h, also available in liquid form.)

✦ Doxycycline, ciprofloxacin, levofloxacin, ofloxacin, amoxicillin, ampicillin, azithromycin, or clarithromycin are appropriate and cost effective for community-acquired pathogens. Ciprofloxacin, levofloxacin, ofloxacin, and ampicillin are available for IV dosing if indicated.

✦ For extended care and hospital acquired: consider third-generation cephalosporins (such as Claforan [cefotaxime] 1 g IV q8h, Cefobid [cefoperazone sodium] 1–2 g q12h, or Fortaz [ceftazidime] 1 g IV q8–12h; or piperacillin plus an aminoglycoside IV). CAUTION: aminoglycosides such as amikacin, gentamicin, and tobramycin can be ototoxic and nephrotoxic and must be dosed according to renal function.

✦ Consider Rocephin (ceftriaxone sodium) 1 g IM q12–24h as an alternative to parenteral infusing of third-generation cephalosporin.

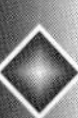

DISPLAY 5-1. *Common Causative Pathogens in the Elderly (identified by Gram stain of sputum)*

Hemophilus influenzae—a gram-negative coccobacillus
Streptococcus pneumoniae—a gram-positive cocci in pairs/chains
Aerobic gram-negative bacilli—mixed gram-negative organisms
Staphylococcus aureus—gram-positive cocci in clusters
Klebsiella pneumoniae—gram-negative rods
Moraxella catarrhalis—gram-negative diplococci
Mixed flora is suggestive of anaerobic organisms
Respiratory viruses, *Mycoplasma pneumoniae*, Legionella, and *M. tuberculosis*—DEMONSTRATE NO GRAM-STAINABLE PATHOGENS, but there may be leukocytes

It is common to find more than one pathogen in the elderly (colonization is prevalent in smokers and in COPD).

✦ If *Pseudomonas aeruginosa* is suspected, consider coverage with Cefobid (cefoperazone sodium), which is metabolized by the liver (1–2 g/IV q12h), or Fortaz (ceftazidime), adjusted according to renal function (1 g/IV q8–12h).

✦ Treatment in the elderly should span 10–21 days; 7 of the treatment days should include parenteral administration when indicated, with close therapeutic monitoring.

✦ Colonized MRSA in sputum can be treated effectively (colonization often delays disposition): Albuterol 0.3 ml in 5 ml NaCl 0.9% per aerosol (prevents bronchoconstriction secondary to vancomycin) followed by vancomycin 120 mg q6h by face mask in room air (120 mg = 1 ml of solution of vancomycin 500 mg diluted in 3 ml sterile water). Two drops of the vancomycin solution may be instilled in each nostril q6h. Treatment continues for 4 days then reculture (sputum or pharyngeal). If culture returns positive, re-treat using same dosing schedule.

KEY ISSUES

Patient/Caregiver Education

Patient/caregiver should be able to:

✦ Identify appropriate preventive measures.

✦ Demonstrate correct use of oral inhalers, as appropriate.

✦ Demonstrate proper feeding techniques to minimize aspiration in high-risk elderly.

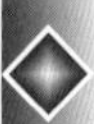

DISPLAY 5-2. *Common Causative Pathogens Based on Environmental Setting*

Acute/Inpatient (Nosocomial)

Gram-negative (*Pseudomonas aeruginosa* is common)
Pneumococcus
Oral anaerobes/mixed flora (associated with aspiration)
Multimicrobial (gram negative plus gram positive)
Staphylococcus aureus (MRSA: Methicillin-resistant *Staphylococcus aureus*)
Legionella pneumophila

Extended Care Facility

Streptococcus pneumoniae
Pneumococcus
Gram-negative rods (*Klebsiella* species)
Hemophilus influenzae
Oral anaerobes/gram negatives (associated with aspiration)
Staphylococcus aureus (MRSA)
Viruses

Community Acquired

Streptococcus pneumoniae (most common cause)
Hemophilus influenzae
Mycoplasma pneumoniae
Oral anaerobes and mixed flora (associated with aspiration)
Gram-negative bacilli (less often in healthy, community-dwelling elderly)
Staphylococcus aureus (especially in elderly diabetics and those with recent influenza)
Klebsiella pneumonia (in EtOH abusers)
Legionella pneumophila
Viruses
Moraxella catarrhalis

- ✦ Identify prescribed medications and demonstrate medication compliance.
- ✦ Verbalize understanding that antibiotics should not be discontinued prematurely as symptoms subside.
- ✦ Discuss hazards of immobility such as deep vein thrombosis, functional loss, urinary tract infection, calcium loss, joint discomfort, myalgia, and orthostasis.
- ✦ Demonstrate appropriate/safe mobilization techniques.

Economic Considerations

✦ Select from formulary. Prior authorization may be required for selective agents.

✦ Monotherapy is least expensive and is optimal coverage for usual pathogens. Avoid unnecessary additional antibiotics to cover for all potential pathogens—this practice alleviates potential for pathogen resistance.

✦ Oral/IM antibiotic administration is less expensive than IV administration. Make switch from IV to oral route as quickly as clinically feasible.

Psychosocial Considerations

✦ Be alert to fear/depressed mood associated with perceived/real threat of loss of independence secondary to functional decline.

✦ Patient/caregiver may need support in understanding return to baseline function requires extended time in the elderly.

Acute/Inpatient Setting

✦ Appropriate antibiotic therapy based on setting and pathogen patterns of institution.

✦ Isolate patient with resistant pathogens according to facility policy.

✦ Consider patient's desires regarding treatment of pneumonia if associated with terminal illness.

✦ Consider referral to PT/OT to prevent further functional decline and promote optimal function.

✦ Mobilize patient as quickly as condition allows.

✦ Request nutritionist's involvement to optimize nutritional status.

✦ Suspect *Clostridium difficile* in the presence of diarrhea.

✦ Consult respiratory therapy regarding aerosol treatments/chest physiotherapy if indicated.

✦ Monitor and correct for dehydration; assess for fluid volume overload in elderly with known cardiovascular disease/CHF.

Extended Care Setting

✦ Base empiric antibiotic therapy on known pathogen patterns and formulary options of the facility.

✦ Consider the patient's advance directives: does patient request withholding antibiotics in the treatment of pneumonia?

✦ Hospitalize those who demonstrate signs of sepsis.

✦ Consider use of oral antibiotics when patient is not severely ill.

✦ Consider use of Rocephin (ceftriaxone sodium) IM to prevent unnecessary hospitalization and ramifications of relocation (such as agitation, confusion/acute delirium).

✦ Be suspect of *Clostridium difficile* in presence of diarrhea and antibiotic usage.

✦ Mobilize patient (frequent position changes in bed/out of bed, in chair/ambulate as appropriate to prevent further functional loss).

✦ If patient is terminal and hospice care is in place, consider low-dose morphine or Duragesic (fentanyl) transdermal patch, 25 μg/hr every 3 days to decrease dyspnea/anxiety.

✦ Provide frequent mouth care.

Home Setting

✦ Emphasize hydration/nutrition.

✦ Consider home health care to monitor medication compliance and clinical progress.

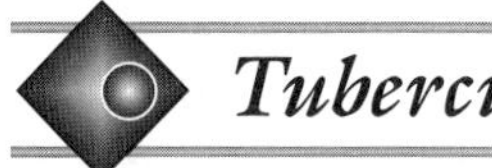

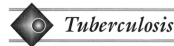

Tuberculosis

HISTORY

✦ Onset and duration of symptoms? **Symptoms are often insidious and of long duration.**

✦ Presence of respiratory symptoms, i.e., cough, shortness of breath, chest pain? **Most frequent manifestation in the elderly, although with long-standing infection TB can occur in almost any organ.**

✦ Sputum? Amount, character, color, presence of blood?

✦ Systemic symptoms, i.e., fever, chills, weight loss, anorexia, night sweats, fatigue?

✦ Exposure to TB (recent or remote)?

✦ Risk factors: chronic disease such as diabetes mellitus, COPD, end-stage renal disease (ESRD), HIV; resides in a congregate living situation, homeless, or immigrant; history of EtOH abuse; or poor nutrition?

✦ Previous history of TB or previously positive skin test? When? How treated? **The elderly represent a large potential population for TB. 80% of active TB found in elders is secondary (reactivated) TB.**

✦ Last TB skin test? Chest x-ray? Results?

✦ History of respiratory infections (recent or remote)? History of recurrent or persistent respiratory infections?

✦ Smoking history?

✦ Recent travel to other countries?

✦ History of bacille Calmette-Guérin (BCG)? **Previous immunization does not totally protect from infection; routine screening procedures are recommended.**

PHYSICAL EXAMINATION

✦ Weight, vital signs, general appearance.

✦ Assess for adenopathy.

✦ General examination including head, eyes, ears, nose, throat (HEENT), cardiac, abdomen.

✦ Respiratory system: assess, thoroughly noting respiratory rate and effort, use of accessory muscles, breath sounds, adventitious sounds. **Tuberculosis classically affects upper lobes.**

DIAGNOSTIC TESTS

✦ PPD (Mantoux 5 TU-PPD) administered intradermally and read in 48–72 hr. **Booster testing is more sensitive (within 1–2 weeks) and is recommended if the first test is negative. Perform in individuals suspected of active TB; those in whom preventive therapy would be considered; and in all elderly nursing home residents. Do not place PPD in patients if known previous positive reaction.**

✧ Induration ≥ 15 mm: positive in general population.

✧ Induration ≥ 10 mm: positive in high prevalence group, i.e., residents of a long-term care facility.

✧ Induration ≥ 5 mm: positive in patients with history of recent close contact with active TB, chest x-ray consistent with TB, or HIV positive.

✦ Chest x-ray. **X-ray findings may be variable, including upper or lower lobe infiltrates, adenopathy, and pleural effusions.**

✦ Sputum for acid fast bacillus (AFB) smear and culture (three specimens). **Collect sputum specimen first thing in the morning to increase yield. Have patient remove dentures and rinse mouth before beginning to cough. May use inhaled saline mist to help stimulate cough. Examine secretions to make sure they contain sputum not saliva. Cultures require 4–6 weeks.**

✦ Consider electrolytes, BUN if suspected dehydration.

✦ Consider serum albumin or prealbumin for nutritional assessment.

✦ Consider referral for bronchoscopy, biopsy, or gastric aspiration when TB suspected but sputum/smears inadequate to make diagnosis; Consult with physician.

PREVENTION

✦ Maintain adequate nutrition and hydration.

✦ Prevent spread with appropriate personal protective devices per OSHA standards.

✦ Prevent respiratory infections with proper hand washing and hygiene techniques.

✦ Consider preventive therapy with INH (isoniazid) 300 mg/daily for 6–12 months in selected patients with positive PPD but without active disease. Consult with physician.

✦ **See Protocol on Prevention and Health Maintenance.**

MANAGEMENT

✦ Avoid EtOH with drug treatment.

✦ Respiratory isolation during diagnosis and first 2 weeks of treatment or until sputum cleared of infectious agent. Isolation rooms must meet CDC ventilation guidelines.

✦ Baseline laboratory testing prior to initiation of drug therapy: liver enzymes, bilirubin, serum creatinine, CBC with platelets, serum uric acid.

✦ Monitor laboratories monthly for toxicity; monitor for clinical symptoms of toxicity, i.e., nausea and vomiting.

✦ Baseline audiogram and vestibular tests if initiating streptomycin.

✦ Monitor visual acuity and color vision with use of ethambutol.

✦ Repeat chest x-ray at 2–3 months and at completion of treatment. **X-ray changes/improvements are slow to manifest.**

✦ Monitor for clinical indicators of improvement: decreased cough, decreased sputum.

✦ Referral/follow-up of contacts for testing/treatment.

✦ Report new case(s) to appropriate infection control units, i.e., hospital infection control, local and state health departments.

✦ Direct observed therapy (DOT) twice weekly is suggested when noncompliance is likely. **Several regimens are available.**

✦ **There is a high incidence of drug–drug interactions with antituberculosis agents. Monitor closely.**

✦ For active TB, consult with physician in prescribing drug regimen and duration of treatment; generally recommend a three- to four-drug regimen customized for patient and based on prevalence of multi-drug resistance in area.

✦ Four-drug regimen usually consists of INH (isoniazid), rifampin, and pyrazinamide with either streptomycin or ethambutol.

✧ **INH (isoniazid)** 5 mg/kg daily (maximum 300 mg daily) or 15 mg/kg two to three times weekly (maximum 900 mg daily) bactericidal for *M. tuberculosis.* **Side effects:** liver toxicity, peripheral neuropathy, increased risk with increased age.

✧ **Rifampin** 10 mg/kg daily or two to three times weekly (maximum 600 mg daily): 75% protein bound; bactericidal for *M. tuberculosis.* **Side effects:** GI upset; colors bodily fluids orange.

✧ **Pyrazinamide** 15–30 mg/kg daily (maximum 2 g daily) or 50–70 mg/kg two times weekly (maximum 4 g daily) or 50–70 mg/kg three times weekly (maximum 2.5 g daily): bactericidal. **Side effects:** liver toxicity, hyperuricemia, may alter insulin requirements.

✧ **Ethambutol** 15–25 mg/kg daily (maximum 2.5 g daily) or 50 mg/kg two times weekly (maximum 2.5 g daily) or 25–30 g/kg (maximum 2.5 g daily): bacteriostatic, possibly bactericidal in higher doses. **Side effects:** ocular effects, i.e., decreased acuity, blurred vision, central scotomata, red–green color blindness.

✧ **Streptomycin** 15 mg/kg daily (maximum 1 g daily) or 25–30 mg/kg two times weekly (maximum 1.5 g daily) or 25–30 mg/kg three times weekly (maximum 1 g daily). **Side effects:** Eighth cranial nerve damage (ototoxicity), nephrotoxicity.

✧ **Pyridoxine:** 25–50 mg daily; should be given as a supplement with INH to prevent peripheral neuropathy especially in conditions in which neuropathy is more common, i.e., diabetes, alcoholism, malnutrition, and in persons with seizure disorders.

✦ When multi-drug resistant TB is suspected, a five- to six-drug regimen is recommended. Additional medications include capreomycin, ciprofloxacin, ethionamide, kanamycin, amikacin, para-aminosalicylic acid (PAS), rifabutin, erythromycin, or cycloserine.

KEY ISSUES

Patient/Caregiver Education

Patient/caregiver should be able to:

✦ Describe treatment regimen and importance of completing full course of therapy as prescribed.

✦ Identify adverse effects and report immediately to care provider.

✦ Describe infection control precautions to prevent spread of TB, i.e., wearing appropriate mask, covering mouth with tissue, disposing of tissues appropriately, good hand washing.

Economic Considerations

✦ Medications are costly; many health departments provide medications at no charge to increase compliance.

Psychosocial Considerations

✦ Patients and families often are reluctant to discuss diagnosis or history of infection/previous treatment.

Acute/Inpatient Setting

✦ Maintain a high degree of suspicion in at-risk patients with respiratory symptoms admitted to acute hospital.

✦ Consider TB among differential diagnosis in patient with persistent pulmonary infiltrates.

✦ Isolate patients appropriately using rooms that meet CDC ventilation guidelines.

✦ Use OSHA-approved respiratory masks when in contact with patient.

✦ Notify infection control service as well as local and state health departments.

Extended Care Setting

✦ **Higher incidence of TB in long-term care (LTC) population than in community-dwelling elderly.**

✦ Screen all new residents on admission using two-step PPD testing.

✦ Screen all residents at least every 2 years with PPD.

✦ Avoid PPD in residents with documented positive reaction; chest x-ray prior to admission is recommended.

✦ Perform PPD testing on all previously negative residents immediately and at 12 weeks if an active case is documented in the facility.

✦ Collect sputum for AFB if previously positive patients develop cough, bronchitis, pneumonia, or unexplained weight loss.

✦ Perform chest x-ray on admission and if PPD turns positive or suggestive symptoms are present.

✦ Notify local and state health departments as indicated.

Home Setting

✦ Assist with setting up medication schedule to enhance compliance with regimen.

✦ Arrange for testing and follow-up of contacts in the home.

✦ Notify local and state health departments as indicated.

Chapter 6

Gastrointestinal System

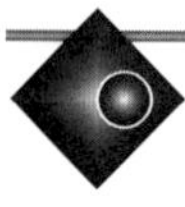

Management of the Enterally Fed Patient

HISTORY

✦ Reason for tube? When was tube placed?

✦ Type: nasogastric, gastrostomy, jejunostomy (j-tube), or gastro-jejunostomy (g-j tube)? Size, condition of tube?

✦ **Nasogastric tubes are generally used for short-term feedings only.**

✦ Problems with displacement, clogging, poor repair?

✦ Name, amount of formula? Intermittent or continuous? Calorie/protein prescription? **Jejunostomy feedings must be given continuously. There is no reservoir for intermittent feedings. Cannot check residual volume (RV) with jejunostomy tube or small-bore nasogastric tube.**

✦ Any missed or held feedings? Why?

✦ Amount, frequency of free water? Schedule for free water; flushing?

✦ Oral intake? Consistency, amount, any difficulty swallowing?

✦ Tolerance to feedings? Nausea, vomiting, diarrhea, constipation? RV, abdominal distention, discomfort?

✦ Change in mental status, functional status, weight, skin condition? **Subtle mentation changes may be the first indication of fluid/electrolyte imbalance and aspiration pneumonia in the elderly.**

✦ Status of underlying conditions (specific questions as applicable)?

✦ Signs of infection? Fever, chills, cough, change in respirations, redness/draining at tube site? **Nasogastric feeding tubes act as obstruction, may lead to sinusitis. With jejunostomy tube, assess how tube is held in place. Often j-tubes are surgically stitched in place, a poor long-term solution because of skin irritation. Drainage tube attachment devices (DTADs) are available.**

✦ Medications: prescription, OTC? Route, form, administration schedule? **Medications given via tube are a frequent cause of obstruction, especially with small-bore nasogastric tubes. Flush tubes well before and after medications.**

✦ Social situation: place of residence, caregiver? How is caregiver coping with care? Home health agency? Home equipment company?

PHYSICAL EXAMINATION

✦ Vital signs, weight.

✦ General appearance/condition: hydration status, nutrition status, skin turgor, pressure ulcers, oral hygiene.

✦ HEENT: Assess frontal, maxillary sinuses. Tenderness is specific for sinusitis.

✦ Condition and patency of tube.

✦ Condition of tube site. **Nasogastric tubes should be secured without pressure to the nose; pressure ulcers in this area are difficult to heal. Gastrostomy tubes should have both internal and external bumpers to prevent tube from sliding in and out.**

✦ Lungs: **increased risk of aspiration pneumonia, which may present atypically in an elderly or debilitated patient.** If aspiration suspected, consider addition of methylene blue to formula and examine for blue stain in respiratory secretions.

✦ Cardiac: note signs of volume overload.

✦ Rectal: stool for guaiac, presence of impaction.

DIAGNOSTIC TESTS

✦ Consider drawing a serum albumin or prealbumin (reference range may vary from laboratory to laboratory) and electrolytes if:

- ✧ Patient with newly initiated feedings.
- ✧ Change in weight since last visit.
- ✧ Reports of frequently missed or held feedings.
- ✧ Long-term tube-fed patient (consider every 6 months to assess ongoing nutritional and hydration status).

✦ Consider serum electrolytes, creatinine, and blood urea nitrogen (BUN) levels if signs/symptoms of dehydration or fluid overload.

✦ **Monitor electrolytes, magnesium, phosphorous, prealbumin with initiation of tube feedings. The patient who is extremely malnourished is at risk for "refeeding syndrome" and increased mortality.**

- Consider CBC if signs/symptoms of infection.
- Consider PA and lateral chest x-ray if signs/symptoms of aspiration pneumonia.
- Consider videofluroscopy to assess swallowing function.
- Abdominal flatplate x-ray to assess tube placement with newly placed or dislodged nasogastric tube; to assess tube placement with jejunostomy tube, order x-ray with dye injection (gastrogaffin).

PREVENTION

- Maintain mouth care.
- Consider that high protein/high fiber enteral formulas are generally well tolerated by the elderly population.
- Provide skin care, especially around feeding tube site.
- Maintain bowel regimen.
- Assess for social isolation, depression, and grieving because feeding tubes may cause change in body image and loss of independence.
- Maintain aspiration precautions: Elevate head of bed at least 30 degrees, preferably 45 degrees, during and 2 hr after bolus feedings and at least 30 degrees during continuous tube feedings.
- **See Chapter on Legal and Ethical Issues.**
- **See Protocol on Prevention and Health Maintenance.**

MANAGEMENT

Patient on Long-Term Maintenance

If following conditions exist, proceed to Interventions.

- Tolerating formula.
  - Low RV: ≤ hourly rate or ≤ 100 cc if bolus feedings.
  - ≤ 4 stools/day.
  - No nausea, vomiting, abdominal distention.
- Adequate nutrition (stable or increasing weight; albumin/prealbumin within normal limits or increasing toward normal range).
- Adequate hydration (good skin turgor, moist mucous membranes, electrolytes/BUN within normal limits).

Interventions:

- Review care/administration with caregiver as needed.
- Continue prescribed formula, rate, free water.

✦ Check albumin/prealbumin every 3–6 months.

✦ Consider need for replacement tube. **Do not replace gastrostomy, j-tube, or g-j tube within first 2–3 weeks of placement. Must allow tract to epithelialize. J-tube can be replaced at bedside with red rubber catheter.** Do not inflate an inner bulb with j-tube; can cause obstruction. Gastrostomy tube can be replaced at bedside with replacement tube.

✦ Follow-up every 3–6 months.

Patient With Poor Tolerance/Complications

If following conditions exist, proceed to Interventions.

✦ RV > hourly rate or > 100 cc if bolus feedings.

✦ Constipation or > 4 stools/day.

✦ Reports of nausea, vomiting, abdominal distention.

✦ Obstructed tube.

✦ Recurrent aspiration events.

Interventions:

✦ Review handling/administration of formula with caregiver, i.e., amount placed in bag, amount hanging ≥ 6 hr, storage of unused formula.

✦ Review bowel regimen:

✧ With constipation, consider adding stool softener, laxative, suppository. Consult with nutritionist. **See Protocol on Constipation.**

✧ With diarrhea, consider adding Metamucil (psyllium) 1 rounded tbsp or 1 30-mg packet (1 tsp sugar-free formulation).

✧ Consider adding prokinetic agent: Reglan (metoclopramide HCl) syrup 5–10 mg qid or Propulsid (cisapride) suspension 10 mg/10 ml qid. **Propulsid is contraindicated in patients taking ketoconazole, itraconazole, or miconazole (systemically). Prokinetic agents may reduce gastric absorption of drugs.**

✦ Consider changing formula. Consult with nutritionist recommended.

✦ Reassess tolerance after addressing underlying problems.

Patient With Inadequate Nutrition/Hydration

If following conditions exist, proceed to Interventions.

✦ Weight decrease? How much? Over what time period?

✦ Albumin/prealbumin decreasing or not increasing. If patient is receiving adequate protein, prealbumin should increase by approximately 1 mg/dL daily.

✦ Abnormal electrolytes/BUN. Suggest dehydration.

✦ Poor skin turgor, dry mucous membranes.

Interventions:

- Review care/administration with caregiver. Is formula or H_2O being held for periods of time and why?
- Consider need for short-term intravenous fluids and/or hospitalization if severe dehydration.
- Consider factors that might increase calorie/protein needs:
  - wounds
  - pressure ulcers
  - increased activity
  - fever.
- Consider increasing rate, changing formula or adding modular protein powder (Promod) to formula. Consult with nutritionist.
- Reassess status in 2 weeks. Recheck prealbumin every 3–5 days.

Patient on Short-Term Tube Feeding for Rehabilitation

Goal: reinstitute oral feedings. If swallowing function improves:

- Consider consult with speech pathologist.
- Consider repeat fluoroscopy.
- Consider night-time feedings to allow oral feeds during day. Perform calorie counts to assure adequate nutrition.
- Consult nutritionist for adjustment of calorie/protein prescriptions as oral feedings progress.
- When adequate oral intake is achieved, discontinue tube feeding.

KEY ISSUES

Patient/Caregiver Education

Patient/caregiver should be able to:

- Explain purpose and expected duration (if appropriate) of tube feeding.
- Identify placement of tube and type of tube feeding.
- Demonstrate safe formula preparation and administration.
- Demonstrate correct medication administration via tube.
- Demonstrate proper tube care and equipment use.
- Describe how to monitor nutritional status.
- Describe how to prevent and manage complications.

✦ Describe aspiration precautions.

Economic Considerations

✦ Is the tube feeding reimbursable under patient's insurance? Note guidelines that must be met for tube feedings to be covered under Medicare.

✦ **Will tube feeding change level of care? New feeding tube will "skill" a patient under Medicare. Patients with long-standing tube feedings are no longer considered eligible for skilled care.**

✦ Is specific tube feeding formula available on formulary?

Psychosocial Considerations

✦ Be alert for grieving due to loss of body image with tube placement.

✦ If possible, allow patient to have small amount of favorite foods orally for pleasure.

Acute/Inpatient Setting

✦ Enteral feeding requirements will likely be affected by acute illness. Reevaluate.

Extended Care Setting

✦ Be aware of potential for social isolation secondary to inability to participate in group meals and activities.

Home Setting

✦ Initiate orders that include:
  - ✧ Formula and free water requirements.
  - ✧ Care of tube site.
  - ✧ Plan for advancement to target feeding.
  - ✧ Plan for eventual wean, if appropriate.
  - ✧ Frequency of weights.
  - ✧ Laboratory monitoring.

✦ Advise primary care provider if poor tolerance or inadequate nutrition occurs.

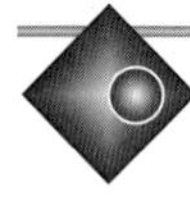

Gastroesophageal Reflux Disease (GERD)

HISTORY

✦ Heartburn, sensation of burning, or warmth behind the sternum with or without radiation to neck? **Elderly may present with milder symptoms secondary to less acidic reflux.**

✦ Chest pain? **Reflux can precipitate esophageal spasm, mimicking angina. Incidence of GERD increases after the age of 40, with increased incidence of esophageal mucosal disease after the age of 60.**

✦ Dyspepsia/indigestion? **Due to delay in gastric emptying; may be accompanied by heartburn and/or regurgitation. Usually associated with irritable bowel, esophagitis, peptic ulcer disease, cholecystitis, gastritis, or gastric malignancy.**

✦ Hiccups? Belching? Vomiting? Bloating? **Symptoms are common following a meal.**

✦ Regurgitation into throat? Warm fluid coming up in the mouth? Sour or bitter taste? When does this occur? **Tends to occur when lying down or bending over from the waist. Symptoms may be milder in elderly.**

✦ Halitosis?

✦ Increased salivation or water brash? **Salivary production and bicarbonate concentration normally decrease with aging. Acid in the esophagus produces an increase in saliva production.**

✦ Sore throat? Painful swallowing?

✦ Difficulty swallowing or sensation of food sticking in the esophagus? Location: pharynx, upper, middle, or lower esophagus? **Pharyngeal dysphagia may be related to CNS disease, diabetes mellitus, thyroid disease, or cervical osteophyte (unique to the elderly). Consider pill esophagitis due to decreased saliva and motility disorders in the elderly and recumbent position in the bedridden patient.**

✦ Constipation? Black stools?

✦ Fatigue? Hemoptysis or hematemesis? **Common with erosive esophagitis and secondary anemia.**

✦ Weight loss? Amount/over what time period?

✦ Hoarseness? Cough? Wheezing? **Reflux can irritate vocal cords and is a common, often unrecognized cause of asthma, recurrent pneumonia, and interstitial fibrosis.**

✦ Onset/duration of symptoms? **Barrett's esophagus (squamous epithelium replaced by columnar epithelium) is a complication of chronic reflux and may progress to esophageal adenocarcinoma.**

✦ History of alcohol (EtOH) or nicotine abuse? History of long-term use of NSAIDs? **EtOH and nicotine reduce lower esophageal pressure. Structural disease must be ruled out.**

✦ How do symptoms interfere with life-style?

✦ Alleviating/aggravating factors?

✦ History of hiatal hernia? **There is an increased incidence of GERD in the presence of a hiatal hernia; however, many with hiatal hernia do not have GERD.**

✦ History of diabetes mellitus, cerebrovascular accident (CVA), Parkinson's disease, or dementia? **Can cause gastroparesis, which can increase the risk of reflux.**

✦ Medications? **Lower esophageal sphincter (LES) pressure is decreased by nitrates, calcium channel blockers, theophylline, anticholinergic agents, antidepressants, and benzodiazepines, which in turn increase the risk of reflux.** Do antacids provide relief? **Antacids maintain/increase LES pressure.**

✦ Nasogastric tube interferes mechanically with LES closure. **See Protocol on Management of the Enterally Fed Patient.**

✦ **GERD may be secondary to one or more of the following conditions:**

- ✧ **Decreased LES tone.**
- ✧ **Esophageal mucosal irritation from acid.**
- ✧ **Delayed esophageal peristalsis.**
- ✧ **Delayed gastric emptying.**

PHYSICAL EXAMINATION

✦ Vital signs, weight.

✦ Assess for icterus and pale mucous membranes, yellow or white oropharyngeal plaques or ulcerations. Assess for inflamed pharynx, dental caries, and gingivitis. **May indicate secondary changes from acid reflux. Absence of gag reflex does not necessarily mean there is dysphagia.**

✦ Palpate for cervical or supraclavicular lymphadenopathy. **May be present with esophageal malignancy.**

✦ Assess lung fields for crackles, rhonchi, or wheezes. **Abnormal findings, especially on the right side, may indicate acute aspiration pneumonia.**

✦ Assess abdomen for diminished bowel sounds, abdominal distention, tenderness, organomegaly, and abdominal masses.

✦ Rectal: stool for guaiac.

✦ Assess skin for changes suggestive of scleroderma. **Scleroderma is known to alter esophageal motility.**

DIAGNOSTIC TESTS

✦ Clinical history of symptoms and risk factors provides the best noninvasive diagnosis.

✦ Consider liver function tests, amylase, and drug levels as appropriate.

✦ Hemoglobin/hematocrit if hemocult positive stool.

✦ Consider serum for *Heliobacter pylori.*

✦ Chest x-ray. **A dilated esophagus with retained food and an air-fluid level suggests achalasia, a common motility disorder in the elderly, presenting with symptoms of progressive dysphagia of solids and liquids, weight loss, and recumbent nocturnal coughing in the absence of chest pain.**

✦ Refer to speech pathologist for swallow study/video fluoroscopy.

✦ Upper GI.

✦ Consider gastric empty study in refractory conditions.

✦ Consider 24-hr ambulatory pH monitoring if endoscopic examination is normal. **Consult physician.**

✦ Refer to gastroenterologist for upper GI endoscopic examination/biopsy to rule out esophagitis, strictures, Barrett's esophagus, Zenker's diverticulum, Schatzki's ring and malignancy. **Consult physician.**

PREVENTION

✦ See Stage 1 Management.

✦ **See Protocol on Prevention and Health Maintenance.**

MANAGEMENT

Stage I

✦ Ask patient to keep a diary of factors triggering, aggravating, or alleviating symptoms.

✦ If unresponsive after 2–3 weeks, precede to stage 2.

Modifications of life-style and diet:

✦ Avoid bending over from the waist.

✦ Avoid straining to lift or defecate.

✦ Avoid tight-fitting clothes around the waist, abdomen.

✦ Discontinue tobacco.

✦ Avoid recumbency and left-lying positions for 2–3 hr after eating.

✦ Elevate head of bed 6–8 inches.

✦ Avoid eating and drinking (other than sips of fluid) 2–3 hr prior to bed time.

✦ Avoid esophageal irritants (citrus juices, caffeine, chocolate, EtOH).

✦ Decrease fried or fatty food intake and spicy foods.

✦ Avoid peppermint, which lowers LES pressure.

✦ Weight reduction program if indicated.

✦ Eat small meals several times a day.

Pharmacologic interventions:

✦ Consider altering or discontinuing medications known to decrease LES pressure (nitrates, theophylline, anticholinergic agents, benzodiazepines, calcium channel blockers, alpha-adrenergic antagonists, beta-adrenergic agonists, narcotics, and hormones).

✦ **Antacids.** Use after meals and bed time; can decrease esophageal acidity for 1 hr and maintain or increase LES pressure. **Use with caution in elderly, monitor potential drug–drug interactions, renal function, constipation, diarrhea, hypercalcemia, and sodium overload. Advise to take 2 hr before or after other medication to avoid drug–drug interactions.**

✦ **Mucosal protectants such as Carafate (sucralfate). May cause constipation.** Advise to take 2 hr before or after other medications to avoid potential malabsorption of other medications. Avoid in renal disease.

Stage 2

✦ Continue Stage 1 interventions and add a histamine-antagonist (H_2 blocker).

✦ **H_2 blocker: Can alter mental status in the elderly; be alert to theophylline, warfarin, and benzodiazepine drug–drug interactions; reduce dose for renal insufficiency.**

✧ Zantac (ranitidine HCl) 150 mg PO bid.

✧ Axid (nizatidine) 150 mg PO bid for maximum of 12 weeks.

✧ Pepcid (famotidine) 20 mg PO bid.

✧ Tagamet (cimetidine) 300–400 mg PO qid for maximum of 12 weeks. Should not be taken with antacids due to decreased absorbency of Tagamet. Can interfere with B_{12} absorption. Has increased drug–drug interaction profile; and has antiandrogen effects (gynecomastia, impotence).

✦ If addition of H_2 blocker is ineffective after 3–4 weeks, proceed to Stage 3.

✦ If gastric emptying is prolonged, consider adding prokinetic agent at this time. Follow instructions in Stage 4.

Stage 3

✦ **Continue Stage 1 interventions and discontinue H_2 blocker 3 days after initiating a proton pump inhibitor.**

✦ **Proton pump inhibitor: Reduces gastric acid secretion.**

✧ Prilosec (omeprazole) 20 mg PO daily for 4 weeks (for erosive or resistant esophagitis, treat 4–12 weeks). **Can increase blood levels of diazepam, warfarin, and phenytoin. May be taken with antacids; capsule should not be crushed.**

✧ Prevacid (lansoprazole) 15–30 mg PO daily for 8 weeks (for erosive esophagitis) and 15–30 mg PO daily for maintenance.

✦ Consider addition of Carafate (sucralfate) 1 g PO qid if esophagitis is suspected. Administer on empty stomach.

✦ **If patient remains symptomatic after 3–4 weeks, proceed to Stage 4.**

Stage 4

✦ **Continue Stage 1 interventions.**

✦ **Continue proton pump inhibitor and add a prokinetic agent.**

✦ **Prokinetic agent: Increases LES pressure and gastric emptying.**

✧ Reglan (metoclopramide HCl) 5–10 mg tid–qid. **Be alert for CNS symptoms: restlessness, tardive dyskinesia, and extrapyramidal effects.**

✧ Propulsid (cisapride) 10 mg tid–qid 15 min before meals and at bed time (acts directly on mucosa; does not have CNS effects). **Avoid use with systemic antifungal agents, erythromycin, and clarithromycin.**

✦ **Refer to gastroenterologist. Consult physician.**

KEY ISSUES

Patient/Caregiver Education

Patient/caregiver should be able to:

✦ Identify factors contributing to symptoms of GERD (refer to stage 1 management).

✦ Discuss which interventions they have found to be effective in reducing symptoms (refer to stages 1 through 4). **Avoid unnecessary restrictions.**

✦ Identify prescribed medications and describe their action.

✦ Identify contraindications and potential drug–drug interactions.

Economic Considerations

✦ H_2 blockers, proton pump inhibitors, and prokinetic agents are expensive and often require prior authorization in a managed care organization.

✦ Some insurance/managed care organizations may require presence of *H. pylori* before authorizing these agents.

Psychosocial Considerations

✦ Assess for fear regarding source of chest discomfort.

✦ Social dining is often avoided when symptoms are pronounced.

Acute/Inpatient Setting

✦ H_2 blockers may need to be given IV during acute phase; change to oral route as soon as possible.

✦ Dysphagia is common problem. If regurgitation occurs, assess for fever spikes, consider CBC and differential along with chest x-ray to rule out aspiration pneumonia.

Extended Care Setting

✦ Proton pump inhibitors are meant for oral use and may lose effectiveness if administered through feeding tubes. May obstruct tube as well. **See Protocol on Management of the Enterally Fed Patient.**

Home Setting

✦ Assess properly adapted environment such as elevated head of bed or hospital bed and provision for proper infusion of enteral feedings when appropriate.

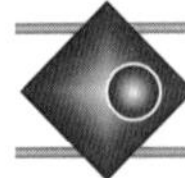

Gastrointestinal (GI) Bleeding

HISTORY

✦ Associated/presenting symptoms: Hematemesis, melena, or hematochezia; color of lost blood? Estimated volume of blood loss? Vomiting prior to hematemesis? Pain: location and intensity? Presence of hemorrhoids? Altered mental status?

✦ Onset of symptoms: sudden or gradual bleeding? **In cases of gradual bleeding, the elderly may present with nonspecific GI complaints.**

✦ Past medical history/comorbid conditions (see Display 6-1): **Elderly with comorbidity may be severely compromised by shock and blood loss from acute bleed** (see Display 6-2). Previous GI bleed, ulcer disease? **GI bleed may be initial presentation of peptic ulcer disease (PUD) because symptoms of PUD may be markedly reduced in the elderly. See Protocol on Peptic Ulcer Disease.** Previous abdominal surgery? Constipation, inflammatory bowel disease, ulcerative colitis, gastric cancer, colon cancer? Renal disease (**increases prevalence of upper GI abnormalities**). Musculoskeletal pain, rheumatoid arthritis? **It is estimated that 2,600 deaths result per year from NSAID-associated gastropathy in patients with rheumatoid arthritis.** Bleeding disorder? Previous aortic surgery? AIDS, CNS disorders, pulmonary, hepatic disorders?

✦ Medication history: especially NSAIDs, aspirin, corticosteroids, anticoagulants?

✦ Family history of cancer in GI tract?

✦ EtOH use?

✦ Tobacco use?

DISPLAY 6-1. *Common Causes of GI Bleeding*

COMMON CAUSES OF UPPER GI BLEEDING

Duodenal ulcer
Gastric ulcer
Varices
Mallory–Weiss tear
Gastroesophageal reflux (GERD)

COMMON CAUSES OF LOWER GI BLEEDING

Colon cancer
Diverticula
Polyps
Inflammatory bowel disease
Angiodysplasia
Ischemic colitis

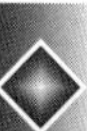

DISPLAY 6-2. ***Conditions Increasing Mortality from GI Bleeding***

Cardiac disease (arrhythmias, arteriosclerotic cardiovascular disease [ASCVD], congestive heart failure [CHF])
Chronic liver disease
Pneumonia
Sepsis
Hemodialysis
Delirium and dementia
CVA

PHYSICAL EXAMINATION

✦ Vital signs. Assess BP in supine and upright positions and pulse for signs of volume depletion, shock. **In the elderly, the pulse may be normal despite volume depletion because of the cardiovascular system's decreased ability to compensate for volume loss. Be aware that usual signs of compromised volume (orthostasis, tachycardia) may be unreliable in elderly patients with baseline autonomic dysfunction.**

✦ Skin: Inspect for pallor. Assess for jaundice, palmar erythema, spider angiomas (suggestive of liver disease).

✦ Abdomen: Note ascites, scars. Auscultate for hyperactive bowel sounds (blood in gut may stimulate gut motility). Palpate for tenderness, hepatomegaly, splenomegaly.

✦ Rectal: stool for guaiac.

DIAGNOSTIC TESTS

✦ CBC including platelet count.

✧ Hemoglobin < 10 or a 3-g/dL decrease from baseline is suggestive of hemorrhage.

✧ Acute decrease in hematocrit may not be seen for 24–48 hr due to body fluid redistribution.

✦ Prothrombin and partial thromboplastin time; international normalized ratio (INR) if on warfarin.

✦ Serum electrolytes and glucose.

✦ Digested blood in GI tract raises BUN. BUN-to-creatinine ratio $> 25{:}1$ suggests upper GI bleed; $< 25{:}1$ suggests lower GI bleed.

✦ Type and cross-match when transfusion may be needed.

✦ Arterial blood gas or oxygen saturation if hemodynamically compromised.

✦ Further diagnostic work-up is dependent on suspected source of bleeding. **See Section on Management.**

PREVENTION

✦ Review medications (prescribed and OTC) of all patients at every visit to avoid iatrogenic causes of GI bleeding.

✦ Refer for alternative therapies (PT, OT) for arthritis patients to avoid NSAID-associated gastropathy.

✦ **See Protocol on Prevention and Health Maintenance.**

MANAGEMENT

✦ GI bleeding is considered emergent until proven otherwise.

✦ Nasogastric aspirate may be performed to distinguish upper from lower GI bleeding. Positive aspirate and/or hematemesis indicates upper GI bleeding. Aspirate may be negative in the presence of duodenal ulcer bleed.

✦ Patients with prosthetic valve or artificial joint will require prophylactic antibiotics if invasive or surgical intervention is necessary.

✦ Hematochezia (bright red blood in stool) usually indicates bleeding in the colon but may be seen in brisk upper GI bleeding.

✦ Melena (black, tarry stools) is usual result of upper GI bleeding but also seen in lower GI bleeding.

Upper GI Bleeding

✦ On acute presentation, initial intervention is stabilization: establishment of adequate airway, monitoring of cardiac rhythm, fluid balance/hemodynamic stabilization, correction of severe anemia. Emergency endoscopic therapy may be performed to locate site, stop bleeding, and prevent recurrent bleeding.

✦ If melena and hematemesis are present, suspect **esophageal varices** caused by portal hypertension. Seen in cirrhotic patients (most frequent single cause of death); also occur with hepatic tumors or mesenteric and central venous thrombi. May be precipitated by coughing, vomiting, straining or heavy lifting, and drinking irritating fluids. Following endoscopic diagnosis, treatment options consist of vasoconstrictive agents, balloon tamponade, injection sclerotherapy, banding ligation, and shunt procedures.

✦ Selected nonemergent patients may be managed on outpatient basis with endoscopic location and treatment of bleeding site.

✦ Consult physician on medical management (H_2 blockers, proton pump inhibitors, treatment of *H. pylori* infection). **See Protocols on Gastroesophageal Reflux Disease and Peptic Ulcer Disease.**

Lower GI Bleeding

✦ May present acutely as severe, life-endangering bleeding or as gradual bleed found only by occult blood testing of the stool.

✦ Consult physician in cases of emergent lower GI bleeding.

✦ Evaluation of lower GI bleeding:

✧ Digital rectal examination and anoscopy/sigmoidoscopy for identification of anorectal bleeding site.

✧ During active bleeding, radiolabeled RBC scan or angiography may be useful to identify bleeding site.

✧ Colonoscopy has high diagnostic yield and is procedure of choice for intermittent lower GI bleeding and asymptomatic patients (positive results on fecal occult blood testing). Adequate preparation is crucial to remove stool and clotted blood from colon. Treatment of some sources of bleeding is possible during colonoscopy.

✧ Barium enema has lower diagnostic yield than colonoscopy and does not permit intervention at site of bleeding. Barium in GI tract can complicate urgent surgery.

✦ Source may be colonic neoplasms, angiodysplasia (arteriovenous malformations), vascular ectasias, colonic ischemia, diverticula, infectious bowel disease, hemorrhoids, or inflammatory bowel disease.

✦ Vascular ectasias occur as a result of dilated and tortuous submucosal veins in the cecum and proximal ascending colon. Two-thirds of patients are over the age of 70. Secondary iron-deficiency anemia and occult blood in stool are usual presenting symptoms. Bleeding stops spontaneously in most cases, although some patients may experience massive hemorrhage.

✦ Bleeding from diverticula usually occurs in the right colon, is not severe, and stops spontaneously. Some may experience recurrent hemorrhage that requires surgical intervention. **See Protocol on Abdominal Pain.**

✦ Ischemic colon is a common cause of lower GI bleeding in the elderly resulting from vascular degeneration (atherosclerosis) or obstruction (volvulus, stricture, or clot). Usually characterized by minimal blood loss and sudden onset of mild pain in left lower quadrant, followed by bright red blood from rectum. Surgical resection is required for infarcted bowel.

✦ Bleeding from angiodysplasia is usually not severe but frequency of rebleeding is high. Diagnosis is by colonoscopy and treatment by endoscopic electrocoagulation.

✦ Most hemorrhoids are managed with band ligation coagulation or surgical excision.

✦ Consult physician/refer patients for colonoscopy if positive results on fecal occult blood testing.

KEY ISSUES

Patient/Caregiver Education

Patient/caregiver should be able to:

✦ Verbalize understanding of diagnostic procedures.

✦ Verbalize importance of correct preparation for diagnostic procedures.

✦ State need to avoid lifing heavy objects and straining to defecate.

Economic Considerations

✦ Evaluation/treatment for GI bleeding frequently results in hospitalization.

Psychosocial Considerations

✦ Fear of poor prognosis may prevent some elderly from seeking treatment for gradual GI bleeding.

✦ Refer for counseling for EtOH abuse if indicated. **See Protocol on Substance Abuse.**

✦ Massive GI bleeding is a frightening experience. Provide emotional support for patients and families.

✦ Be aware that a patient's religious beliefs may prohibit transfusion of blood from others. Refer to pastoral service for counseling if indicated.

Acute/Inpatient Setting

✦ Postoperative upper GI bleeding increases risk for morbidity and mortality in cardiovascular patients.

✦ Monitor cardiopulmonary status closely during transfusions; may result in symptoms of congestive heart failure (CHF).

Extended Care Setting

✦ Minor rectal hemorrhage may occur as a complication of manual removal of fecal impaction. Stercoral ulcers may form under masses of hard, impacted stool. **See Protocol on Constipation.**

✦ Educate staff to report possible signs of GI bleeding: altered mental status, subtle changes in baseline behavior, and changes in gait.

Home Setting

✦ Recommend screening with at-home fecal occult blood testing.

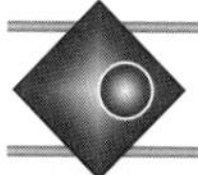

Nausea and Vomiting

HISTORY

✦ Onset and duration of symptoms?

✦ Episodic or continuous?

✦ Timing and number of episodes? Relationship to eating?

✦ Character of emesis: undigested food, coffee ground, bile?

✦ Associated symptoms: anorexia, abdominal pain (note location, character, duration), constipation or diarrhea (last bowel movement [BM]), flatus, lethargy, change in mental status, change in functional status, halitosis, respiratory symptoms (cough, dyspnea, orthopnea), cardiac symptoms (chest pain, dyspnea, palpitations, diaphoresis), urinary symptoms (dysuria, frequency, hematuria, incontinence)?

✦ Weight loss? Number of pounds over what time period?

✦ Comorbid conditions: cholecystitis, hepatitis, diverticulitis, pancreatitis, hiatal hernia, ulcer disease, GI bleed, esophageal strictures, abdominal surgeries, bowel obstruction/ileus, diabetes mellitus, cardiac disease, cancer?

✦ Medications, prescription/OTC? EtOH use?

✦ Diet? Any recent change in diet? Enteral feedings?

✦ Anyone else in family ill? Recent travel outside of country?

PHYSICAL EXAMINATION

✦ Vital signs, weight, general appearance. **Note usual temperature; even slight elevations in elderly may be significant.**

✦ Skin: color (note presence of jaundice or pallor), hydration status. Assess skin turgor on forehead or sternum.

✦ Mouth: assess dentition, condition of oral mucosa, presence of mouth lesions.

✦ Abdomen: assess contour and for presence of distention, ascites, surgical scars; auscultate bowel sounds; assess for organomegaly, masses, pain on palpation, rebound tenderness

✦ Anorectal: assess sphincter tone, presence of stool or impaction, guaiac.

✦ Focused examination based on comorbid conditions.

DIAGNOSTIC TESTS

✦ Serum electrolytes, BUN to assess for dehydration and electrolyte abnormalities; creatinine to assess renal function; CBC for possible anemia and infection; urinalysis to rule out urinary tract infection (UTI); albumin or prealbumin to assess nutritional status.

✦ Consider: liver profile for possible liver disease; serum amylase for possible pancreatitis.

✦ Consider checking therapeutic drug levels, e.g., Lanoxin (digoxin), Dilantin (phenytoin), theophylline.

✦ Consider *H. pylori* with symptoms of GERD or if suspected PUD.

✦ Consider abdominal flatplate and upright x-ray if suspected obstruction.

✦ Consider chest x-ray if suspected respiratory process. **Elderly are at high risk for aspiration with nausea and vomiting.**

✦ Consider gastric emptying study.

✦ Consider abdominal ultrasound for possible gallstones, hydronephrosis.

✦ Consider upper GI series for possible esophageal stricture, PUD, or hiatal hernia.

✦ Consider CT scan of abdomen for possible abdominal mass, abscess, or retroperitoneal bleed.

PREVENTION

✦ Educate on good oral hygiene especially during episodes of vomiting.

✦ Refer for regular dental examinations.

✦ Maintain normal bowel regimen to prevent constipation. **See Protocol on Constipation.**

✦ Encourage well-balanced diet, adequate hydration.

✦ If bedbound patient, maintain proper positioning to decrease risk of aspiration. Head of bed should be elevated 30 degrees at all times.

✦ **See Protocol on Prevention and Health Maintenance.**

MANAGEMENT

✦ Review and adjust medication regimen as appropriate. Consider alternate routes of administration during acute episodes of vomiting. Discontinue or decrease dose of medications if outside of therapeutic range. **Elderly may experience symptoms of toxicity even with therapeutic drug levels of digoxin.**

✦ Recommend dietary adjustments to maintain nutrition and hydration. Hold enteral feedings or reduce rate. In general, elderly persons need 1 oz fluids per kilogram body weight. **See Protocol on Management of the Enterally Fed Patient.**

✦ Instruct diabetics to continue insulin and oral hypoglycemic regimen when ill. Monitor blood glucose more frequently (q 2–3 hr) and maintain hydration. Notify NP if persistent hyperglycemia or if unable to eat. **See Protocol on Diabetes Mellitus.**

✦ Treat associated constipation or diarrhea. **See Protocols on Constipation and Diarrhea.**

✦ Treat associated abdominal pain as indicated. Refer for possible surgical problems. **See Protocol on Abdominal Pain.**

✦ Consider use of antacids with associated dyspepsia.

✦ For symptom management, consider antiemetics. **Use antiemetics cautiously and at lowest dose possible in elderly; may cause sedation or altered mental status.**

✧ Phenergan (promethazine HCl) 12.5–25 mg q 4–6 hr prn, available in tablets, suppository, and injectable.

✧ Compazine (prochlorperazine maleate) 5–10 mg tablets tid or qid, 25 mg suppository bid, or 5–10 mg IM q 4–6 hr prn.

✧ Tigan (trimethobenzamide HCl) 250 mg capsules tid or qid, 200 mg suppository tid or qid, or 200 mg tid or qid IM.

✦ For resistant cases, consider:

✧ Ativan (lorazepam) 0.5 mg q 4 hr prn.

✧ Zofran (ondanestron HCl) 0.15–0.3 mg/kg IV q 4 hr prn or 32 mg q 4 hr PO.

✦ **See Chapter on Palliative Care** for other pharmacological options in terminally ill patient.

✦ If suspected gastroparesis or GERD, a prokinetic agent may be useful:

✧ Reglan (metoclopramide HCl) 5–10 mg tid or qid; **for short-term use.**

✧ Propulsid (cisapride) 10 mg qid, before meals and at bed time.

✦ Consider use of an H_2 blocker for acid suppression. **See Protocols on GERD and GI Bleeding.**

✦ Consider short-term use of a proton pump inhibitor for acid suppression:

✧ Prilosec (omeprazole) 20 mg PO daily.

✧ Prevacid (lansoprazole) 15–30 mg PO daily.

✦ If dehydration or electrolyte abnormalities present, replace orally or intravenously. Patient with intractable vomiting or severely dehydrated patient may require hospitalization. **See Protocol on Fluid and Electrolyte Abnormalities. Dehydration is a poorly understood syndrome in the elderly, but is known to increase mortality in hospitalized patients.**

✦ Manage comorbid conditions as indicated.

✦ Treat underlying infections if present. **See Protocols on Pneumonia and Urinary Tract Infection.**

✦ Consider referral to gastroenterologist for further evaluation. Consult physician.

KEY ISSUES

Patient/Caregiver Education

Patient/caregiver should be able to:

✦ Identify signs and symptoms that warrant contacting health care professional.

✦ Recognize adverse effects of medications prescribed.

✦ Describe dietary adjustments recommended to maintain nutrition and hydration.

✦ Describe alterations of medication regimen recommended during acute episodes of nausea and vomiting.

Economic Considerations

✦ Zofran and proton pump inhibitors are expensive, may require prior authorization for patients on managed care formularies.

Psychosocial Considerations

✦ Persistent or prolonged nausea and vomiting can be debilitating and result in an alteration in functional status.

Acute/Inpatient Setting

✦ Antiemetics and H2 blockers may need to be given IV during acute hospitalization.

✦ Monitor serum electrolytes, BUN as indicated.

✦ Administer fluids IV to maintain hydration.

✦ Correct electrolyte abnormalities.

✦ Assess nutritional status; consult nutritionist.

Extended Care Setting

✦ Be alert to medications, constipation, and infection as common causes of nausea/vomiting.

✦ Maintain state of hydration during acute episodes of nausea and vomiting. Short-term IV fluids may be needed.

✦ Consider schedule for offering fluids, especially for the patient with dementia. **Sensation of thirst is decreased in elderly.**

✦ Manage care in the extended care facility when possible.

Home Setting

✦ Early intervention before dehydration occurs may prevent the need for IV fluids and/or hospitalization.

✦ Consider home health assessment and intervention for administration of IV fluids in the home setting.

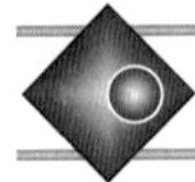

Abdominal Pain

HISTORY

✦ Onset? Duration? Quality of pain: intermittent or constant? Severity (rate on scale of 1 to 10)? Location; specify quadrant(s), other sites? Alleviating/exacerbating factors?

✦ Associated symptoms: nausea, vomiting, constipation, diarrhea, bloody stool, change in normal bowel routine, early satiety, bloating, fever, chills? **The elderly may not present with classic associated symptoms of nausea, vomiting, and diarrhea. Abdominal pain may be absent, mild, or not localized.**

✦ Comorbid conditions: Gastrointestinal disease, gallbladder disease, history of abdominal surgery, history of gynecologic surgery (ovarian/uterine disease), history of recurrent UTI, renal calculi, liver disease, diabetes mellitus, Parkinson's disease, cardiac disease, vascular disease (may lead to ischemic bowel)?

✦ Medications including OTC? Note especially NSAIDs, theophylline, phenothiazines, oral hypoglycemic agents, colchicine, digoxin, erythromycin, salicylates, diuretics, anticholinergics?

✦ EtOH use? **EtOH abuse may impair ability to relate history.** Tobacco use?

✦ Diet: any recent changes; history of lactose intolerance?

✦ Functional status: ability to take in food/fluids; inactivity (may predispose to bowel obstruction)?

✦ Anyone else in family or facility ill?

PHYSICAL EXAMINATION

✦ Vital signs. **The elderly are more likely than younger patients to present with hypothermia rather than a febrile response.** Orthostatic blood pressure evaluation to assess for dehydration.

✦ Eyes: Inspect conjunctiva and sclera for icterus.

✦ Cardiac: **Tachycardia of volume compromise may be absent in the elderly.**

✦ Skin: Inspect for dry mucous membranes; icterus.

✦ Neuro: Absent peripheral reflexes may suggest neuropathy that may accompany gastroparesis.

✦ Abdomen: Palpate for tenderness (see Table 6-1), masses, organomegaly, and bladder distention. A palpable mass may be found in diverticulitis and

TABLE 6-1. Differential Diagnosis of Abdominal Pain

Location	Differential diagnosis
Right upper quadrant	Cholecystitis Duodenal ulcer, gastric ulcer Pancreatitis Pyelonephritis, stones Pleurisy Hepatitis
Right lower quadrant	Appendicitis Crohn's disease, ulcerative colitis Ovarian cyst, ovarian cancer
Left upper quadrant	Ruptured spleen Pyelonephritis, stones
Left lower quadrant	Diverticulitis Colon carcinoma Ovarian cyst, ovarian cancer
Epigastric or central	Duodenal ulcer, gastric ulcer Gastroenteritis Hiatal hernia Aneurysm Mesenteric thrombosis/embolism
Suprapubic	Cystitis Uterine masses Prostatitis

high fecal impaction. Presence of a pulsatile mass may be suggestive of aortic aneurysm. Percuss liver size.

✦ Pelvic examination in females.

✦ Rectal: Palpate for fecal impaction; obtain stool for guaiac.

DIAGNOSTIC TESTS

✦ CBC with differential.

✦ Liver function tests—**See Gallstone Disease.**

✦ Guaiac testing of stool—If positive, may be caused by diverticulosis but should not be assumed cause of bleeding. **See Protocol on Gastrointestinal Bleeding.**

✦ Abdominal flatplate and upright films detect obstruction, perforation, ileus.

✦ Abdominal ultrasound detects presence of gallstones.

✦ CT evaluates the abdominal vascular system, identifies diverticula, and differentiates causes of abdominal obstruction.

PREVENTION

✦ Utilize bowel regimen to avoid constipation. Avoid use of stimulant laxatives. **See Protocol on Constipation.**

✦ **See Protocol on Prevention and Health Maintenance.**

MANAGEMENT

✦ See Display 6-3 for differential diagnoses.

Chronic Gastritis

ATROPHIC

✦ Affects the mucosa of the stomach body and fundus and is probably caused by autoimmune processes.

✦ Patients usually remain asymptomatic, but weight loss, malnutrition, nutrient malabsorption may occur.

✦ Initial symptoms may be sequela of pernicious anemia. **See Protocol on Anemia.**

INFLAMMATORY

✦ **Prevalence rates in the United States increase with aging, reaching almost 80% by age 75.**

✦ Symptoms may include nausea, upper abdominal pain, distention, or anorexia, and physical findings are nonspecific.

✦ May be caused by medications, EtOH or *H. pylori* infection. Affected site is the antral mucosa.

✦ Strong association exists between *H. pylori* infection and PUD. **See Protocol on Peptic Ulcer Disease.**

✦ May require endoscopy for diagnosis. Consult physician.

Diverticula

✦ Diverticula (balloon-like sacs) develop in the colon as a result of decreased colonic motility; most likely cause is insufficient dietary fiber.

✦ **Incidence increases with aging.**

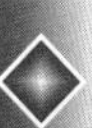

DISPLAY 6-3. ***Possible Causes of Abdominal Pain in the Elderly***

Gastritis, acute or chronic
Diverticula, diverticulitis
Gastropathy/gastroparesis
Bowel obstruction
Peritonitis
Perforated viscus
Ruptured abdominal aortic aneurysm
Gallstone disease
Acute cholecystitis
- Gallstone ileus
- Acalculous cholecystitis
- Suppurative cholangitis

Intra-abdominal cancer
Muscular strain
Atypical presentation of myocardial infarction, congestive heart failure
Intestinal tuberculosis
Pneumonia, pulmonary emboli
Addisonian crisis
Iatrogenesis (medication related)
- NSAIDs
- Oral hypoglycemic agents
- Tricyclic antidepressants
- Diuretics
- Phenothiazines
- Erythromycin

✦ Most diverticula are located in the sigmoid colon and remain asymptomatic. When symptoms occur, most common complaints are colic-type pain in the abdomen and constipation.

✦ Identified by barium radiographs of colon or colonoscopy.

✦ Recommend dietary intake rich in high-fiber foods such as cereals, whole grains, bran, vegetables, fruits, and plenty of water.

✦ Consider Metamucil (psyllium) 1 Tbsp. (1 tsp. sugar-free formulation) in 8 oz of water qd–tid.

✦ Diverticulitis is a potential complication that presents with acute abdominal pain eventually localized to the left lower quadrant, nausea, vomiting, mild fever, leukocytosis, and (occasionally) a palpable mass. Consult physician. **See Acute/Inpatient Setting.**

✦ In the elderly, bleeding from diverticula is the most common source of lower GI hemorrhage. **See Protocol on Gastrointestinal Bleeding.**

Gallstone Disease (GSD)

✦ **Approximately 9 million Americans over age of 60 have GSD or have had a cholecystectomy.**

✦ Increased prevalence in Native Americans and Hispanics and decreased prevalence in African Americans compared with the total population in the United States.

✦ No definitive measures are available for preventing gallstones.

✦ **Most GSD remains asymptomatic.**

✦ Symptomatic GSD is characterized by episodes of biliary colic, acute attacks of steady, intense pain that last from several minutes to several hours and resolve spontaneously. Pain may occur in the epigastric area or right upper quadrant and radiate to the upper back with accompanying diaphoresis. Fever may be present, but peritoneal signs are rarely evident unless examination is performed during a painful episode.

✦ Even during episodes of biliary pain, laboratory results may be normal, although leukocytosis may be seen.

✦ Ultrasound is diagnostic test of choice for detecting gallstones and measuring gallbladder wall.

✦ Consult physician for appropriate management referral (surgical or gastrointestinal specialist consult). Elders should be advised of available treatment options:

✧ Surgery is usual treatment of choice for symptomatic GSD. Elective cholecystectomy is associated with less mortality in the elderly than emergency surgery. Elective surgery may prevent complications of later emergency surgery for acute cholecystitis, especially in patients with diabetes mellitus who have greater mortality.

✧ Laparoscopic cholecystectomy provides short hospital stays but requires general anesthesia and carries increased risk of common bile duct injury.

✧ Many elderly with a single episode or rarely occurring episodes may decline surgical treatment. 20–30% of patients with GSD have rare episodes.

✧ Stone dissolution with oral medications is an alternative for nonsurgical candidates.

✧ Shock wave lithotripsy fragments stones so they can be passed easily and does not require routine sedation or analgesia. Qualification criteria for use of this technology, which is widely available in the United States, are: 1–3 stones with a combined diameter not larger than 3 cm, history of biliary colic, and a functional gallbladder.

✦ Most common complication of GSD is acute cholecystitis (inflammation of the gallbladder). Pain that begins in the epigastrium, shifts to the right upper quadrant, and lasts longer than 8–10 hours is suggestive, especially if accompanied by fever, vomiting, or dark urine. **Symptoms may be less severe than in the younger population and may be nonspecific.** Mild elevations of bilirubin (rarely > 4 mg/dL), alkaline phosphatase, amylase, and hepatic transaminases may be found. Consult physician.

✦ Less-frequent complications of GSD include:

✧ **Acalculous cholecystitis**—surgery, major illness, parenteral hyperalimentation predispose elders—most commonly seen in elderly men with peripheral vascular disease.

✧ **Suppurative cholangitis** (inflammation of the bile ducts)—rare in patients before the seventh decade, associated with high mortality rates.

✧ **Gallstone ileus**—results in high mortality probably due to late diagnosis and treatment in the elderly.

Gastroparesis

✦ Caused by delayed gastric emptying. Patients with Parkinson's disease encounter delayed gastric emptying and commonly complain of early satiety and epigastric distress.

✦ Occurs most often as a neuropathic complication of diabetes mellitus.

✦ Characterized by abdominal pain, bloating, nausea, vomiting of undigested food, early satiety, anorexia, or high residuals in the tube-fed patient. **Elderly diabetics often do not report symptoms without specific questioning because they may have multiple concerns or consider symptoms to be normal consequences of aging.**

✦ Most sensitive diagnostic test is radionuclide scintigraphy that quantifies how long it takes for food to leave the stomach. Retention will be longer than 1 hr in patients with gastropathy.

✦ Gastroparesis should be considered when good blood glucose control deteriorates. Postprandial hypoglycemia and wide fluctuations in blood glucose control are key indicators of delayed gastric emptying and absorption of carbohydrates. **Elderly patients taking insulin may suffer serious consequences from these complications.**

✦ **Stress the importance of good blood glucose control. See Protocol on Diabetes Mellitus.** Patients should be instructed regarding the correlation of hyperglycemia and delayed gastric emptying. Blood glucose levels should be monitored to judge the effects of different meals on glycemic levels.

✦ Refer to nutritionist/diabetes educator for instruction in meal planning and measures to avoid postprandial hypoglycemia and delayed hyperglycemia:

✧ Eat small, frequent meals.

✧ Avoid high-fiber and high-fat foods. Eat foods that are digested easily.

✦ Monitor for failure or fluctuating effects of oral medications (digoxin, levodopa) that may result from delayed/reduced drug absorption.

✦ Monitor/limit use of medications that delay gastric emptying: tricyclic antidepressants, anticholinergics, calcium channel blockers, opioids, tranquilizers, antacids that contain aluminum.

✦ Prokinetic agents for management of gastroparesis:

✧ Propulsid (cisapride) 10 mg PO before meals and at bedtime; speeds gastric emptying and intestinal motility but has little antiemetic effect; potential side effects include diarrhea and abdominal cramping. **Contraindicated in combination with antifungals, certain antiarrhythmics, erythromycin, clarithromycin, nefazodone, indinavir, and ritonavir (increased poten-**

tial for cardiac dysrhythmias) and for patients with renal failure, CHF, ischemic heart disease, prolonged QT intervals.

✧ Reglan (metoclopramide HCl) 5–10 mg PO before meals and at bedtime; **potential for dystonic reactions and depression especially in the elderly.**

✧ Motilium (domperidon) is an investigational drug that has been shown to be effective in increasing gastric emptying and preventing nausea and vomiting, with few side effects except breast tenderness and galactorrhea. Dosage is 10–20 mg PO qid.

✦ Venting gastrostomy and jejunostomy for enteral feeding may be indicated for patients refractory to diet and pharmacological therapy.

Obstruction

SMALL BOWEL

✦ Obstruction of small bowel occurs as a result of cancer, adhesions from previous abdominal surgery, or hernia.

✦ Signs/symptoms include abdominal pain and distention followed by nausea and vomiting.

✦ Order abdominal flatplate and upright x-ray.

✦ Consult physician/refer to emergency department for IV fluids and nasogastric decompression. Surgical intervention is required if decompression fails or bowel strangulation is suspected.

LARGE BOWEL

✦ Predominant cause in the elderly is colon cancer; also caused by diverticulitis and sigmoid volvulus.

✦ Elderly may present with complaints of vomiting, diarrhea, constipation, or obstipation.

✦ **Elders using tranquilizers, anticholinergic medications, anti-Parkinsonian drugs, or frequent laxatives may be predisposed to sigmoid volvulus.** Symptoms may have gradual onset.

✦ Order abdominal flatplate and upright x-ray.

✦ Consult physician for referral for sigmoidoscopy (with barium enema or passage of rectal tube) for decompression. Surgical intervention is required if decompression fails or bowel strangulation is suspected.

KEY ISSUES

Patient/Caregiver Education

Patient/caregiver should be able to:

- ✦ Verbalize dietary recommendations.
- ✦ Verbalize timing and dosing of medications.
- ✦ Identify potential side effects of medications.

Psychosocial Considerations

✦ **Fear of a loss of independence may cause elderly to under-report symptoms.**

✦ Screen elders with gastroparesis for depression and anxiety that can cause hopelessness and lack of motivation for good blood glucose control.

Acute/Inpatient Setting

✦ Diverticulitis may require admission for IV hydration, antibiotics, and bowel rest. Fewer than one-fourth of patients will require surgical intervention for perforation to the peritoneal cavity.

✦ Prompt diagnosis and early treatment of acute cholecystitis may prevent surgical complications.

Extended Care Setting

✦ Increased frequency of abdominal pain as a manifestation of intestinal tuberculosis is seen in extended care settings.

Home Setting

✦ For patients with gastroparesis, advise caregive to monitor eating habits.

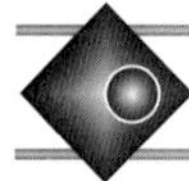

Constipation

HISTORY

✦ Bowel habits: last BM, color, size, consistency, frequency of stools, normal routine?

✦ Onset and duration of symptoms?

✦ Associated symptoms: straining, blood in stools, pain with defecation, abdominal pain, nausea, vomiting, flatus, urinary or fecal incontinence, decreased appetite, lethargy, change in mental status, halitosis?

✦ Dentures? Fit of dentures? Quality/adequacy of dentition? Last dental examination?

✦ Weight loss or gain in past 6 months? Past month? **Further evaluation is recommended if patient has lost 5% of weight in past month, 7 1/2% in 3 months, or 10% in 6 months. Any unintentional weight loss can be significant.**

✦ Past medical history for conditions associated with abdominal discomfort/dysfunction: abdominal surgery, hemorrhoids, diverticulitis, bowel obstruction, hypothyroidism, CVA, diabetes mellitus, CHF, Parkinson's, spinal cord lesions/injuries, myasthenia, multiple sclerosis, enlarged prostate, or GI bleed?

✦ History of depression or dementia?

✦ Medications: especially note those that may contribute to constipation, i.e., analgesics, antacids, diuretics, anticholinergics, calcium channel blockers, iron supplements; habitual use of laxatives or enemas?

✦ Diet: 24-hr recall, type of diet, fluid intake, change in dietary pattern, access/availability to food, use of enteral feedings/type of formula?

✦ Level of activity/exercise?

✦ Functional status?

✦ Social situation/support?

PHYSICAL EXAMINATION

✦ Vital signs, weight, general appearance.

✦ Skin integrity and color, hydration status, dentition, oral mucosa, tongue.

✦ Abdomen: assess for contour, bowel sounds, organomegaly, masses, pain, urinary retention.

✦ Anorectal: assess for sphincter tone, presence of stool, impaction, hemorrhoids, fissure, enlarged prostate/stool for guaiac.

✦ Consider sensory/motor neurological examination.

✦ Assess cognitive and functional status.

DIAGNOSTIC TESTS

✦ Stool for occult blood; consider further GI work-up if positive. **See Protocol on GI Bleeding.**

✦ Consider an abdominal flatplate and upright x-ray if ileus, obstruction, or high impaction suspected.

✦ Consider: serum electrolytes, BUN to rule out dehydration and electrolyte abnormalities; thyroid function tests; CBC to assess for anemia, infection.

PREVENTION

✦ Identify normal bowel function and encourage patient to establish normal routine of toileting. Establish bowel training in dependent patient.

✦ Maintain adequate fluid intake (goal: at least six to eight 8-oz glasses of water daily), modify goal for patient with fluid restriction; for patient with tube feeding, assess fluid needs and provide adequate free water. **See Protocol on Management of the Enterally Fed Patient.**

✦ Increase dietary fiber (goal: 20 g/day); if enterally fed, consider change to a higher fiber formula; consider high-fiber oral supplements/recipes.

✦ Review medications, eliminate potentially anorectic or constipating medications if possible.

✦ Increase activity/mobility as tolerated.

✦ Provide privacy for toileting.

✦ Improve access to toileting if applicable, i.e., bedside commode, raised toilet seat, scheduled toileting.

✦ Order suppository for occasional use: glycerin or Dulcolax (bisacodyl).

✦ **See Protocol on Prevention and Health Maintenance.**

MANAGEMENT

Chronic Constipation

For patient who requires frequent use of laxatives for bowel movements:

✦ Customize bowel regimen for each patient.

✦ Begin with a stool softener (emollient), which softens and lubricates fecal mass: Dialose or Colace (docusate sodium) 100–250 mg 1 bid (capsule or liquid preparation). **Recommend for bedbound patient with hard, dry stools.**

✦ Consider addition of a bulk-forming agent, which absorbs water and increases fecal mass: Metamucil (psyllium) 1 rounded tsp. or Tbsp. in 8 oz of water one to three times daily; comes in a powder, an effervescent, and a wafer, in a variety of flavors and sugarless; Fiber Con (calcium polycarbophil) 2 caplets once daily up to 2 caplets qid. **May cause bloating, encourage patient to drink large glass of water with each dose. Avoid bulk-forming agents in bedbound patients.**

✦ Consider addition of or change from stool softener to a stimulant laxative or combination stool softener/stimulant (which increases intestinal motor activity) if stool softener alone not effective: Peri-Colace (docusate sodium 100 mg and casanthranol 30 mg) or Dialose Plus (docusate sodium 100 mg and phenolphthalein 65 mg) 1–2 tablets daily; Senekot (senna concentrate) 2 tablets daily: or Senekot-S (senna concentrate and docusate sodium 50 mg) 2 tablets daily; Dulcolax (bisacodyl) 2 tablets daily or suppository qod prn. **Avoid excessive and prolonged use of stimulant laxatives that contain phenolphthalein.**

✦ Consider prn use of an osmotic laxative, which stimulates colonic motility: Milk of Magnesia, lactulose, magnesium citrate. **Use magnesium-containing laxatives with caution in patients with renal insufficiency.**

✦ Avoid routine enema use in chronic constipation.

✦ For patients with history of laxative or enema abuse/chronic use, attempt to add nonpharmacological strategies to bowel routine and gradually decrease use of laxatives/enemas.

Acute Constipation/Impaction

✦ Consider the possibility of impaction in the patient at risk for constipation who has small amounts of liquid stool leakage.

✦ Perform a digital rectal examination.

✦ Assess and manage underlying cause.

✦ Initiate stool softener, stimulant laxative, or bulk-forming agent to prevent recurrence.

✦ Initiate an osmotic laxative, which stimulates colonic motility.

✦ Consider enemas for initial management:

✧ Fleet enema (available as saline enema, bisacodyl, or mineral oil preparations)—softens feces, stimulates evacuation, easily administered, may be repeated if no results.

✧ Mineral oil—lubricates and softens hard feces.

✧ Tap water enema—acts as a stimulant.

✧ **Enemas may result in electrolyte abnormalities, rectal bleeding. Administer with caution.**

✦ May require digital disimpaction, followed by enemas or laxatives as needed; consider use of lidocaine gel lubricant to reduce discomfort during procedure.

KEY ISSUES

Patient/Caregiver Education

Patient/caregiver should be able to:

✦ Identify important nonpharmacological strategies in maintaining normal bowel function.

✦ Explain proper use of medications.

✦ Demonstrate understanding of care of feeding tube if appropriate; **See Protocol on the Management of the Enterally Fed Patient.**

Economic Considerations

✦ Medications are often OTC and not covered by insurance plans.

Psychosocial Considerations

✦ Patient with altered bowel function may be at risk for social isolation.

✦ Patients with dementia or depression are at high risk for constipation.

✦ Management of constipation problems can add to caregiver stress especially if constipation is chronic and associated with bowel incontinence. May contribute to decision for nursing home placement.

Acute/Inpatient Setting

✦ Consider factors that increase the risk of constipation in the acute care setting: NPO or liquid diets, radiological procedures using barium with no follow-up bowel cleansing, decreased activity, irregular or altered schedule, narcotic analgesics, environmental barriers to toileting, and tethers (IV lines, restraints, Foley catheters, oxygen).

✦ Prevention and early intervention is vital. **15–25% of acutely ill and chronically hospitalized elderly patients become constipated.**

✦ Identify and address iatrogenic risk factors.

✦ Assess nutritional status; refer to a nutritionist.

✦ Assess functional status; consider OT and PT evaluations to increase activity and maintain function.

✦ Consider speech pathology assessment if evidence of dysphagia.

✦ Initiate a bowel regimen early in a hospital stay.

✦ Resume normal diet and activity as quickly as possible.

Extended Care Setting

✦ Identify and address iatrogenic risk factors.

✦ Initiate a bowel regimen/bowel training program when appropriate.

✦ Monitor bowel function closely.

✦ Be alert to atypical presentations of constipation in elderly, i.e., altered mental status, decreased appetite, decreased function, resistive/combative behaviors, or a change in baseline behavior in the presence of dementia and fever.

Home Setting

✦ Identify and address iatrogenic risk factors.

✦ Initiate educational and preventive strategies.

✦ Consider a bowel regimen for patients at high risk for chronic or acute constipation.

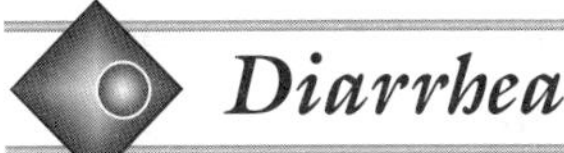

Diarrhea

HISTORY

✦ Onset and duration of diarrhea? Acute or chronic?

✦ Number of stools per day? **Diarrhea is defined as a change in normal pattern or > 3 stools/day.**

✦ Characteristics of stools? Watery, "small stool"?

✦ Associated symptoms: cramping, abdominal pain, nausea/vomiting, fever, chills, anorexia, malaise, myalgias, weight loss, rectal pain, tenesmus, fecal incontinence, mental status changes?

✦ Previous history of constipation or diarrhea?

✦ Medications: note recent antibiotics, change in medication regimen, laxative use?

✦ Others in the family or in same living environment sick?

✦ Recent travel outside the country?

✦ Usual diet, any changes? Tube feeding? **Up to 5 stools/day are considered acceptable for patients receiving tube feedings.**

✦ Any relationship of diarrhea to food intake?

✦ Allergies to medications or food?

✦ History of cholecystitis, gastritis, ulcerative colitis, PUD, malabsorption, past/recent GI surgery?

✦ EtOH intake? History of pancreatitis?

✦ History of diabetes mellitus, cardiac disease, CHF, diffuse vascular disease, connective tissue disease?

✦ Functional status? Risk for falls?

PHYSICAL EXAMINATION

✦ Vital signs, weight. Note orthostatic hypotension or tachycardia, which may indicate volume depletion.

✦ Assess for signs of dehydration: dry mucous membranes, poor skin turgor, coated tongue, altered mental status. Assess skin turgor over forehead or sternum.

✦ Abdominal examination: bowel sounds, tenderness to palpation. **Generalized tenderness is common in benign infectious diarrhea. Localized right lower quadrant tenderness is suspicious for acute appendicitis, Crohn's disease, diverticulitis or cecal carcinoma. Localized left lower**

quadrant tenderness suggests acute diverticulitis, fecal impaction, or colon cancer. See Protocol on Abdominal Pain.

✦ Rectal examination: assess sphincter tone, note presence of hemorrhoids, check for occult blood, fecal impaction. **Fecal impactions may present as watery stools around the impaction.**

✦ Focused examination as indicated by patient's overall condition and history.

DIAGNOSTIC TESTS

✦ Stool culture: indicated when bacterial cause suspected or in prolonged acute diarrhea (> 1 week).

✦ Three stool collections for ova and parasites: indicated for suspected acute dysentery or proctitis, in the case of foreign travel, or in prolonged acute diarrhea.

✦ Stool for *Clostridium difficile* toxin: indicated in hospitalized patient, patient with recent hospitalization, or patient with recent course of antibiotics.

✦ Consider lactose tolerance test.

✦ Consider upper GI series with small bowel follow-through and barium enema. Consult with physician.

✦ Consider CBC, BUN, electrolytes, thyroid function tests.

PREVENTION

✦ Maintain optimal nutrition and hydration.

✦ Encourage regular bowel routine; avoid chronic use of laxatives.

✦ Consider using yogurt or Lactinex to promote normal flora colonization during course of antibiotics.

✦ Protect skin from contact with fecal material; prevent skin breakdown. **See Chapter on Special Hygiene Needs.**

✦ **See Protocol on Prevention and Health Maintenance.**

MANAGEMENT

Acute Diarrhea

✦ Benign infectious diarrhea usually resolves spontaneously and requires only supportive, symptomatic treatment. **Usually due to food-borne tox-**

ins (occurs within hours of ingestion) or viral gastroenteritis (rotovirus).

✦ Maintain fluid intake; consider need for electrolyte replacement.

✦ Avoid lactose-containing foods; adjust diet as tolerated.

✦ Consider referral for hospitalization in acutely ill, debilitated, or severely dehydrated older patient. **Risk for dehydration may be greater in elderly and may increase morbidity and mortality. See Protocol on Fluid and Electrolyte Abnormalities.**

✦ Consider use of antidiarrheal medications:

✧ Adsorbents such as Kaopectate.

✧ Antisecretory drugs such as Pepto Bismol (bismuth sabsalicylate).

✧ Antimotility drugs such as Lomotil (diphenoxylate HCl-atropine sulfate) or Imodium (loperamide HCl).

Acute Dysentery

✦ Common bacterial infections causing acute dysentery include *Campylobacter,* toxogenic *Escherichia coli, Shigella,* and *Salmonella.*

✦ Pseudomembranous colitis due to *C. difficile* should be considered in the hospitalized patient or in the patient with recent course of antibiotics. May occur up to 2 weeks after the drug is discontinued.

✦ Antibiotic therapy should be deferred until stool culture results are available. Consult with physician on antibiotic choice. Cipro (ciprofloxacin HCl), Bactrim (trimethoprim-sulfamethoxazole), and E.E.S. 400 (erythromycin ethylsuccinate) are often used.

✦ For suspected positive *C. difficile,* oral Vancocin (vancomycin HCl) 250–500 mg qid or oral Flagyl (metronidazole) 250 mg tid for 7–10 days may be begun presumptively. Consult physician.

Chronic Diarrhea

✦ Assess for and manage chronic systemic illnesses that can cause chronic diarrhea: diabetes mellitus, liver disease, diffuse vascular disease/mesenteric ischemia, malabsorption, connective tissue disease, hyperthyroidism.

✦ Discontinue any potentially offending medications.

✦ If laxative use/abuse is a problem, eliminate offending laxatives. Work with patient toward an effective bowel regimen. **See Protocol on Constipation.**

✦ Have patient keep a food diary for review. Consider referral to nutritionist.

✦ Consider trial of lactose-free diet.

✦ Consider referral to gastroenterologist for further evaluation. Consult with physician.

✦ Consider empiric treatment for irritable bowel (after appropriate work-up for underlying pathology), especially if constipation and diarrhea are present intermittently: **Irritable bowel syndrome should never be a presumptive diagnosis in the elderly.** High-fiber diet, sufficient liquids, and hydrophilic colloid preparation (Metamucil) daily; brief trial of a lactose-free diet may also be helpful.

✦ Consider use of:

✧ Anticholinergics: Levsin (hyoscyamine sulfate) or Bentyl, Antispas (dicyclomine HCl). Use with caution in elderly patients. May cause confusion, urinary retention.

✧ Combination agents: Librax (clidinium-chlordiazepoxide), Donnatal (hyoscyamine, atropine, scopolamine, phenobarbital).

✧ Antidiarrheal: Lomotil (diphenoxylate HCl-atropine sulfate) or Imodium (loperamide HCl).

KEY ISSUES

Patient/Caregiver Education

Patient/caregiver should be able to:

✦ Verbalize understanding of role of diet, medication and/or infection in cause of diarrhea.

✦ Verbalize need to increase oral or enteral fluids during episodes of diarrhea.

✦ Recognize signs of dehydration.

✦ Demonstrate appropriate infection control measures.

✦ Demonstrate appropriate skin care measures.

Economic Considerations

✦ If diarrhea is associated with fecal incontinence, hygiene products may be costly and are generally not covered by insurance.

Psychosocial Considerations

✦ Chronic diarrhea or fecal incontinence may limit activities and result in social isolation.

✦ Chronic diarrhea or fecal incontinence may place increased stress on the caregiver in any setting.

Acute/Inpatient Setting

✦ Monitor for dehydration and electrolyte imbalance (potassium, bicarbonate) with acute diarrhea. **See Protocol on Fluid and Electrolyte Abnormalities.**

✦ Consider need for isolation and enteric precautions.

✦ Provide frequent toileting, bedside commode, close observation to meet increased toileting needs and prevent falls.

✦ Consider short-term use of a fecal incontinence bag if diarrhea is profuse and watery.

✦ Be aware that standard colon cleansing techniques for diagnostic studies may result in diarrhea of several days' duration.

Extended Care Setting

✦ Chronic diarrhea may contribute to malnutrition, dehydration, decline in functional status, and changes in mental status.

✦ Infectious diarrhea may affect other patients and staff; follow infection control policies.

✦ For tube-fed patients, consider nutrition consult to reassess nutritional and free water requirements during acute diarrhea.

✦ Increase fluids (oral, enteral, or intravenous) to prevent dehydration and avoid hospitalization.

✦ Initiate strategies to maintain skin integrity. **See Chapter on Special Hygiene Needs.**

✦ Be alert to increased risk for falls in elderly patient with diarrhea.

Home Setting

✦ Diarrhea greatly increases caregiver burden.

✦ Increase fluids (oral, enteral, or intravenous) to prevent dehydration and avoid hospitalization.

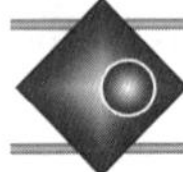

Peptic Ulcer Disease (PUD)

HISTORY

✦ Symptoms? Substernal pain, dysphagia, left upper or lower quadrant pain, vertigo, dizziness? **Elders present atypically, often with absence of classic burning epigastric pain that is relieved by eating. Maintain a high index of suspicion on vague, minor complaints such as lack of appetite, weight loss, and gas pains. Major gastrointestinal bleeding, perforation, CVA, transient ischemic attacks, anemia-induced angina, or myocardial infarction are frequently initial presentations of PUD in the elderly.**

✦ Gender? **There is increased incidence of PUD complications in elderly women, possibly related to increased NSAID use and lower body mass-to-dose ratio in females.**

✦ Associated risk factors: NSAID use, smoking, presence of *H. pylori* infection?

✦ Comorbidities? Cardiovascular, renal, hepatic, and pulmonary disease frequently seen in the elderly decrease compensatory capabilities when PUD complications occur.

✦ Medications? **NSAIDs (predispose to PUD and may mask symptoms, making serious complications the initial presentation)**, corticosteroids. Initiation of anticoagulants may precipitate bleeding from PUD.

✦ Mental status? **Confusion may be the only sign of PUD complication in the elderly.**

PHYSICAL EXAMINATION

✦ Vital signs. Assess for orthostasis. Initial presentation may be bleeding.

✦ Neuro: mental status examination.

✦ Cardiac: auscultate for tachycardia.

✦ Abdomen: assess for tenderness in epigastric area, although presentation is often painless.

✦ Rectal: stool for guaiac.

DIAGNOSTIC TESTS

✦ **Upper GI endoscopy is best diagnostic method if history of PUD, previous GI surgery, or tracheoesophageal fistula.** Antral biopsy for *H.*

pylori and pH measurement of gastric juice can be obtained during endoscopic procedure.

✦ **Double-contrast barium meal** can be used to identify PUD in patients with dysphagia, symptoms of early satiety, motility disorders, or impaired cardiorespiratory function (without aspiration).

✦ Further diagnostic studies that may be used if pharmacotherapy fails:

- ✧ Acid secretory studies.
- ✧ Measurement of serum gastrin level.
- ✧ Serum calcium.
- ✧ Serum salicylate level.

PREVENTION

✦ Recommend alternative therapies to avoid NSAID use. GI hemorrhage often occurs within first 4 weeks of NSAID therapy.

✦ Use acetaminophen (up to 1,000 mg q 6 hr) for pain relief.

✦ If NSAIDs are unavoidable, use the smallest dose possible of least-potent formulation (e.g., ibuprofen).

✦ Avoid combination of NSAIDs and steroids.

✦ Monitor all patients on NSAID therapy for anemia. **See Protocol on Anemia.**

✦ **See Protocol on Prevention and Health Maintenance.**

MANAGEMENT

✦ **PUD is primarily a disease of the elderly in developed countries. Peak incidence in the United States occurs in the sixth decade.**

✦ **Increased incidence of PUD in the elderly compared with younger generations may be due to high rates of childhood exposure to *H. pylori.***

✦ **Duodenal ulcers are the most frequent cause of upper GI bleeding in the elderly.**

✦ Gastric ulcers require biopsy to rule out carcinoma.

✦ Acute therapy includes H_2 blockers, proton pump inhibitor, misoprostol, sucralfate, or antacids.

✦ If *H. pylori* is detected (endoscopic sampling, breath test, or by serology), combination therapy is indicated for eradication. See Table 6-2.

✦ Suppressive therapy for PUD includes long-term use of acute therapy agents at 50% dose, with the exception that H_2 blockers are not effective in

TABLE 6-2. Treatment for *Helicobacter pylori* Infection

Medications	Dosage	Duration
Bismuth subsalicylate	2 chewable tabs before meals and at bedtime	14 days
Metronidazole	250 mg PO qid	14 days
Tetracycline or amoxicillin	500 mg PO qid	14 days
OR		
Clarithromycin	250 mg PO bid	14 days
Omeprazole	20 mg PO bid	14 days
Metronidazole	500 mg PO bid	14 days
OR		
Bismuth subsalicylate	2 chewable tabs before meals and at bedtime	7 days
Tetracycline	500 mg PO qid	7 days
Metronidazole	500 mg PO tid	7 days
Omeprazole	20 mg PO bid	7 days

preventing gastric ulcers. Proton pump inhibitors are especially helpful in GERD.

✦ Antacids are effective in healing PUD, but may pose problems for the elderly due to:

✧ sodium content (fluid retention)

✧ frequent dosing

✧ decreased bioavailability of concomitant medications used frequently in the elderly

✧ diarrhea with preparations containing magnesium

✧ constipation with preparations containing calcium.

✦ Single daily doses of H_2 blockers appear to be as effective for ulcer healing as divided doses:

✧ Tagamet (cimetidine HCl) 800 mg PO at bed time.

✧ Zantac (ranitidine HCl) 300 mg PO at bed time.

✧ Pepcid (famotidine) 40 mg PO at bed time.

✧ Axid (nizatidine) 300 mg PO at bed time.

✧ Reduction of H_2 blocker dose is recommended in patients with renal impairment, liver impairment, or altered mental status.

✧ Duration of therapy:

✧ Gastric ulcer: 12 weeks; healing should be assessed with repeat endoscopy.

✧ Duodenal ulcer: 8 weeks; repeat endoscopy not necessary after treatment.

✦ Monitor for drug interactions and altered mental status with use of H_2 blockers and for increased bioavailability of theophylline and warfarin with Tagamet therapy.

✦ Maintenance therapy with H_2 blockers is necessary for those with history of relapse or as prevention of the serious outcomes of PUD complications. Usual maintenance dose is equal to therapeutic dose.

✦ Carafate (sucralfate) requires more frequent dosing than H_2 blockers and must be taken 1 hr before meals. An advantage of its use in the elderly is that the drug is not absorbed systemically, but constipation is a frequent side effect.

✦ **High-risk patients** older than 65 years may receive maintenance therapy with a proton pump inhibitor: Prilosec (omeprazole) 10–20 mg PO qd or Prevacid (lanisopazole) 15 mg PO qd.

NSAID-Associated Ulcers

✦ **Consider discontinuing NSAIDs, initiating acetaminophen therapy.**

✦ **Factors associated with increased risk for ulcer complications during NSAID therapy:**

✧ High dosage of NSAID.

✧ Use of more than one NSAID.

✧ Combined NSAID and steroid therapy.

✧ Comorbidities.

✦ Both H_2 antagonists and high-dose antacids have been shown to heal 80% of existing gastric and duodenal ulcers during concomitant NSAID therapy.

✦ Consider Cytotec (misoprostol) as prophylaxis for elders with previous or active PUD while on NSAIDs, especially in the presence of NSAID-related risks for ulcer complications. Usual adult dose: 200 μg PO qid; reduce geriatric starting dose to 100 μg PO qid to avoid diarrhea.

✦ Consider Arthrotec (diclofenac sodium and misoprostol) in patients at high risk for developing NSAID-induced ulcers.

KEY ISSUES

Patient/Caregiver Education

Patient/caregiver should be able to:

✦ List medications, doses, timing, and potential side effects.

✦ **Verbalize the importance of complying with medication regimen to ensure healing of ulcers and/or eradication of *H. pylori.***

✦ State that many OTC pain relievers contain NSAIDs and verbalize the importance of avoiding their use.

✦ State recommended limitations on caffeine and EtOH and importance of smoking cessation.

Economic Considerations

✦ Misoprostol and proton pump inhibitor therapy are costly. Check managed care formularies for availability.

✦ Antibiotic therapy for *H. pylori* is costly. Documentation of *H. pylori* infection may be required prior to authorization of medications by managed care/insurance organizations.

Psychosocial Considerations

✦ Stress and depression may contribute to PUD.

✦ Provide reassurance to increase compliance with *H. pylori* eradication regimen.

Acute/Inpatient Setting

✦ Hospitalization and GI consultation are appropriate for acute GI bleeding and GI consultation.

✦ Routine prophylaxis with H_2 blockers for hospitalized patients or patients in ICU is not indicated.

Extended Care Setting

✦ PUD is a frequent occurrence in individuals taking aspirin, NSAIDs, steroids.

✦ H_2 blockers may cause CNS alteration.

✦ Staff education should emphasize reporting possible indicators of GI bleeding: subtle changes in baseline behavior, gait abnormality, and/or altered mental status (especially in the patient with dementia).

Home Setting

✦ Dietary modification is seldom required in patients with PUD.

✦ Avoidance of EtOH is important in healing PUD.

Chapter 7

Genitourinary System

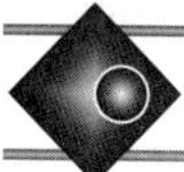

Urinary Tract Infection (UTI)

HISTORY

✦ Acute signs or symptoms: burning, dysuria, frequency, nocturia, urgency, strong odor, cloudy urine, hematuria, fever, chills, low back or abdominal pain? **In the elderly, classic signs and symptoms are often absent. Atypical presentations may occur: change in mental or functional status, new onset of urinary incontinence or increase in incontinent episodes, falls, or fatigue. Demented patients may exhibit unexplained increased agitation.**

✦ Onset and duration of symptoms?

✦ Vaginal or urethral discharge?

✦ Comorbid conditions: enlarged prostate, chronic prostatitis, renal stones, renal disease, diabetes mellitus, cerebrovascular accident (CVA), neurogenic bladder, or immobility?

✦ Previous urinary tract infections (UTIs)? Urinary retention?

✦ History of genitourinary surgery?

✦ Presence of acute or chronic constipation?

✦ Chronic indwelling catheter? Duration?

✦ Intermittent catheterization? By whom? Frequency? Clean or sterile? **Clean technique is generally taught for patients/caregivers who do intermittent catheterization.**

✦ Condom catheter in place or used intermittently?

✦ Age at menopause? Hormone replacement therapy?

✦ Resident of a long-term care facility? Recent hospitalization?

✦ Medications: prescription/OTC? **Anticholinergics, alpha-adrenergic agonists, calcium channel blockers, beta-adrenergic agonists, tricyclic antidepressants, and decongestants may produce urinary retention and contribute to risk of infection.**

✦ Medication allergies?

✦ Functional status? Immobility contributes to urinary retention.

PHYSICAL EXAMINATION

✦ Vital signs. **Hypothermia in the elderly may be a sign of sepsis.**

✦ General appearance, hygiene, skin turgor, mucous membranes, presence of pressure ulcers or macerated skin.

✦ Functional status; limitations to self-toileting.

✦ Abdominal examination: assess for suprapubic distention, tenderness or dullness to percussion.

✦ Assess for costovertebral angle tenderness.

✦ Assess external genitalia for irritation, discharge, tenderness, edema.

✦ Consider a pelvic examination in females: assess for cystocele or rectocele, atrophic vaginitis, urethral or vaginal discharge, erosion, vesicles.

✦ Rectal examination: assess for sphincter tone, fecal impaction, enlarged prostate.

DIAGNOSTIC TESTS

✦ Urine dipstick test for screening; first morning specimen is best. Positive leukocyte esterase test is an indirect test for pyuria/bacteriuria; positive nitrite test strongly suggests infection.

✦ Urinalysis with microscopic on a clean catch midstream or catheterized specimen: levels higher than 100,000 CFU/ml indicate significant bacteriuria.

✦ Urine culture and sensitivity. In community elders, urine culture is generally reserved for infection failing to respond to empiric therapy.

✦ Consider a post-void catheterization for residual if questionable urinary retention or patient with neurogenic bladder. More than 50–75 cc collected indicates urinary retention.

✦ Consider saline and KOH wet mount of any discharge.

✦ Consider abdominal flatplate x-ray.

✦ Consider CBC with differential, blood cultures if sepsis suspected.

✦ Consider electrolytes, blood urea nitrogen (BUN) if dehydration suspected; serum creatinine to assess renal function.

✦ Consider renal ultrasound, CT of abdomen for evaluation of upper tract sources of infection and hydronephrosis. Consult with physician.

PREVENTION

✦ Avoid chronic suppressive antibiotics—promotes resistant organisms.

✦ Avoid chronic indwelling catheter. **The risk of asymptomatic bacteriuria increases 3–10% with each day of catheterization; in nursing home residents, 50% of UTIs associated with bacteremia are in patients with chronic Foley catheter. Colonization occurs after 4 weeks.**

✦ Teach clean technique intermittent catheterization for patients with urinary retention.

✦ Avoid condom catheters; colonization occurs within 7 days.

✦ Promote regular bowel function.

✦ Teach incontinence prevention techniques. **See Protocol on Urinary Incontinence.**

✦ Encourage adequate fluid intake. Goal: six to eight 8-oz glasses of water per day unless otherwise restricted. Increase fluid intake while symptomatic.

✦ Teach perineal hygiene and toileting techniques; void after intercourse.

✦ Consider trial of an alpha-adrenergic antagonist such as Minipress (prazosin HCl) 1–2 mg PO bid–qid or Hytrin (terazosin HCl) 1–5 mg PO at bed time to reduce post-void residual and improve outlet resistance and urinary flow rate. **May lower blood pressure, be associated with syncope, orthostasis; use with caution in patients with history of falls and those receiving other antihypertensive agents.**

✦ In females, consider intravaginal estrogen cream or hormone replacement therapy (HRT). **See Chapter on Management of the Postmenopausal Woman.**

✦ Manage comorbid conditions that may predispose to UTI.

✦ **See Protocol on Prevention and Health Maintenance.**

MANAGEMENT

✦ Consider referral to urologist if outlet obstruction and urinary retention present or to further evaluate urinary incontinence.

✦ If patient with a chronic indwelling catheter becomes symptomatic, change the catheter before obtaining a specimen for culture to better differentiate between bacterial colonization and infection.

✦ Be alert to drug allergies to sulfa and penicillin, as these drugs are used commonly to treat UTIs.

✦ Antibiotic therapy should be specific to the identified organism. In elderly females, gram-negative *Escherichia coli* cause 50–60% of UTIs (compared with 80% in younger population). In men, the most common organism is Gram negative *Proteus.* Nosocomial UTIs are often due to Gram positive *Enterobacter,* and Gram negative *Klebsiella, Proteus,* and/or *Pseudomonas.* **Patients with chronic indwelling catheters have bacteriuria, often polymicrobial, and may be associated with a high incidence of antibiotic resistance especially if antibiotics are used frequently.**

✦ In ambulatory setting for elders with uncomplicated UTIs: initiate treatment with Bactrim (trimethoprim-sulfamethoxazole 160/800 mg) one double-strength tablet bid or suspension 40/200 mg per 5 ml. In frail or underweight patients or those with reduced renal function, reduce dosage of Bactrim to one double-strength tablet daily or one single-strength tablet (80/400 mg) bid or Augmentin (amoxicillin with clavulanic acid) 250–500 mg every 8 hr (also available in suspension 125–250 mg/5 ml).

✦ For patients with recurrent infections, chronic indwelling catheters, or recently hospitalized, initiate treatment with a fluoroquinolone antibiotic: Noroxin (norfloxacin) 400 mg daily/bid, Cipro (ciprofloxacin HCl) 250–500 mg bid; may be dose adjusted to every 18 hr or every 24 hr with renal impairment, or Floxin (ofloxacin) 200 mg bid.

✦ In most older patients, asymptomatic bacteriuria should **not** be treated with antibiotics. Patients with chronic indwelling catheters have persistent asymptomatic bacteriuria and should be treated only when symptoms develop or there is a decline in functional status unexplained by other factors. Treatment usually leads to the emergence of resistant organisms.

✦ Duration of treatment will vary. For community-dwelling, ambulatory elders with uncomplicated UTI, 3-day regimen is often effective with fewer side effects. If failure on 3-day regimen, culture and treat for 2 weeks.

✦ If suspected bacterial prostatitis, treat 4–6 weeks with a fluoroquinolone or sulfamethoxazole-trimethoprim. **See Protocol on Prostatism.**

✦ Consult with physician if suspected sepsis. Will likely require hospitalization.

KEY ISSUES

Patient/Caregiver Education

Patient/caregiver should be able to:

✦ Describe and implement preventive strategies.

✦ Demonstrate correct technique if intermittent catheterization necessary.

✦ Identify action/possible side effects of prescribed medications.

✦ Discuss correct administration and duration of therapy.

Economic Considerations

✦ Consider formulary restrictions and cost for antibiotic selection.

✦ Cost of caring for patients with incontinence is in the billions; most care products are not covered under insurance plans.

Psychosocial Considerations

✦ Management of incontinence and toileting issues adds to caregiver stress and contributes to the decision for nursing home placement.

✦ Urinary problems, including incontinence and infection, are embarrassing and can lead to social isolation or depression.

Acute/Inpatient Setting

✦ Avoid/minimize catheter use. Risk of nosocomial UTIs is increased with short-term catheter use in acute setting; **UTI is most common nosocomial infection.**

✦ Nosocomial UTIs may be caused by more resistant organisms.

✦ Frail elderly may require hospitalization for UTI with bacteremia. **Urine is most common source of infection in elderly and most common cause of sepsis.**

✦ For elderly patient admitted for UTI and possible bacteremia, obtain urine and blood cultures before initiating treatment. Begin empiric treatment with IV ampicillin and gentamicin unless contraindicated by penicillin allergy and/or impaired renal function. Adjust dose of gentamicin based on age, weight, and renal function. Follow peak and trough levels. Consider IV cephalosporin or fluoroquinolone as alternative therapy.

✦ Calculate creatinine clearance and adjust dosage of antibiotics appropriately. Consult pharmacist.

Extended Care Setting

✦ Be alert to atypical presentation of infection in frail elderly.

✦ Avoid catheter (condom, indwelling); limit use of incontinence undergarments.

✦ Implement incontinence program. **See Protocol on Urinary Incontinence.**

✦ Generally do not treat asymptomatic bacteriuria; consider treatment if patient has been hospitalized recently.

Home Setting

✦ Consider medication administration system to ensure compliance with prescribed antibiotics.

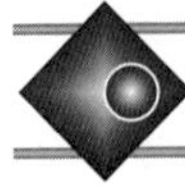

Urinary Incontinence (UI)

HISTORY

✦ **Perform routine screening in the elderly for UI. UI is not a normal consequence of aging. Consider asking, "Do you have trouble holding your water (urine)?" 80% of incontinent persons receive no treatment largely due to the patient's reluctance to discuss the problem.**

✦ Initial onset of incontinence? Number of incontinent episodes/24 hr?

✦ Ability to remain dry during the night?

✦ Exacerbating factors: sneezing, coughing, laughing, lifting, sudden urge to empty bladder?

✦ Volume of urine leakage: small, large, dribble?

✦ Characteristics of urine: odor, color?

✦ Associated symptoms/accompanying problems: nocturia, dysuria, hesitancy, frequency, urgency, hematuria, changes in urine stream, constipation, sexual dysfunction?

✦ Any previous treatment for incontinence? Expectations from treatment?

✦ Use of incontinence products (pads, adult incontinence briefs)?

✦ Gender? In elderly males, UI usually results from an enlarged prostate or as a result of prostatectomy. Stress incontinence is the most common type of UI seen in elderly females.

✦ Past medical history: hernia repair, surgery for ruptured disc? Females: childbirth history, onset of menopause, hysterectomy, Cesarean section, cystocele repair? Males: prostatic hypertrophy, prostatectomy?

✦ Comorbidities: multiple sclerosis, CVA, spinal cord injury, obesity, diabetes mellitus, dementia, renal calculi, dehydration? Are conditions present that contribute to functional UI (degenerative joint disease, Parkinson's disease, rheumatoid arthritis)?

✦ Allergies: **antihistamine use may contribute to UI by causing atonic bladder.**

✦ Medications: **diuretics, tranquilizers, narcotics, hypnotics?**

✦ Diet: daily fluid intake? **The age-associated decrease in thirst leads to diminished bladder capacity in the elderly.** Caffeine use?

✦ Functional status: Is UI interfering with ability to work or perform activities of daily living or instrumental activities of daily living (ADL/IADLs)? **Is there impaired ability to reach the toilet before urinating? Are sensory deficits present (decreased vision)? Is there impaired ability to communicate the need to urinate? Are physical or chemical restraints being used?**

✦ Is UI interfering with sleep?

✦ Living arrangements? If elder is not independent, who is the caregiver and how involved is the caregiver?

✦ Social situation: **Elderly with UI are at high risk for social isolation.**

PHYSICAL EXAMINATION

✦ Neurological: Note anxiety. Evaluate gait, manual dexterity, and reflexes. Assess cognitive status. Mental status examination if indicated. Screen for depression.

✦ Eyes: assess visual acuity, type of corrective lenses, depth perception, peripheral vision.

✦ Cardiovascular: assess for peripheral edema.

✦ Musculoskeletal: assess muscle strength and tone.

✦ Abdomen: Percuss for bladder distention. Palpate bladder for tenderness, distention, or masses.

✦ Genital: Females: Note atrophy, skin breakdown, or vaginal discharge. Bimanual examination: palpate for muscle tone and contraction, tenderness, masses, cystocele, urethral prolapse. Perform Bonney test—while bladder is full, support with examiner's finger on either side of the urethral opening. Ask patient to cough. If no urine leakage, test is positive, which indicates patient may be able to be continent if the urethra is supported (by surgical means). Males: Inspect and palpate foreskin, glans penis, and perineum.

✦ Rectal: Evaluate anal sphincter tone. (The urethral and anal sphincters are ennervated by the same nerves. Evaluation of the anal sphincter provides clue to competency of the urethral sphincter.) Assess for masses and fecal impaction. Palpate prostate in males for size, consistency, masses.

DIAGNOSTIC TESTS

✦ Urinalysis, culture and sensitivity to assess for UTI. **Asymptomatic bacteriuria is often seen in the elderly but no association between asymptomatic bacteriuria and incontinence has been found. See Protocol on Urinary Tract Infection.**

✦ Serum creatinine and BUN to evaluate renal function.

✦ Serum glucose to assess for hyperglycemia.

✦ Prostate-specific antigen (PSA) for males with obstructive symptoms.

✦ **Observation of normal voiding** to detect straining, hesitancy, dribbling, dexterity problems, or intermittent stream.

✦ **Post-void residual (PVR) urine volume** is determined by catheterization or pelvic ultrasound 5–10 min following voiding. If difficulty is experienced in passing catheter, suspect obstruction. PVR < 50 cc = adequate emptying; PVR 50–199 cc = clinical judgment necessary; PVR > 200 cc = inadequate emptying and obstruction or bladder contractility problem should be suspected (urge or overflow UI). More than 50–75 cc indicates abnormality.

✦ **Provocative stress testing** assesses for involuntary urine loss due to stress incontinence. Ask patient to assume standing or lithotomy position and cough vigorously while the bladder is full.

✦ A **voiding diary** kept by the patient (or caregiver for cognitively impaired) may provide clues for differentiation of the type of incontinence and should include:

✧ Time, frequency, and amount of voids.

✧ Record of incontinent episodes and what activity was taking place at the time of each episode.

✧ Record of type and amount of fluid and food intake.

PREVENTION

✦ Advise patients to maintain normal body weight because obesity contributes to UI.

✦ Consider changing times of diuretic dosages if necessary to avoid UI.

✦ Indwelling catheter use should be reserved for cases of intractable UI.

✦ **See Protocol on Prevention and Health Maintenance.**

MANAGEMENT

✦ Nonpharmacological (behavioral), pharmacological, and surgical treatments are available for management of UI. Options available to the individual elderly patient should be discussed, and the patient's decision regarding preferred treatment respected.

✦ The least invasive modality should be first choice. Behavioral interventions are often effective for most types of UI.

✦ Referral to a urologist is needed for patients refractory to nonpharmacological and pharmacological measures and for those with complicating comorbidity:

✧ Prostate abnormality.

✧ Severe pelvic prolapse.

✧ Recurrent urinary tract infections.

✧ Hematuria without urinary tract infection.

TABLE 7-1. Transient or Reversible Causes of Urinary Incontinence in the Elderly

Co-existing conditions	Pharmacological agents
Symptomatic urinary tract infection	Sympatholytics (prazosin, terazosin)
Diabetes mellitus	Diuretics
Congestive heart failure	Antihistamines
Hypercalcemia	Opiates
Excessive or inadequate fluid intake	Antidepressants
Limited mobility	Benzodiazepines
Fecal impaction	Antipsychotics
EtOH use	Decongestants
Caffeine intake	Calcium channel blockers

- ✧ Persistent symptoms of difficulty with emptying bladder.
- ✧ Abnormal PVR.
- ✧ Multiple sclerosis or spinal cord injury.

Transient or Reversible Incontinence

✦ **UI in the elderly often is related to reversible or transient causes.** See Table 7-1.

✦ Manage co-existing conditions and discontinue offending pharmaceutical agents, if possible, to correct UI. If UI continues, further evaluation for other type of UI is needed.

✦ Refer to nutritionist for education on appropriate food and fluid intake and dietary modification to avoid constipation.

Functional Incontinence

✦ Characterized by involuntary loss of urine resulting from impaired functional status, environmental barriers, or impaired cognitive or psychological status.

✦ Refer to physical therapist (PT) or occupational therapist (OT) for assessment of environmental barriers that can be corrected by the following measures:

- ✧ Relocation of toilet for easier access.
- ✧ Raised toilet seat.
- ✧ Toilet substitutes (urinals, bedpan) if indicated.
- ✧ Improved lighting.
- ✧ Installation of grab bars.

✧ Clearing obstacles from the pathway to the toilet.

✧ Providing privacy.

✧ Assistive ambulatory devices.

✧ Nonslip footwear.

✧ Clothing that facilitates toileting: Velcro fasteners, flap-open undergarments, elastic waistbands.

✦ Nonpharmacological interventions:

✧ Habit training—patient toilets on a schedule (determined by a voiding diary) that mirrors his or her individual pattern. Function is not improved but patient remains dry.

✧ Prompted voiding—patient is provided opportunity to toilet at regular intervals. Time between intervals is gradually extended so that urge is suppressed. Normal bladder function can be restored. Patient is given positive feedback each time he or she remains dry until the next scheduled voiding.

✧ Absorbent pads or briefs—use the smallest product possible to reduce costs and the risk of skin breakdown.

✧ External collection devices.

Stress Incontinence

✦ Characterized by urine leakage that occurs as a result of an increase in intra-abdominal pressure (coughing, lifting, laughing, sneezing, exercising) or atrophic vaginitis.

✦ Often occurs following abdominal or pelvic surgery.

✦ Nonpharmacological treatments:

✧ **Kegel exercises** to strengthen pelvic muscles.

✧ **Urethral devices** that are inserted or applied externally (i.e., Cunningham clamp) to occlude the urethral opening and are removed for voiding; may cause discomfort or UTI.

✧ **Electrical stimulation**—uses electrical impulses to artificially contract the pelvic floor muscles. Stimuli are delivered by probe, needle, or sensor and may be associated with pain or discomfort.

✧ **Vaginal weights** placed in the vagina to strengthen pelvic muscles.

✧ **Biofeedback** to increase perception and function of pelvic muscles.

✧ **Pessaries** support the bladder and urethra in case of pelvic prolapse.

✦ Pharmacological interventions:

✧ Premarin (conjugated estrogen) improves closure of the urethra. **See Chapter on Management of the Postmenopausal Woman.**

✧ Alpha-adrenergic agonists to increase bladder outlet resistance:

✧ Ornade (chlorpheniramine maleate 12 mg/phenylpropanolamine HCl 75 mg) 1 tablet PO bid.

        - Sudafed (pseudoephedrine HCl) 15–30 mg PO tid.
        - Tofranil (imipramine HCl) 25–50 mg PO bid or tid.
- Surgical treatments:
    - Sling to correct sphincter deficiency in females.
    - Artificial sphincter to correct sphincter deficiency in males.
    - Needle or retropubic suspension corrects urethral hypermobility.

Urge Incontinence

- Characterized by abrupt urine loss preceded by a strong feeling of urgency.
- Most commonly caused by involuntary detrusor muscle contraction.
- Associated with CVA, Parkinson's disease, dementia, or other disorders of the CNS.
- Nonpharmacological interventions:
    - Kegel exercises.
    - Bladder retraining—schedules voiding times with delays between episodes to suppress the urge to urinate. Individualized schedule is based on a voiding diary.
    - Electrical stimulation.
- Pharmacological interventions:
    - Anticholinergics/antispasmodics:
        - Ditropan (oxybutynin chloride) 2.5–5 mg PO bid or tid.
        - Urispas (flavoxate HCl) 100–200 mg PO bid or tid.
        - Tofranil (imipramine HCl) 25–50 mg PO bid or tid.
        - Detrol (tolterodine tartrate) 1–2 mg PO bid.
- Surgical treatment is rarely used for urge incontinence.

Overflow Incontinence

- Characterized by frequent leakage (dribbling) caused by obstruction of the bladder outlet (enlarged prostate, urethral stricture), atonic bladder, or chronically full bladder (diabetes mellitus, spinal cord injury).
- May also be caused by anticholinergic medications.
- Surgical treatment is indicated for relief of obstruction.
- Self intermittent catheterization (SIC) is indicated for patients who are not surgical candidates and for those with a chronically full bladder. Many elderly are eager to learn SIC rather than spend great lengths of time trying to empty their bladders. **See Patient/Caregiver Education.**

✦ Pharmacological intervention for patients **without** obstruction:

✦ Urecholine (bethanechol chloride) 10–30 mg PO bid or tid.

✦ Pharmacological intervention for patients **with** obstruction: **See Protocol on Prostatism.**

Mixed (Stress and Urge) Incontinence

✦ **Elderly women present frequently with a combination of symptoms of stress and urge incontinence.**

✦ Symptoms of one type of UI are usually more problematic for the patient than the other type.

✦ Begin with treatment of predominant symptom. **See Management.**

KEY ISSUES

Patient/Caregiver Education

Patient/caregiver should be able to:

✦ Discuss bladder function and UI without experiencing feelings of reluctance or shame.

✦ State the expected outcomes and risks of treatment options.

✦ State the importance of keeping complete records in voiding diary.

✦ Verbalize medication doses, timing, and potential side effects.

✦ Demonstrate proper use of urethral devices or external collection devices.

✦ Verbalize technique for performing Kegel exercises.

✦ If indicated, demonstrate technique for SIC and state recommended frequency. Verbalize understanding that clean technique is usually recommended except for immunocompromised patients.

Economic Considerations

✦ Incontinence products and pads are costly and often not covered under insurance.

✦ UI is a risk factor for skin breakdown and formation of pressure sores that require costly treatment. **See Chapter on Pressure Ulcers.**

✦ The annual cost of UI in the United States is more than $16 billion.

Psychosocial Considerations

✦ Social stigma associated with UI may lead to isolation from family, friends, and usual activities.

Acute/Inpatient Setting

✦ Environmental barriers posed by hospitalization (bed rails, restraints) may precipitate transient incontinence. Provide scheduled toileting.

✦ A small number of male patients suffering from UI after prostatectomy may receive artificial urinary sphincter implantation.

✦ Hospitalized elders may be labeled "incontinent" during acute illness; obtain information on baseline.

Extended Care Setting

✦ **UI is a major determinant of institutionalization in the elderly.**

✦ The U.S. Department of Health and Human Services has published a caregiver's guide entitled "Helping People with Incontinence" designed for training certified nursing assistants about UI. A companion "Alert" is also available for Directors of Nursing. Both may be ordered at no charge (up to 250 copies of each) by calling toll-free (800) 358-9295. The caregiver's guide is available in both English and Spanish.

Home Setting

✦ Refer to PT/OT for evaluation of home toileting environment.

✦ Maintain voiding diary.

✦ Provide information on adaptive equipment to promote self-toileting.

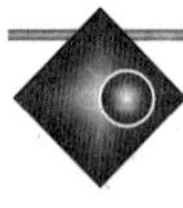

Prostatism: Benign Prostatic Hyperplasia (BPH)/Prostatitis

HISTORY

- ✦ Decrease in the force or caliber of urinary stream?
- ✦ Hesitancy or straining to initiate urinary stream?
- ✦ Interruption of urinary stream or dribbling after urination?
- ✦ Painful urination?
- ✦ Frequency of urination?
- ✦ Nocturia? How many times? Is this an increase or decrease?
- ✦ Urgency? Incontinence? Sensation of incompletely emptied bladder?
- ✦ Symptoms can be categorized as shown below:

Obstructive symptoms	Irritative symptoms
Hesitancy	Urgency
Straining	Frequency
Interrupted stream	Pain/burning
Dribbling	Nocturia
Retention	Incontinence

More than half of men over the age of 60 have significant prostatic enlargement. This hyperplasia is not necessarily progressive. Not all have obstructive symptoms.

- ✦ Change in characteristics of urine? Cloudy? Hematuria?
- ✦ Onset/duration of symptoms? Alleviating/aggravating factors?
- ✦ Low back, testicular, perineal, low abdominal, or rectal pain? Onset? Painful defecation or ejaculatory pain? **More common in chronic prostatitis than BPH. Symptoms may be subtle or absent in older men.**
- ✦ Malaise, myalgia, anorexia, nausea, chills, fever? Onset? **Suggestive of UTI and/or prostatitis.**
- ✦ Urinary tract infections, onset/recurrence? Stones? Strictures?
- ✦ Previous urinary tract surgeries?
- ✦ Diabetes mellitus, CVA, cardiovascular disease, Parkinson's disease or other neurological disorders?
- ✦ Medications, prescription/OTC?

PHYSICAL EXAMINATION

- ✦ Height, weight, vital signs. Assess for orthostasis.

✦ Inspect abdomen for distention. Percuss for bladder distention (dull, drum-like sound). Palpate for suprapubic fullness and tenderness as well as abdominal masses and organomegaly.

✦ Percuss costovertebral angle for tenderness (may indicate hydronephrosis or pyelonephritis).

✦ Inspect external genitalia for erythema, rash or lesions, swelling, drainage, and phimosis.

✦ Palpate inguinal areas for enlarged lymph nodes.

✦ Inspect for facial and dependent edema.

✦ Focal neurological examination as appropriate to rule out neurological disease.

✦ Digital rectal examination of prostate: normally consistency is soft or rubbery-firm but smooth and irregular; a hard prostate is suggestive of malignancy, not BPH. In prostatitis, gland is usually softer/boggy and may be tender to palpation. **Prostate size assessed by digital examination does not correlate with severity of symptoms, degree of obstruction, or treatment outcomes.** Rule out perirectal abscess.

DIAGNOSTIC TESTS

✦ Urinalysis, culture and sensitivity to rule out UTI secondary to BPH; recurrent UTIs of the same organism are characteristic of chronic bacterial prostatitis, culture will be negative in nonbacterial prostatitis. Hematuria requires further work-up to rule out malignancy.

✦ PVR (normal is < 50–75 cc).

✦ BUN (hydration variable), creatinine (to determine renal insufficiency due to obstruction), glucose, electrolytes, hemoglobin, and hematocrit.

✦ Ultrasound of kidneys to rule out hydronephrosis (in presence of elevated BUN and creatinine, history of urinary tract stones, hematuria, and recurrent UTIs). Transrectal ultrasound (measures bladder volume, prostate size and consistency, as well as residual urine and presence of prostatic stones). May require physician consult.

✦ PSA is controversial in men over the age of 50 years, because the serine protease is produced by both benign and malignant prostatic epithelium. If tested, obtain prior to digital rectal examination or instrumentaion such as catheterization. Levels > 10 ng/ml are suggestive of malignancy.

✦ Evaluation of prostatic secretions produced by prostatic massage. >10 WBCs per high powered field is characteristic of prostatitis. Do not obtain if acute prostatitis is suspected; massage can induce bacteremia. Chronic bacterial prostatitis is most common in older men and is usually caused by gram-negative organisms. In nonbacterial prostatitis, WBCs are elevated as above, and urine culture is negative.

PREVENTION

✦ **See Protocol on Prevention and Health Maintenance.**

MANAGEMENT

Benign Prostatic Hyperplasia

✦ Symptoms often get better over time with or without intervention. Exceptions: severe obstructive symptoms, chronic urinary retention, and/or renal insufficiency. Consider quantitative symptom assessment using scales such as the American Urological Association Symptom Score Index or the International Prostate Symptom Score initially and over time. The symptom scores are not diagnostic for BPH but can assist in evaluating interventions and management.

✦ Pharmacological management:

✧ **Alpha-adrenergic blockers** decrease tone of smooth muscle, decreasing symptoms of urethral obstruction. **Decrease PVR by 50%. Examples:** Minipress (prazosin HCl) range 1–5 mg twice daily. Give test dose of 1 mg at bed time (can cause orthostasis/syncope). Cardura (doxazosin mesylate) range 1–4 mg daily. Hytrin (terazosin HCl) usual range is 1–5 mg daily but may require 10 mg daily. May lower cholesterol and triglycerides. All can cause weakness, dizziness, orthostasis, hypotension, tachycardia, headache, and nasal congestion. Flomax (tamsulosin) 0.4 mg daily. Flomax is not indicated for hypertension; can be used with antihypertensive agents without potential adjustments required with other alpha blockers. Alpha-adrenergic blockers may be more effective than antiandrogens for obstructive symptoms.

✧ **Antiandrogens** decrease prostatic size, thereby decreasing obstructive symptoms. Proscar (finasteride) 5 mg daily may take 6 months to reach peak effect. May decrease serum PSA. Can use alpha-blocker and hormonal therapy together.

✦ **Avoid decongestants (sympathomimetics)**, which lead to obstructive symptoms. Increase urinary retention by increasing contractile tone in the bladder neck and prostate, increasing pressure on the urethra.

✦ **Avoid anticholinergic agents:** antipsychotic agents, tricyclic antidepressants, and antihistamines lead to obstructive symptoms. Increase urinary retention by decreasing bladder contraction.

✦ **Avoid bladder irritants:** caffeine, alcohol (EtOH), spicy foods can lead to irritative symptoms and cause bladder spasms.

✦ Limit fluid intake after last evening meal of the day but maintain at least 1½–2-liter intake throughout the day, unless otherwise contraindicated.

✦ Avoid delay of urge to urinate.

✦ Avoid prolonged exposure to cold environmental temperatures; can cause urinary retention.

✦ **Surgical management** is considered if patient has refractory urinary retention, has failed at least one voiding trial after catheter removal, has recurrent UTIs, has gross hematuria, bladder stones, or renal insufficiency. Refer to urologist. May include urethral stenting, transurethral resection or incision, laser resection, open prostatectomy, or microwave therapy. (Reduces PVR by 60–80%.)

Acute Bacterial Prostatitis

✦ **Seen less frequently in older males.**

✦ Empiric antibiotic therapy for gram-negative organisms should be initiated, awaiting results of culture and sensitivity. Bactrim or Septra (trimethoprim-sulfamethoxazole) 160/800 mg 1 double-strength tablet daily to bid for 30 days. Use renal dosing in presence of elevated BUN and creatinine; closely follow BUN and creatinine to ensure renal function is not deteriorating.

✦ Alternative antibiotics include Noroxin (norfloxacin) 400 mg PO bid for 4 to 6 weeks or Cipro (ciprofloxacin HCl) 250–500 mg PO every 12 hr for 4–6 weeks. Use renal dosing in the presence of renal insufficiency. If patient appears seriously ill, refer for hospitalization and broad-spectrum IV antibiotics.

✦ NSAIDs and analgesics for comfort. Follow BUN and creatinine levels closely due to possibility of renal toxicity.

✦ Colace (docusate sodium) or Peri-Colace (docusate sodium-casanthranol) to alleviate painful defecation. Follow management of BPH in controlling obstructive and irritative symptoms.

✦ Encourage 1½–2 liters PO fluid daily; sitz baths several times a day.

Chronic Bacterial Prostatitis

✦ **Seen most frequently in older males.**

✦ Bactrim or Septra (trimethoprim-sulfamethoxazole) 1 double-strength tablet daily to bid for 12–16 weeks (prostatic stones may be source of gram-negative organisms that are difficult to eradicate). Alternatives include Cipro (ciprofloxacin HCl) 250–500 mg twice daily, Geopen (carbenicillin) 382–764 mg qid or Minocin (minocycline HCl) 100 mg bid. All require renal dosing.

✦ **Surgical management** for removal of prostatic calculi in resistant conditions.

Nonbacterial Prostatitis

Not common in older male. When present, often due to chlamydia.

✦ Minocin (minocycline HCl) 100 mg bid, Vibramycin (doxycycline hyclate) 100 mg daily for 2–4 weeks. **Refer to obstructive and irritative symptom relief listed in Management of Benign Prostatic Hyperplasia.**

✦ Control bladder spasticity to prevent urine reflux into the prostatic ducts and increasing symptoms of nonbacterial prostatitis.

✦ Consider Hytrin (terazosin HCl) or Cardura (doxazocin mesylate), if bladder outlet obstruction is suspected.

✦ NSAIDs, sitz baths, and avoidance of irritants to bladder.

KEY ISSUES

Patient/Caregiver Education

Patient/caregiver should be able to:

✦ Identify medications causing bladder retention.

✦ Identify irritants causing bladder spasms.

✦ Enter data in a voiding diary.

✦ Verbalize techniques to promote urination.

✦ Verbalize benefits of double voiding technique, and steps involved in double voiding technique.

✦ Describe potential side effects from alpha-adrenergic blockers.

✦ Verbalize need to take prostate reducing drugs a life-time.

✦ Demonstrate proper technique of SIC.

✦ Verbalize symptoms prompting emergency care (anuria with distention and bladder fullness) when unable to perform SIC.

✦ Verbalize symptoms of UTI.

Economic Considerations

✦ Consider whether patient can afford medications prescribed. Take into consideration multiple tablets per day and compliance issues. Newer antibiotics tend to be more expensive. Prostate-reducing medications are expensive and are used indefinitely.

✦ PSA is a screening test not covered by Medicare, although it is covered by some supplemental policies. Patient must be informed that he will be financially responsible for the test if not covered by insurance.

Psychosocial Considerations

✦ Evaluate for depression, social withdrawal/isolation secondary to:

 ✧ urgency, frequency, incontinence

 ✧ exacerbations despite compliance.

✦ Assess for fears of prostate cancer and impotency secondary to prostatism.

Acute/Inpatient Setting

✦ Acute obstructive symptoms may develop after Foley catheterization and may signify infection or underlying BPH.

✦ Relief of acute obstruction may produce hypotension, excessive diuresis.

Extended Care Setting

✦ Institute 3-day voiding diary to develop prompted or scheduled voiding program.

✦ Be alert to changes in behavior and mental status in the cognitively impaired patient. **This may be the only sign of UTI.**

✦ Avoid chronic indwelling Foley catheter to decrease risk of antibiotic resistant bacteria and sepsis.

✦ Assess environment for accessible toileting, which could prevent functional incontinence.

✦ Limit fluid intake during the evening hours. Encourage 1½–2 liters of PO fluid per day if not otherwise contraindicated (sense of thirst is decreased in the older adult).

Home Setting

✦ Avoid chronic catheterization.

✦ Educate patient/caregiver concerning anticholinergic effects of OTC drugs (cold/sinus preparations, sleeping medications).

Renal Disease

HISTORY

✦ Symptoms: hematuria, dysuria, oliguria (<30 cc/hr), proteinuria, nocturia, frequency, hesitancy, dribbling, incontinence, cloudy urine, dark urine?

✦ Associated symptoms: flank pain, abdominal pain, suprapubic pain, pruritis, dry skin, nausea, vomiting, confusion, lethargy, intractable hiccups, peripheral edema, orthopnea, paroxymal noctural dyspnea (PND)?

✦ Onset, duration, course of symptoms?

✦ Comorbid conditions: known renal or hepatic dysfunction, hypertension, diabetes mellitus, congenital kidney problems, renal calculi, hyperlipidemia, anemia, heart disease, congestive heart failure (CHF), aneurysm, CVA, peripheral vascular disease?

✦ Previous renal evaluation?

✦ Family history of renal problems, hypertension, diabetes mellitus, CVA, or hyperlipidemia?

✦ EtOH or tobacco use?

✦ Medications? Note any recent nephrotoxic medications, i.e., NSAIDs, angiotensin-converting enzyme (ACE) inhibitors, penicillin antibiotics, aminoglycosides, IV contrast dye.

✦ Cognitive status?

✦ Functional status?

✦ Social situation? Supports?

PHYSICAL EXAMINATION

✦ Vital signs. Assess for orthostasis.

✦ Weight on each visit.

✦ Note general appearance; assess for asterixis.

✦ Assess skin for color, turgor, excoriations related to pruritis and scratching.

✦ Assess cognitive and functional status throughout the examination. Use standardized tools to establish baseline if impairment present.

✦ Cardiovascular: auscultate for bruits in carotids, over renal and femoral arteries; auscultate heart sounds, assess for murmurs; palpate peripheral pulses; palpate for abdominal aneurysm.

✦ Respiratory: assess respiratory function and note signs of pulmonary edema.

✦ Abdomen: note presence of ascites or organomegaly.

✦ Assess for peripheral edema.

✦ Rectal: assess for prostatic hypertrophy in males.

DIAGNOSTIC TESTS

✦ Urinalysis with microscopic, culture and sensitivity if suspected UTI. **Pyuria and hematuria are common in UTI.**

✦ If protein noted on dipstick, obtain a spot urine protein-creatinine ratio. **Higher than 3 mg/dL is consistent with nephrotic range proteinuria. A 24-hr collection of urine for protein is an alternative method of measuring proteinuria. Normal level is < 150 mg/24 hr; nephrotic range is > 3 g/24 hr. An abnormal amount of protein in the urine is frequently the first sign of significant renal or systemic disease.**

✦ First morning urine specimen for cytology, if painless microscopic hematuria.

✦ In and out catheterization to assess PVR. **>50–75 cc is considered abnormal.**

✦ CBC with differential, serum electrolytes, BUN, creatinine, albumin, prothrombin time, partial thromboplastin time, and international normalized ratio (INR) to assess for anemia, fluid/electrolyte disturbances, renal failure, hypoalbuminemia, or an associated coagulopathy. **Calculate creatinine clearance for an estimate of renal function corrected for age and muscle mass. There is a linear decline in creatinine clearance with age. See Chapter on Medication Issues** for formula.

✦ Consider checking phosphorus, calcium, magnesium, uric acid, creatine phosphokinase, erythrocyte sedimentation rate, PSA.

✦ Consider chest x-ray to assess for presence of granulomatous disease.

✦ Consider 12-lead electrocardiogram (ECG) to assess for associated cardiovascular abnormalities.

✦ Consider echocardiogram if evidence of heart failure.

✦ Consider ultrasound of kidneys and ureters to assess size, presence of renal parenchymal lesions, nephrolithiasis, or hydronephrosis secondary to obstruction.

✦ Consider CT of kidneys if any abnormality is found on ultrasound to assess internal structure of masses.

PREVENTION

✦ Optimal management of hypertension and diabetes mellitus. **Hypertension and diabetes mellitus are the two most common systemic diseases**

in the U.S. that lead to renal dysfunction. See Protocols on Hypertension and Diabetes Mellitus.

✦ Follow renal function of patients with use of potentially nephrotoxic agents, i.e., NSAIDs, ACE inhibitors, penicillin antibiotics, aminoglycosides, IV contrast dye. Adjust dosages of medications based on calculated creatinine clearance.

✦ **See Protocol on Prevention and Health Maintenance.**

MANAGEMENT

Microscopic or Gross Hematuria

✦ Assess for and treat underlying infectious process if present. May be associated with painful hematuria. **See Protocol on Urinary Tract Infection.**

✦ Assess for renal calculi with renal ultrasound; advise patient to strain all urine; manage pain/nausea acutely; monitor fluid intake and output; refer to nephrologist for acute management and for further evaluation of type of calculi with recommendations for chronic management. Consult with physician.

✦ If history of trauma, refer immediately to emergency department or to a nephrologist. Consult with physician.

✦ If suspected coagulopathy, refer to hematologist. Consult with physician.

✦ **Painless microscopic hematuria may be a sign of early transitional cell carcinoma of the bladder, prostate cancer, or adenocarcinoma of the kidney.** Get first morning urine specimen for cytology. Perform rectal examination and obtain PSA. **See Protocol on Prostatism.** Refer to urologist or nephrologist as appropriate. Consult with physician.

✦ Refer any patient with unexplained hematuria.

✦ Massive hematuria, evidence of pyelonephritis, concurrent renal failure, or evidence of obstruction is indication for hospitalization.

Proteinuria

✦ Non-nephrotic range proteinuria ($<$ 3 g of protein lost in 24 hr or $<$ 3 mg/dL spot urine protein-to-creatinine ratio) is usually asymptomatic unless associated with a UTI. Most common causes are hypertension and diabetes mellitus. Treat underlying cause. **See Protocols on Hypertension, Diabetes Mellitus, and Urinary Tract Infection.**

✦ Nephrotic range proteinuria ($>$ 3 g protein lost in 24 hr or $>$ 3 mg/dL spot urine protein-to-creatinine ratio). Most common causes are hypertension and diabetes mellitus. Other possible causes include membranous glomerulonephritis (GNP), systemic lupus erythematosus (SLE), amyloidosis, exposure to heavy metals, and monoclonal gammopathies such as multiple myeloma. Refer if suspected vasculitis or glomerulonephritis. **See Protocols on Hypertension and Diabetes Mellitus** for management recommendations.

Pre-Renal Azotemia

✦ Symptoms include: orthostasis, volume changes, oliguria, increased concentration of urine, decreased weight, dry mucous membranes, dry skin.

✦ Modestly elevated creatinine is seen, although increase in BUN is proportionately greater.

✦ Caused by decreased fluid in the intravascular system and decreased blood flow to the kidneys. The most common cause is volume depletion (dehydration) secondary to deficient fluid intake; fluid losses from diarrhea, nasogastric suction, vomiting, hemorrhage, or burns; or third-spacing of fluids due to sepsis, pancreatitis, or ascites.

✦ Management includes: fluid replacement; withholding of diuretics; monitoring of weight, creatinine, BUN, electrolytes, and urine output. Evaluate for source of bleeding if suspected. Evaluate for concurrent acute or chronic process in the elderly. Dehydration associated with a co-existing process increases risk of mortality. Observe for signs of volume overload or CHF with fluid replacement. **See Protocol on Fluid and Electrolyte Abnormalities.**

Acute Renal Failure

✦ Symptoms may include: edema, oliguria, encephalopathy, and hypertension. Other symptoms of underlying disease may be present, i.e., hypotension, sepsis, or CHF.

✦ Proportional increases in BUN and creatinine are seen; urine sodium < 1 mEq/L.

✦ Patient is clinically euvolemic and may have evidence of metabolic acidosis and hyperkalemia.

✦ Caused by direct damage to the kidneys. See Display 7-1.

✦ Treatment includes: management of underlying disease process; discontinuation of potentially offending agents; relief of obstruction if present; supportive fluid management; and correction of electrolyte abnormalities.

✦ Indications for emergency dialysis include: volume overload that is resistant to aggressive diuretic therapy; severe hyperkalemia that is resistant to treatment; severe, refractory acidosis; uremic encephalopathy; uremia-induced pericardial friction rub; bleeding due to uremic platelet dysfunction; severe rhabdomyloysis; or dialyzable toxins, i.e., theophylline, ethylene glycol, aspirin.

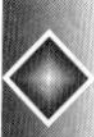

DISPLAY 7-1. *Common Causes of Acute Renal Failure (ARF)*

Ischemic disorders

Sepsis	Transfusion reactions	Burns
Hemorrhage	Trauma	Pancreatitis

Nephrotoxins

Heavy metals	Ethylene glycol
IV contrast dye	Chemotherapeutic agents
Antibiotics	NSAIDs

Diseases of glomeruli and small blood vessels

Acute poststreptococcal glomerulonephritis
Systemic lupus erythematosus (SLE)
Polyarteritis nodosa
Wegener's granulomatosis
Drug-related vasculitis

Major blood vessel disease

Dissecting aortic aneurysm
Renal artery thrombosis, embolism, or stenosis
Bilateral renal vein thrombosis

Interstitial nephritis associated with infection, granulomas, crystals

Tuberculosis	Hyperuricemia	Hypercalcemia

Insterstitial nephritis associated with drugs

Penicillins	Allopurinol	Warfarin
Tetracyclines	Cimetidine	Thiazides
Rifampin	Sulfonamides	Phenytoin
Furosemide	Cephalosporins	

✦ Kayexalate sodium (polystyrene sulfonate) 15 g PO/PR to acutely lower dangerously elevated potassium level. Repeat as indicated.

✦ Follow weight, urine output, serum creatinine, potassium, phosphorus, magnesium, and BUN frequently.

✦ Consult with physician. Consider referral to nephrologist.

✦ Consult with nutritionist for recommendations for dietary modifications, i.e., potassium, protein, sodium, and fluid restrictions.

Post-Renal Azotemia

✦ Symptoms may include: edema, oliguria, encephalopathy, and hypertension. History may be significant for recent UTI and symptoms of urinary obstruction.

✦ Patient is usually euvolemic, but may be hypervolemic.

✦ Caused by obstruction to the flow of urine between the kidneys and the external environment. Common etiologies include: renal calculi; bladder obstruction with urinary retention related to prostatic hyperplasia or use of anticholinergic agents; retroperitoneal lesions such as lymphoproliferative disorders, fibrosis, or sarcomas; or an obstructed Foley catheter.

✦ Assess presence of hydronephrosis with renal ultrasound.

✦ Place (or replace) Foley catheter; refer to a urologist for further evaluation. Consider referral to nephrologist. Consult with physician.

Chronic Renal Failure

✦ Most common causes include: hypertension, diabetes mellitus, chronic glomerulonephritis, and polycystic kidney disease. Acute worsening of chronic renal insufficiency can occur in the setting of acute renal insult. **See Acute Renal Failure.**

✦ Reduced creatinine clearance, elevated serum creatinine and BUN, anemia, hyperphosphatemia, osteoporosis, and platelet dysfunction often coexist. Symptoms of uremia progress slowly to end-stage renal disease (ESRD).

✦ Identify potentially reversible factors, initiate measures to slow progression, monitor renal function (creatinine and BUN), and treat metabolic consequences.

✦ Management may include erythropoietin, phosphate binder, calcium with vitamin D, and bicarbonate buffers. Routine medications may require dose adjustment.

✦ **See Protocols on Hypertension and Diabetes Mellitus** for management recommendations.

✦ Discuss treatment options with patient and family.

✦ Consult with physician or refer to nephrologist if dialysis or transplantation is being considered.

✦ Consult with nutritionist for dietary modifications.

KEY ISSUES

Patient/Caregiver Education

Patient/caregiver should be able to:

✦ Verbalize understanding of disease processes affecting kidney function and identify signs of progression.

✦ List medications, dosages, effect, and potential side effects.

✦ Demonstrate compliance with prescribed diet.

✦ Verbalize role and mechanism of dialysis in treatment of renal failure.

Economic Considerations

✦ Dialysis costs approximately $40,000 annually per patient; majority of cost is covered by Medicare.

✦ Transplantation is often less successful in the elderly.

Psychosocial Considerations

✦ As many as 25% of chronic dialysis patients choose to discontinue treatment; mortality for dialysis patients is approximately 25% annually. Provide support to the patient adjusting to a chronic disease or with end-of-life issues.

✦ Hemodialysis is required three times a week for 2–3 hr each session, and is often difficult physically and psychologically for patients and families.

✦ Consult social worker to assess social situation and supports, counsel patient/family regarding chronic disease issues, assist with arrangement for dialysis when appropriate.

Acute/Inpatient Setting

✦ Drug-induced acute renal failure is common in hospitalized elderly patients, especially in those with diabetes and underlying renal insufficiency. Monitor renal function closely. Adjust medication dosages based on calculated creatinine clearance.

Extended Care Setting

✦ Not all long-term care facilities can accommodate patients who require peritoneal or hemodialysis.

✦ Transportation must be arranged for patients who are receiving hemodialysis.

Home Setting

✦ Peritoneal dialysis can be performed at home if a caregiver is available. Must be performed daily, often overnight.

Chapter 8

Musculoskeletal System

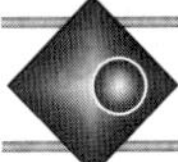

Musculoskeletal Pain

HISTORY

✦ Location of pain? Does it radiate?

✦ Does the pain involve a joint? If so how many?

✦ Description of pain?

✦ Onset, duration of pain?

✦ What were you doing when it started?

✦ Aggravating/alleviating factors?

✦ Is the pain acute or chronic (6 weeks or longer)? Is it intermittent or constant?

✦ Associated symptoms: swelling, limited motion, or increased heat in the area? Numbness or tingling in hands/feet? Fever? Malaise? Fatigue? Weakness, generalized or localized? Change in bowel or bladder function?

✦ Recent fall? Trauma?

✦ Weight gain or loss?

✦ Medications: prescription/OTC? Note especially anticoagulants, corticosteroids, analgesics, muscle relaxants, NSAIDs.

✦ History of cancer, diabetes mellitus, peripheral vascular disease, hypertension, rheumatoid arthritis, osteoarthritis, systemic lupus erythematosus, gout, fracture, polymyalgia rheumatica, thyroid disease, chronic obstructive pulmonary disease (COPD), renal disease, neurologic disorder, or B12 deficiency?

✦ Occupation? Recreational activities?

✦ Exercise program? Form of exercise?

✦ Functional status? How has the pain affected functional status? How has the pain affected quality of life? **Musculoskeletal conditions are the leading cause of functional decline.**

✦ Social situation? Social support?

PHYSICAL EXAMINATION

✦ Vital signs, weight.

✦ Observe general appearance. Observe ability to sit down, get up from a chair, maintain balance, ambulate using assistive aide if indicated, turn around and sit down.

✦ Assess ability to doff and don clothing.

✦ Assess ability to raise arms above head. Assess ability to hold eating utensils, toothbrush, and pen.

✦ Inspect and palpate tissue overlying muscles and joints for tenderness, erythema, swelling, crepitations, and increased warmth. Note limitations in active and passive range of motion of major joints and related muscle groups. Note movement or positioning reproducing symptoms and number of joints involved. **Periarticular pain in the absence of joint inflammation is suggestive of bursitis, tendinitis, tenosynovitis, and myositis. Articular pain and swelling is suggestive of gout, pseudogout, infection, and inflammatory arthritis.**

✦ Palpate the entire spinal process. Percuss for tenderness.

✦ Assess for muscle atrophy. Assess for decreased muscle tone and strength.

✦ Neurological examination to access for focal deficits. Assess for absent or decreased deep tendon reflexes. Assess perception of pain, temperature, position, vibration, and light touch.

✦ Assess for tophi.

DIAGNOSTIC TESTS

✦ CBC and differential.

✦ Uric acid, glucose (HgbA1c in diabetic), electrolytes, magnesium, phosphorus, and albumin.

✦ Consider thyroid function tests.

✦ Consider B12 and folate.

✦ Consider erythrocyte sedimentation rate (ESR), although results are nonspecific. Consider serum rheumatoid factor (RF).

✦ Consider aspiration of synovial fluid for cell count, differential, culture and sensitivity including fungus and acid-fast organisms, and presence of crystals. **Most useful diagnostic test especially in new symptom onset. Inflammatory conditions of gout, pseudogout, infection, and rheumatoid arthritis: white count and differential markedly elevated (50,000–200,000 cells/cm^3 with neutrophils $>$ 80%). See Protocol on Rheumatoid Arthritis. Tubercular arthritis: white count $<$ 25,000 cells/cm^3, differential variable.**

✦ Consider x-ray/bone scan.

✦ Consider CT scan to further define etiology of back pain. Consult physician.

PREVENTION

✦ Implement interventions to prevent falls/trauma and eliminate condition-specific causative factors. **See Protocol on Falls.**

✦ Encourage treatment compliance to prevent recurrent conditions.

✦ **See Protocol on Prevention and Health Maintenance.**

MANAGEMENT

Bursitis

✦ Can be caused by acute or chronic strain; injury; infection; or crystal deposits. May be associated with rheumatoid arthritis.

✦ Common sites include: trochanteric bursitis (hip); prepatellar bursitis (knee); anserine bursitis (below the medial aspect of the knee); subdeltoid or subacromial bursitis (shoulder); olecranon bursitis (elbow); medial first metatarsophalangeal (bunion); and Achilles or calcaneal bursitis (heel).

✦ Bursitis at site of trauma accompanied by fever, tenderness, and cellulitis requires aspiration, gram stain, culture and sensitivity to rule out infectious process. Follow with appropriate antibiotic therapy. **Gram-positive organisms are most commonly seen in infected bursae (Staphylococcus aureus and streptococci; pseudomonas and less frequently, pneumococci). Non-infected bursa fluid contains < 1,000 WBC/L.**

✦ Superficial bursitis, often seen in the heel and elbow, may be swollen without pain.

✦ In noninfected bursitis, treatment consists of elimination of etiology; joint rest; cold compresses initially, then heat, chronically; compression dressing to provide comfort where feasible, and a 14-day course of an NSAID. Consider injection of bursa with a corticosteroid (such as methylprednisolone acetate 10–40 mg or triamcinolone diacetate 10–40 mg) and a local anesthetic such as lidocaine 1–2%, 1–2 cc. See Tables 8-1 and 8-2.

✦ Instruct patient to avoid overuse of joint following injection.

✦ Emphasize movement with shoulder bursitis to prevent frozen shoulder.

✦ Suspect rotator cuff tear if there is muscular weakness and associated muscular wasting.

✦ Optimize functional status, refer to physical therapy (PT) or occupational therapy (OT) for progressive range of motion.

Tendinitis

✦ Often difficult to distinguish from bursitis.

✦ Same etiologies exist for bursitis and tendinitis.

TABLE 8-1. Intra-Articular Corticosteroid Injections

Indications	Contraindications
Gout	Systemic or joint sepsis
Pseudogout	Fracture
Osteoarthritis	Prior failure to injection
Psoriatic arthritis	Anticoagulation or clotting disorders
Rheumatoid arthritis	

✦ Usually there is a specific area of exquisite tenderness (trigger point). This is the site of tendon insertion. Common sites include: supraspinatus tendinitis (shoulder); bicipital tendinitis (upper medial humerus); and lateral epicondyle tendinitis (wrist). See Table 8-3.

✦ Follow treatment guidelines for bursitis. Inject trigger point with corticosteroid/anesthetic agent.

Gout

✦ Incidence increases with age. Occurs more frequently in men than women.

✦ Sodium urate crystals are found in the synovial fluid and deposit on the cartilage, causing acutely painful joint.

✦ Usually presents as acute, distal, monarticular arthritis of first metatarsophalangeal joint; can present in any joint, with multiple joint involvement. Trauma, surgery, or illness can trigger a gouty attack.

✦ Thiazide diuretics tend to increase urate levels by inhibiting uric acid excretion. Other agents known to increase urate levels include salicylates and uricosuric agents such as allopurinol and alcohol (EtOH).

TABLE 8-2. Quantities for Intra-Articular Injection (Corticosteroid/Lidocaine)

Joint	Quantity
Interphalangeal joint Metacarpophalangeal	0.1–0.5 cc
Elbow Wrist	0.5–1.0 cc
Shoulder Hip Knee Ankle	1.0–2.0 cc

TABLE 8-3. Nonarticular Corticosteroid Injections

Location	Indications	Signs/symptoms
Shoulder	Rotator cuff tendinitis (subacromial bursitis)	Pain in subdeltoid area Pain increases with arm abduction
	Bicipital tendinitis	Pain in anterior shoulder Pain increases with elbow supination or flexion against resistance Onset with overuse
	Capsulitis or frozen shoulder	Pain within shoulder, especially nocturnally Limited motion
Elbow	Tennis elbow (lateral epicondylitis)	Pain over humerus lateral epicondyle Pain increased with dorsiflexion of wrist against resistance Decreased grip strength Onset with overuse
	Golfers elbow (medial epicondylitis)	Pain over humerus medial epicondyle Pain increased with flexion of wrist against resistance Onset with overuse
	Olecranon bursitis	Pain and swelling over olecranon Pain unchanged with movement May be infected
Hand	Locking trigger fingers	Pain over finger flexor tendons Intermittent flexion locking Onset with repetitive gripping
	Dupuytren's contracture	Nodularity within palmar fascia Finger flexion of MCP joints Usually not painful
Hip	Trochanteric bursitis	Pain of lateral hip/thigh Pain is deep/aching Pain increases with activity Pain is position related No limitation of movement
Knee	Prepatellar bursitis	Well-delineated pain/swelling anterior to patella Related to trauma May be infected
	Anserine bursitis	Pain over medial aspect of upper tibia
Foot	Achilles tendinitis/ bursitis	Pain/swelling at Achilles insertion Pain increases with dorsiflexion of ankle
	Plantar fasciitis	Pain over plantar surface of heel when weight bearing Pain increases with dorsiflexion of toes

✦ Tophi are the consequence of slower build up of sodium urate. Tophi are usually not painful. They are typically found on the ear lobe, great toe, olecranon bursa, ankles, heels, wrists, and hands.

✦ Acute gouty attack may mimic rheumatoid arthritis. **See Protocol on Rheumatoid Arthritis.**

✦ Serum uric acid levels support the diagnosis but may be nonspecific or normal during acute event.

✦ Untreated gout usually resolves spontaneously over days to weeks.

✦ Treatment during the acute phase includes rest of the joint(s), and cold compresses. Options in pharmacological management:

✧ NSAIDs: indomethacin 25–50 mg tid–qid with food for 1–3 days, followed by 7–10-day dose reduction. OR

✧ Oral steroids: short course of prednisone 20–40 mg daily, followed by gradual taper over 4–8 days.

✧ Colchicine: (effective in pain control) 0.6 mg every 1–2 hr until acute joint pain is alleviated, GI symptoms develop, or a maximum of 4–6 mg/day has been reached). Must be renal dosed; use with caution in hepatic disease.

✧ Corticosteroid intra-articular injection is often required in monarticular involvement: Methylprednisolone acetate 5–40 mg. Not advisable in anticoagulated patient; avoid if infection is suspected.

✧ Intramuscular corticosteroids: Triamcinolone acetonide 60 mg or methylprednisolone acetate 40 mg IM. Useful if more than one joint is involved.

✦ Allopurinol is used to prevent recurrent attacks and prevent tophi formation. Allopurinol is indicated in hyperuricemia secondary to lymphoma, leukemia, and myeloproliferative conditions being treated with chemo- and radiation therapy. Initial dosing 50–300 mg/day as single dose, usually < 600 mg/day. Must be renal dosed. Can induce acute gouty attack, then add colchicine. Colchicine can be dosed chronically at 0.5 mg daily or bid. Goal: maintain serum uric acid levels at 4–6 mg/dl. Can expect serum uric acid levels to return to normal within 1–2 weeks after initiation of allopurinol.

✦ Refer to nutritionist for low purine diet.

✦ Advise weight reduction program if indicated.

Pseudogout

✦ Incidence increases with age. Occurs more frequently in females than males.

✦ Presentation is similar to gouty event, but usually affects the knee instead of the great toe. Pseudogout typically involves the large joints such as the wrist, ankles, shoulder, hip, or elbow and may affect more than one joint simultaneously.

✦ The joint is usually enlarged with crepitus and discomfort.

✦ Aspirate crystals are calcium pyrophosphate dihydrate and are positively birefringent. The crystals are located in the synovial fluid or seen as chondrocalcinosis on x-ray.

✦ The onset can accompany a metabolic stress such as surgery, gout, hypomagnesemia, hyperparathyroidism, and possibly hypothyroidism. Fever and leukocytosis is common.

✦ A chronic polyarthritis can develop that resembles rheumatoid arthritis.

✦ Treatment includes joint rest, NSAIDs (especially indomethacin) and/or local corticosteroid injection or colchicine.

✦ Joint replacement surgery is successful in advanced disease.

Chronic Lower Back Pain

✦ Establish any change in characteristics of presenting back pain. **Potential for cancer, infection, fracture, and cauda equina syndrome must be ruled out.**

✦ The incidence of compression fracture (especially those requiring chronic steroids) and tumor is higher in the elderly.

✦ Be alert for weight loss, fever, chills, and/or sweats associated with a change in chronic back pain.

✦ Chronic back pain is mechanical (pain related to activity/position and usually alleviated with rest). **Be alert for nonmechanical pain (constantly present, often worse when recumbent).**

✦ PT/OT referral for techniques to decrease pain; increase mobility, flexibility, and strength; and maximize function.

✦ NSAIDs, non-narcotic analgesic agents. Consider muscle relaxant in presence of spasms. Consider trial of antidepressant. **See Chapter on Pain Management.**

✦ Trial of dry heat application (use lowest setting, automatic turn-off heating pad) or use of moist heat (pad or bath tub/shower if feasible).

✦ Encourage maximal functional status. Avoid immobilization.

✦ Consider referral of those resistant to intervention to pain management center. Consult physician.

Spinal Stenosis

✦ Onset usually seen in the elderly 70+.

✦ Lumbar stenosis is most common, although stenosis can occur at other levels. Symptoms correspond to level of stenosis and are the consequence of bone hypertrophy narrowing the spinal canal and neural foramina, causing arterial insufficiency.

- May present as aching or cramping low back pain with/without radiation into buttocks, vague leg pains, and paresthesia. Onset of symptoms occurs with walking or prolonged standing, relieved by rest or by bending forward. Over time, some patients may ambulate, bending forward at the waist.
- Symptoms often mimic claudication of vascular insufficiency.
- Physical examination may be normal early in the disease process except during period immediately following exercise. Abnormal deep tendon reflexes, muscular weakness, and sensory deficits will be present. In chronic disease process, abnormalities may be present without exercise process.
- CT scan or MRI provides definitive diagnosis. Consult physician.
- Consider electromyography (EMG) with sensory-evoked potentials (SEPs) to further define nerve root dysfunction. Consult physician.
- PT/OT referrals to provide instruction on proper back and abdominal strengthening exercises and other indicated interventions to optimize function or prevent functional decline.
- May respond to NSAIDs and rest.
- Bladder and bowel management may be required.
- Surgical intervention (laminectomy or decompression of neural foramina) may be indicated and have fairly high success rate in the elderly. Neurosurgery referral.

KEY ISSUES

Patient/Caregiver Education

Patient and caregiver should be able to:

- Demonstrate an understanding of the underlying condition.
- Identify prescribed medications and verbalize an understanding of their use, possible side effects, and symptoms requiring medical provider contact.
- Demonstrate proper use of assistive devices and associated safety techniques.
- Identify and avoid disease-specific triggers.
- Demonstrate proper application of devices used for "joint rest" and techniques to decrease joint stress.
- Recognize need for life-style modification.
- Verbalize/demonstrate stress reduction techniques where indicated.

Economic Considerations

- **Pharmacological management is costly and not covered by Medicare.**

✦ Insurance coverage for outpatient therapies may be limited. Transportation may be costly.

✦ Home health PT/OT may be limited.

✦ Cost of in-home assistance.

Psychosocial Considerations

✦ Be alert for sign/symptoms of depression. **See Protocol on Depression.**

✦ Social isolation may occur secondary to pain, disfigurement secondary to tophi, and functional decline.

Acute/Inpatient Setting

✦ Timely PT/OT referrals.

✦ Prevent immobilization.

✦ Initiate falls prevention program/strategies.

✦ Initiate bowel and bladder regimen.

Extended Care Setting

✦ Educate staff in nonverbal pain indicators in patients with dementia.

✦ Implement appropriate pain management.

✦ Resources are often limited, patient may require transportation to outpatient setting or require hospitalization for diagnostic evaluation.

✦ Initiate falls prevention program/strategies.

✦ Initiate bowel and bladder program.

Home Setting

✦ Consider home health PT/OT to evaluate environment and make suggestions on interventions to reduce joint stress and improve pain control.

✦ Consider home-delivered meals.

✦ Consider adult day health program/senior center for socialization, exercise/fitness programs.

✦ Suggest other living arrangement as appropriate to functional status.

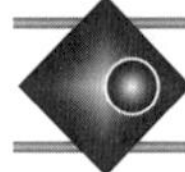

Degenerative Joint Disease (DJD)

HISTORY

✦ Characteristics of pain: dull, sharp, aching, constant, intermittent? Symmetrical or asymmetrical?

✦ Presence of pain that is worse with weight bearing or activity, relieved by rest?

✦ Location of pain? **Pain usually affects knees, hips, cervical and lumbar spine, distal interphalangeal joints, and first carpometacarpal joints.**

✦ Onset and duration of pain? Aggravating and alleviating factors? What remedies have been tried? With what results?

✦ Associated symptoms: joint swelling, deformity, decreased range of motion, redness, morning stiffness, numbness/tingling, leg pains especially at night?

✦ Systemic symptoms: fever, weight loss, prolonged stiffness, muscle pain, skin rash, conjunctivitis, change in vision, headache (temporal), dysuria, bowel or bladder dysfunction? **Systemic symptoms are usually absent in DJD but suggest other rheumatic diseases.**

✦ History of musculoskeletal problems/surgeries: gout, septic arthritis, periarticular syndrome, injury or trauma, rheumatoid arthritis, fractures, osteoporosis, back pain, falls?

✦ History of GI symptoms: gastritis, dyspepsia, history of peptic ulcer disease, GI bleed? **Important in designing an appropriate medication program.**

✦ Family history of DJD?

✦ Current medications? Use of NSAIDs? OTC medications? Topical preparations? Effectiveness?

✦ Medication allergies? History of side effects from NSAIDs?

✦ Use of assistive devices? Home adaptations?

✦ Current functional status? Change in functional status in last 6 months? Impact of symptoms on ability to perform activities of daily living (ADLs)?

✦ Social situation? Residence? Supports/caregiver?

PHYSICAL EXAMINATION

✦ Vital signs, height, weight.

✦ Assess gait and posture; assess spine for kyphosis, lordosis, scoliosis, or restricted movements.

✦ Note any asymmetry of shoulder height.

✦ Inspect and palpate joints comparing right to left sides for signs of crepitus, decreased range of motion, deformities, edema, joint effusion, tenderness.

✦ Assess muscle strength.

✦ Assess deep tendon reflexes.

✦ Consider further neurological examination for decreased sensation, nerve root pain.

✦ Assess functional status and mobility.

DIAGNOSTIC TESTS

✦ Consider x-rays of affected joint(s) to assess severity of disease, rule out fractures, other diseases.

✦ Laboratory blood values are usually normal in DJD. Consider: CBC with differential (if suspected systemic illness or infection); ESR (if suspected polymyalgia rheumatica or temporal arteritis); serum rheumatoid factor (RF) (if suspected rheumatoid arthritis); antinuclear antibody (ANA) (if suspected systemic lupus erythematosus); creatine phosphokinase (CPK) (if suspected polymyositis).

✦ Consider synovial fluid analysis with possible septic or inflammatory arthritis. Consult physician.

PREVENTION

✦ Recommend judicious use of exercise and rest.

✦ Recommend weight bearing exercise as tolerated, e.g., supervised walking program.

✦ Maintain appropriate weight.

✦ Implement fall assessment and prevention program. **See Protocol on Falls.**

✦ Maintain assistive devices in good repair.

✦ Maintain proper positioning to prevent contractures in patients with decreased mobility.

✦ **See Protocol on Prevention and Health Maintenance.**

MANAGEMENT

✦ Apply moist heat to affected joint three to four times daily. ***A*void heating pads, especially with frail elderly who may have decreased sensation and be at risk for burns.**

✦ Exercise to tolerance; encourage weight-bearing exercises; water exercise/swimming may be better tolerated.

✦ Encourage weight reduction and refer to nutritionist if indicated.

✦ Consider PT referral if function, gait, or safety is affected; for adaptation recommendations; or to augment pain management.

✦ Consult with physician for intractable pain; consider referral to rheumatologist, orthopedist, or pain management center.

✦ Consider evaluation by orthopedic surgeon for possible joint replacement.

✦ Scheduled Tylenol (acetaminophen) 650 mg PO qid; may also use prn to supplement NSAIDs. **Do not exceed 4 g daily.**

✦ Aspirin 1.2–2.4 g daily in divided doses; consider enteric-coated pills. **Caution about possible GI side effects; avoid if patient on warfarin or has a diagnosis of congestive heart failure (CHF).**

✦ NSAIDs. Examples include the following:

✧ Motrin (ibuprofen) 400, 600, or 800 mg tablets tid or qid; do not exceed 3,200 mg total daily dose; available in suspension.

✧ Naprosyn (naproxen) 250, 375, or 500 mg tablets in bid dosing; available in suspension.

✧ Relafen (nabumetone) 500 or 750 mg tablets with recommended starting dose 1,000 mg daily in single dose. Maximum dose is 2,000 mg daily in single or divided dose.

✧ Voltaren (diclofenac sodium) 50 mg tablet bid or Voltaren XR 100 mg daily.

✧ Arthrotec (diclofenac sodium 50–75 mg and misoprostol 200 mcg), a combination of an NSAID and a gastrointestinal mucosal protective prostaglandin E1 analog. Dose: 50 mg bid/tid or 75 mg bid.

✧ Celebrex (celecoxib), 100 mg/200 mg tablets, an NSAID which has cyclooxygenase-2 (COX-2) inhibitory properties. Dose: 200 mg daily in single or divided dose.

✧ Arthrotec and Celebrex are useful in patients at high risk for developing NSAID-induced gastric and duodenal ulcers.

Select NSAIDs with shorter half-life and use smaller doses in elderly. See Chapter on Medication Issues.

✦ Consider change to alternate NSAID if no improvement after 2–3 weeks of therapy.

✦ Monitor for potential side effects with NSAIDs: GI upset, GI bleeding, renal failure, hepatic toxicity, sodium retention, peripheral edema, elevated BP, exacerbation of CHF, mental status change. **Side effects are usually reversible when NSAIDs are stopped.**

✦ Topical analgesics: trial of Aspercreme (salicylate cream 15%) or Zostrix cream (capsaicin) applied to affected joint(s) three to four times daily.

Patient may experience burning sensation with capsaicin immediately after application.

✦ Intra-articular injections of corticosteroids and local anesthetic may offer temporary relief. Example: Depo-Medrol (methylprednisolone acetate) 10–40 mg/lidocaine 1–2% 1–2 ml. **Do not repeat more than four times a year; may be useful when only one to two joints are affected. Caution patient not to overdo activity when pain is temporarily improved after injection.**

✦ Follow-up: monitor at least every 3–6 months. Consider follow-up CBC, electrolytes, liver function tests, blood urea nitrogen (BUN), creatinine, stool guaiac at periodic intervals when patient taking aspirin or NSAIDs.

KEY ISSUES

Patient/Caregiver Education

Patient/caregiver should be able to:

✦ Verbalize treatment plan prescribed for DJD.

✦ Demonstrate correct and safe use of assistive devices.

✦ Identify common side effects of prescribed medications.

✦ Identify changes that warrant immediate attention, i.e., change in mental or functional status, dark stools, increased joint pain, swelling or redness, persistent abdominal or epigastric pain, weight gain, or fluid retention.

Economic Considerations

✦ Assistive devices/adaptive equipment may require authorization or may not be covered under the patient's insurance plan.

✦ Cost of medications may be significant.

✦ Change from independent living to assisted living may be necessary with severe functional impairment.

✦ OT and PT assessments in the home may require authorization under the patient's insurance plan.

✦ Severe DJD may affect ability to remain employed/active.

Psychosocial Considerations

✦ Impact of disability may result in social isolation, inactivity, and depression.

✦ Fear of falling may cause the patient to limit mobility resulting in further decline in function.

Acute/Inpatient Setting

✦ Avoid prolonged bedrest/immobility. **Functional decline in the elderly begins within 24–48 hr of hospitalization.**

✦ During hospitalization, consider OT and PT referrals to maximize function, prevent functional decline, assess mobility/safety.

✦ Assess level of pain; provide alternative medications for pain if patient is NPO, i.e., Tylenol suppository, topical treatments, transdermal analgesics: Duragesic (fentanyl) patch every 3 days. Begin at low dose (25 μg) and titrate as needed. Be alert to possible mental status changes.

✦ Individual may benefit from a short stay in a skilled nursing facility (SNF), subacute unit, or inpatient rehabilitation unit to regain mobility and function after an acute hospitalization; refer to social work as needed.

Extended Care Setting

✦ Maintain mobility: have patient out of bed for all meals, encourage participation in ADLs and recreational activities such as chair exercise.

✦ Maintain correct positioning for bed-to-chair patients to prevent contractures.

✦ Consider splinting if indicated to prevent contractures.

✦ Consult OT and PT as needed for recommendations for positioning, splinting, mobility, and function.

✦ Reassess need for assistive devices periodically.

✦ Implement fall assessment and prevention program.

Home Setting

✦ Consider home OT and/or PT for assessment of home environment and recommendations for adaptations to maintain function and promote safety.

✦ Maintain assistive devices in good repair; replace rubber tips on walkers/canes when worn.

✦ A variety of adaptive equipment is available and should be customized to the needs of the patient:

✧ Feeding aids: built-up handles for utensils, special plates.

✧ Dressing aids: button/zipper helpers, sock/stocking aids, reachers.

✧ Bathroom aids: long-handled sponges, tub grab bars, portable hand shower, bath benches, raised toilet seats, bedside commode.

✦ A variety of walking and transfer aids are available and should be fitted to the individual patient: regular cane, quad cane, walker (with or without wheels), wheelchairs.

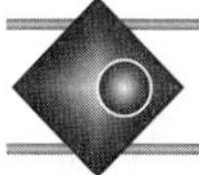

Rheumatoid Arthritis (RA)

HISTORY

✦ Gender? **During the childbearing years, more females are affected than males, but in the elderly there is more equal involvement of males and females.**

✦ Onset and duration of symptoms? **Elders may present with long-standing RA or with initial symptoms. Elderly-onset of RA is usually less severe. Course may be sporadic or insidious.**

✦ Pain and stiffness of joints? Joint involvement is symmetric. Joint inflammation in RA may involve the hands, elbows, shoulders, hips, knees, cervical spine, ankles, metatarsal phalangeal joints of the feet and wrists, and metacarpal phalangeal and proximal interphalangeal joints of the hands. **The distal interphalangeal joints are typically spared. Most commonly affected are the small joints of the hands and feet.**

✦ Swelling, tenderness, or warmth of joints?

✦ Muscle wasting?

✦ Exacerbating/alleviating factors? Stiffness usually is worst on awakening and improves with activity.

✦ Changes in skin? Presence of nodules?

✦ Associated symptoms: fatigue, malaise?

✦ Comorbidities? **Systemic involvement in RA can affect the cardiac, nervous, renal, integumentary, pulmonary, and rediculoendothelial systems.**

✦ Baseline functional status? Decline in functional status?

✦ Does pain disturb sleep?

PHYSICAL EXAMINATION

✦ Skin: Inspect for vasculitic lesions.

✦ Neurological: Inspect for wrist or foot drop indicating vasculitic involvement of peripheral nerves.

✦ Respiratory: Auscultate breath sounds for indication of pulmonary involvement (pneumonitis, interstitial fibrosis). **Pulmonary disease in RA is often asymptomatic.**

✦ Musculoskeletal: Inspect for foot deformities (hammer toe, hallux rigidus, fixation of joints, fibular deviation of toes) and hand deformities (ulnar deviation of the fingers, swan-neck deformity, boutonniere deformity).

DIAGNOSTIC TESTS

✦ CBC with differential may reveal anemia of chronic disease. **See Protocol on Anemia.** WBC count is usually normal except during acute episodes of RA or multiple joint involvement, when platelets may also be elevated.

✦ Urinalysis is useful for monitoring for pharmacological toxicity resulting from treatment for RA. Proteinuria is an early sign in patients taking long-acting agents.

✦ ESR may be elevated.

✦ Rheumatoid factor (RF) is found in 75% of patients with RA.

✦ Aspiration of synovial fluid of affected joints may reveal WBCs 50,000–200,000 cells/cm^3 with neutrophils > 80%. Consult physician.

✦ X-ray of affected joints may show bone erosions, periarticular osteopenia, and joint space narrowing. An early finding is erosion of the lateral aspect of the fifth metatarsal head.

PREVENTION

✦ Advise patients to maintain normal body weight, because obesity places additional stress on joints.

✦ Refer for annual eye exam.

✦ **See Protocol on Prevention and Health Maintenance.**

MANAGEMENT

✦ **RA is a chronic inflammatory disease that affects primarily the synovial-lined joints, but can affect various organ systems.**

✦ Joint deformities are often symmetric, tender, and proximal.

✦ Consider referral to a rheumatologist for patients with potential or existing disability.

✦ **Goals of treatment are:**

- ✧ **Pain relief.**
- ✧ **Reduction of inflammation.**
- ✧ **Early identification of side effects of treatment.**
- ✧ **Preservation/restoration of functional ability.**
- ✧ **Maintenance of quality of life.**

✦ Evaluate the impact of RA on the patient's functional status.

✦ Refer patients to PT for:

✧ A treatment plan that balances exercise (isometric is exercise of choice) and rest.

✧ Assistive ambulatory devices (e.g., canes, crutches, walkers) if indicated.

✧ Splints and braces for local joint rest and support.

✦ Refer patients to OT for:

✧ Evaluation/improvement of ability to perform ADLs.

✧ Task modification to reduce joint stress.

✧ Evaluation/modification of work or home site.

✧ Assistive devices.

✧ Energy-conserving techniques.

✦ Pharmacological therapy (best managed by a rheumatologist) includes:

✧ NSAIDs, which may have no significant effect on underlying disease process.

✧ Disease-modifying antirheumatic drugs (methotrexate, antimalarials, sulfasalazine, minocycline, gold compounds, cyclosporine, azathioprine, and penicillamine), which slow the rate of joint erosion/destruction.

✧ Corticosteroids, which reduce inflammation and symptoms. Potential for adverse side effects, including osteoporosis superimposed on RA, restricts use of corticosteroids to short-term intervention while attaining therapeutic levels of other agents.

✧ Investigational drugs aimed at altering the immunological abnormalities in RA—available to some patients through research trials.

✦ Monitor elderly patients for potential side effects of pharmacological treatment (rash, anemia, GI symptoms, liver disease, renal failure, retinal changes, and osteoporosis).

✦ Consider calcium/hormonal agents for prevention/treatment of osteoporosis. **See Protocol on Osteoporosis.**

KEY ISSUES

Patient/Caregiver Education

Patient/caregiver should be able to:

✦ State the importance of periods of rest therapy in management of RA.

✦ State the importance of continuing daily exercise during periods of remission.

✦ Verbalize the importance of wearing splints and braces as recommended.

✦ Verbalize understanding that braces and splints should not be worn if it causes pain or emotional upset or if it impairs function.

✦ List medications, doses, timing, and potential side effects.

Economic Considerations

✦ Within 10 years of onset of RA, approximately 50% of patients can no longer function in their employment.

✦ Adaptive aids and assistive devices may be ordered from self-help product catalogs.

Psychosocial Considerations

✦ Refer to local support groups and the National Arthritis Foundation for education about disease process and self-care. This knowledge will reduce the patient's sense of helplessness.

✦ Fear of discrimination in the workplace and concerns about body image may prevent patients from wearing braces/splints. Allow patients to verbalize concerns and provide emotional support.

✦ Depression may result from chronic pain, inability to work, loss of independence, life-style changes, and physical losses.

Acute/Inpatient Setting

✦ Chronic steroid use may impair resistance to infection and elevate glucose and white blood cell count values.

✦ Stress doses of steroids may be required for acute illness.

Extended Care Setting

✦ Chronic steroid use may predispose to skin breakdown.

✦ Be alert to chronic pain management issues. **See Chapter on Pain Management.**

Home Setting

✦ Assistance from family members or home health may be required.

✦ RA is a progressive disease with potential to seriously impair functional abilities.

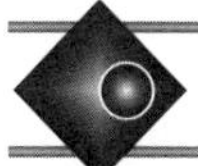

Polymyalgia Rheumatica (PMR)

HISTORY

✦ Age? **PMR almost always occurs in persons > 50.**

✦ Gender? PMR affects females twice as often as males.

✦ Ethnicity? Whites are more frequently affected than African Americans.

✦ Onset and duration of symptoms: aching, myalgia (note affected parts), stiffness (before or after rest)? Sudden or prolonged onset?

✦ Associated symptoms: malaise, fever, night sweats, weight loss, anorexia, fatigue, depression?

✦ Comorbidities: PMR is associated with temporal arteritis in approximately 15% of patients.

✦ Functional status: Is there decreased functional ability related to limited joint mobility, muscle soreness, or stiffness?

PHYSICAL EXAMINATION

✦ Vital signs. Low-grade fever may be present in PMR.

✦ Musculoskeletal: Inspect for muscular atrophy. Palpate for muscular tenderness, especially in areas of neck, shoulders, hips, and lower back. Assess muscle strength. Palpate joints for effusion, tenderness, and warmth. Differentiate symmetry versus nonsymmetry of signs. Assess range of motion of joints.

✦ Focused examination based on comorbidities.

DIAGNOSTIC TESTS

✦ CBC with differential—mild to moderate normocytic, normochromic anemia with elevated platelets is usually present.

✦ ESR is nearly always elevated in PMR but may be normal.

✦ Absence of rheumatoid factor differentiates PMR from rheumatoid arthritis.

PREVENTION

✦ Patients with PMR should be maintained on the lowest possible dose of corticosteroids to avoid complications of steroid therapy—mental status changes, uncontrolled diabetes, osteoporosis, and infections.

✦ **See Protocol on Prevention and Health Maintenance.**

MANAGEMENT

✦ **The cause of PMR is unknown.**

✦ **PMR is characterized by tenderness, stiffness, and pain in the proximal girdle muscles (primarily the hips and shoulders). There is typically no weakness or atrophy. Tenderness may extend to the proximal muscles in the thighs and arms. Pain may be aggravated by joint movement and be severe enough to limit activity. Stiffness classically occurs in the early morning after rest.**

✦ **Synovitis occurs in up to one-third of patients and usually affects the wrists or knees.**

✦ Pain associated with visual changes or jaw claudication may indicate presence of temporal arteritis and should prompt referral for diagnosis and management. **See Protocol on Headache.**

✦ Refer to PT/OT for evaluation/treatment of functional disability.

✦ Pharmacotherapy of choice is corticosteroids (prednisone 10 mg PO qd) until response is evidenced by reduction in ESR. Dose is then tapered with periodic monitoring of ESR and symptom relief. Maintenance therapy (5–10 mg PO qd) may be required for several years.

✦ Prevention of osteoporosis with calcium/hormonal therapy is important. **See Protocol on Osteoporosis.**

✦ A small number of patients' symptoms may be controlled with NSAIDs or salicylates, but symptomatic relief is more rapid with corticosteroids. Rapid improvement confirms the diagnosis of PMR.

KEY ISSUES

Patient/Caregiver Education

Patient/caregiver should be able to:

✦ Verbalize medication regimen including doses, times, and potential side effects.

✦ State the importance of continuing maintenance therapy to avoid relapse.

Economic Considerations

✦ Functional impairment may result in inability to work or maintain independent living.

Psychosocial Considerations

✦ Pain and functional impairment may predispose to social isolation and depression.

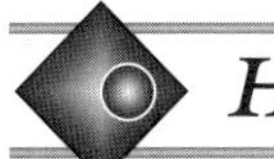

Hip Fracture

HISTORY

✦ Age? **The sequelae of hip fracture increase in severity with age due to comorbidity. The majority of the oldest elderly do not return to baseline level of functioning after hip fracture.**

✦ Gender/ethnicity? **Elderly white females are at high risk for hip fracture.**

✦ Circumstances surrounding injury? Majority of hip fractures in the elderly occur as a result of falls. Stress fractures may occur in the elderly when the usual level of activity is changed (increased walking). Occult fractures can occur with minimal or no trauma.

✦ Associated signs/symptoms: pain with/without ambulation? **With femoral neck fractures there is persistent groin pain on ambulation.** Dizziness, numbness/tingling?

✦ Comorbidities—history of previous fracture, Parkinson's disease, cerebrovascular accident (CVA), transient ischemic attacks (TIAs), history of duplicate fracture, osteoporosis, rheumatoid arthritis, diabetes mellitus? **Hip fracture may be the initial presentation of dementia.** Note conditions that predispose to spontaneous fracture (osteoporosis) or pathological fracture (renal disease, prolonged immobility).

✦ Co-existing conditions that may limit fracture rehabilitation—COPD, CVA, dementia, coronary artery disease (CAD), CHF, Parkinson's disease, peripheral neuropathy, orthostasis, pressure ulcer (especially heel ulcer)? Visual/hearing impairments?

✦ Medications—prescribed/OTC? Note especially antihypertensives, benzodiazepines, tricyclic antidepressants, barbiturates, phenothiazines. Phenytoin and phenobarbital decrease vitamin D absorption.

✦ EtOH use?

✦ Is there potential for malnutrition that may contribute to risk for falls/hip fracture?

✦ Functional status? Pre-fracture mobility is a predictor of ambulation status following hip fracture. Use of assistive device(s): cane, quad cane, walker?

✦ Social support system?

PHYSICAL EXAMINATION

✦ Vital signs. Assess for orthostasis. Note tachycardia, tachypnea, and decreased blood pressure, which may indicate shock.

✦ Weight. Calculate body mass index (BMI) [wt (kg)/height (m^2)]. Low BMI (< 20) is a risk factor for hip fracture.

✦ General: note pallor, diaphoresis.

✦ Eyes: assess visual acuity.

✦ Ears: assess hearing.

✦ Neurological: assess deep tendon reflexes (DTRs); assess for unsteady gait, impaired proprioception, presence of peripheral neuropathy, and altered sensation. Evaluate cognitive status and risk for depression.

✦ Musculoskeletal: Inspect for malalignment, contractures, foot drop. Assess muscle strength, range of motion. Palpate for pain.

✦ Skin: note bruising, swelling, and presence of skin breakdown or pressure ulcers with special attention to sacrum and heels.

DIAGNOSTIC TESTS

✦ Plain x-ray is most helpful diagnostic tool in assessing hip fracture.

✦ Bone scan or MRI is useful if stress or pathologic fracture is suspected or if severe osteoporosis limits quality of plain x-ray.

✦ Complete blood count. Mortality following hip fracture is related to decreased hemoglobin.

✦ Serum albumin or prealbumin to assess for malnutrition.

✦ Consider serum electrolytes, BUN, creatinine, urinalysis to rule out possible underlying cause of falls.

PREVENTION

✦ Encourage regular weight-bearing exercise.

✦ Consider hormone replacement therapy (HRT) in postmenopausal females to prevent osteoporosis-related fractures. **See Protocol on Osteoporosis.**

✦ Consider calcium and vitamin D supplementation.

✦ Implement/recommend fall prevention strategies. **See Protocol on Falls.**

✦ Consider use of protective hip pads for the frail elderly to absorb shock from a fall.

✦ Recommend foam-backed carpeting to absorb shock from a potential fall. Caution patients with shuffling gait that balance may be disturbed by foam-backed carpeting.

✦ **See Protocol on Prevention and Health Maintenance.**

MANAGEMENT

✦ Fracture site, bone character, and comorbidity (rather than age) determine operative treatment, management, and rehabilitation.

✦ Treatment of choice in the elderly for displaced femoral neck fracture is often prosthetic replacement. Nondisplaced femoral neck fractures are usually managed with internal fixation.

✦ Avascular necrosis and nonunion are possible complications of femoral neck fracture and may require total hip replacement.

✦ Goal of treatment for intertrochanteric fracture is stable reduction with sliding hip screw and fast weight-bearing status. Complications include collapse of fracture, infection, avascular necrosis, and nonunion.

Acute Presentation

✦ Consult physician for new fracture (may be accompanied by shock).

✦ Evaluate for accompanying head injury.

✦ Assess for fractures at additional sites. Accompanying wrist fracture is seen less frequently in the elderly than in the young.

✦ Management of acute fracture requires:

✧ Stabilization of fracture.

✧ Prevention of pulmonary emboli and deep vein thrombosis with anticoagulant therapy.

✧ Management of sequelae of fall (dehydration, skin breakdown, delirium, and rhabdomyolysis).

✦ **See Acute/Inpatient Setting.**

Postsurgical Management

✦ Evaluate risk for falls. Consider discontinuation/substitution of medications that may cause hypotension. **See Protocol on Falls.**

✦ Assess for signs of infection, prosthesis dislocation, avascular necrosis, nonunion, and deep vein thrombosis.

✦ Urinary retention, incontinence, and UTI are frequent complications following hip fracture. **See Protocol on Urinary Incontinence.**

✦ Refer to PT/OT for maximization of independence in ADLs, muscle strengthening, gait training, balance exercises, and assistive devices. **See Chapter on Rehabilitation.**

✦ Refer to social worker for assistance with transportation, living situation, Meals on Wheels, and other social supports.

✦ Assess and manage pain level. **See Chapter on Pain Management.**

✦ Monitor risk/recommend management for pressure ulcers. **See Chapter on Management of Pressure Ulcers.**

KEY ISSUES

Patient/Caregiver Education

Patient/caregiver should be able to:

✦ List dosage, timing, and potential side effects of medications.

✦ Identify environmental hazards that contribute to falls.

✦ Verbalize understanding of hip movement precautions.

✦ Verbalize importance of PT/OT for rehabilitation success. State realistic goals for rehabilitation.

✦ Demonstrate proper use of walker or cane. State that cane should be held in the hand opposite the fractured hip.

✦ Demonstrate safe negotiation of stairs, i.e., ascend with unaffected leg first and descend with affected leg first.

Economic Considerations

✦ **More than $10 billion in health care costs is incurred annually in the U.S. as a result of hip fracture.**

✦ Hip fracture may permanently alter level of care for the affected individual.

Psychosocial Considerations

✦ **Fear of falling may limit functional recovery.**

✦ Decreased mobility and functional status may contribute to depression.

Acute/Inpatient Setting

✦ **Institute fall risk precautions.**

✦ Postoperative weight-bearing status is dependent on site of fracture, bone integrity, time since surgery, operative treatment, and patient's cognitive and physical status. Refer to orthopedic surgeon's treatment plan.

✦ Internal rotation, flexion > 90°, and adduction past midline are hip movements that must be avoided for 6–12 weeks following arthroplasty to avoid dislocation. Educate staff and patient regarding hip movement restrictions.

✦ Provide reorientation and monitor cognitive status following operative fracture treatment. There is a high incidence of postoperative delirium in the elderly. **See Protocol on Delirium.**

✦ Cognitively impaired patients may be at greater risk for inadequate pain relief following surgery.

✦ Monitor for urinary incontinence and complications of recumbent status (pneumonia, skin breakdown).

✦ Refer to PT for progressive exercise therapy.

✦ Refer to OT for assistance with ADLs and assistive devices.

✦ Discharge planning should begin immediately on hospitalization. Consider accessibility to rehabilitation services at the patient's planned destination.

✦ Risk for readmission is high. Use an interdisciplinary approach to provide holistic management and discharge planning.

✦ Prophylactic antibiotics may be given to reduce risk of infection following surgical treatment.

✦ Consider a weekend visit prior to discharge home to test patient/caregiver's coping abilities.

Extended Care Setting

✦ **Hip fracture increases risk for institutionalization.**

✦ The prospective payment system has reduced hospital stays for elderly hip fracture patients; much of rehabilitation is being done in extended care settings.

✦ Refer to PT/OT for continued rehabilitation.

✦ Monitor for complications of pain-relieving narcotics (constipation, fecal impaction, altered mental status).

✦ Advise staff of weight-bearing status, risk for falls, and need for assistance with toileting.

✦ Institute measures to reduce risk for pressure ulcers. **See Chapter on Management of Pressure Ulcers.**

✦ Be aware that spontaneous fractures may occur especially in osteoporotic bedbound patients and patients with metastatic cancer to the bone. Educate staff regarding fracture potential.

Home Setting

✦ **The majority of hip fracture patients are discharged home.**

✦ Elderly hip fracture patients have been found to achieve more complete recovery at home than in institutions.

✦ Plan alternate arrangements for those patients who are unable to manage medications independently.

✦ Refer to PT for continued rehabilitation.

✦ Refer to OT for evaluation of meal preparation ability and home safety.

✦ Assess for caregiver burden and unrealistic expectations of recovery.

Chapter 9

Neurological System

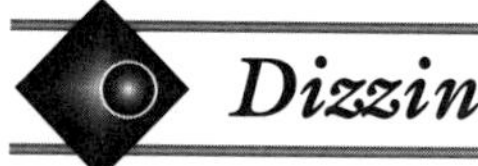

Dizziness

HISTORY

✦ Onset and duration of symptoms?

✦ Episodic or continuous? If episodic, duration of episodes?

✦ Timing of episodes, i.e., upon standing, when turning head, when rolling over in bed, or bending over and then straightening up, sitting quietly or lying in bed?

✦ Sensation: lightheadedness, weakness, or spinning sensation? **Major categories of dizziness are vertigo, presyncopal lightheadedness, disequilibrium, and nonspecific. More than half of older persons with dizziness cannot be placed in a specific category.** See Table 9-1.

✦ History of falls? Change in balance? Fear of falling?

✦ Associated symptoms: loss of consciousness, decreased hearing, tinnitus, visual changes, headaches, change in speech, nausea/vomiting, shortness of breath, chest pain?

✦ Recent eye examination, change in prescription glasses? Change in vision?

✦ Precipitating or aggravating factors, i.e., position change, change in medications, stressful situations, sleep disturbances?

✦ History of heart disease, arrhythmias, hypertension, seizure disorder, cerebrovascular accident (CVA), transient ischemic attack (TIA), peripheral neuropathy, sinusitis, hearing disorders, vertigo?

✦ Anxiety? Depression?

✦ EtOH use? Tobacco use?

✦ Medications: prescription/OTC?

✦ Impact on ability to function, perform activities of daily living (ADLs)?

TABLE 9-1. Categories of Dizziness

Symptom	Definition	Common causes
Vertigo	Sensation of spinning or motion. Usually arises from inner ear, middle ear, brain stem, or cerebellum.	Benign paroxysmal postural vertigo (BPPV); cardiovascular disease; acute labyrinthitis.
Presyncopal lightheadedness	Sensation of impending faint. Due to cerebral ischemia; arises from vascular (vasovagal) or cardiac causes.	Vasovagal episode; postural hypotension; cardiac diseases, i.e., arrhythmias, congestive heart failure.
Disequilibrium	Sensation of being unsteady or off balance. Arises from disturbance of motor control system (vision, vestibulospinal, proprioceptive, somatosensory, cerebellar, or motor function).	Stroke; multiple neurosensory deficits; peripheral neuropathy; cerebellar disease.
Nonspecific	Vague complaints; may be described as "lightheadedness" or "floating."	Anxiety; other psychological disorder.

PHYSICAL EXAMINATION

✦ Head, eyes, ears, nose, throat (HEENT): complete examination including visual acuity and hearing evaluation.

✦ Neurological: cranial nerves, check for nystagmus, Romberg, deep tendon reflexes (DTRs).

✦ Musculoskeletal examination: gait, thorough neck examination, muscle strength.

✦ Cardiovascular examination: Note tachycardia or bradycardia, arrhythmias, abnormal heart sounds.

✦ Hallpike maneuver: **Positive for benign paroxysmal positional vertigo (BPPV) if spinning sensation is brought on by rapid position change, subsides within 60 sec, associated with rotatory nystagmus, 2–10-sec latency for onset of dizziness and nystagmus after the position is assumed and fatigability if maneuver is repeated several times in succession.**

DIAGNOSTIC TESTS

✦ Vital signs including blood pressure (BP) in three positions. **Orthostatic hypotension is defined as 20 mm Hg drop in systolic blood pressure (SBP) or 10 mm Hg drop in diastolic blood pressure (DBP) 2 min after**

changing from recumbent to standing position; elderly may have delayed BP drop 10–30 min after standing or impaired cerebral perfusion without corresponding drop in BP.

- Thyroid function tests, glucose, blood urea nitrogen (BUN), electrolytes, B_{12}, calcium, liver function, hematocrit/hemoglobin.
- Therapeutic monitoring of drugs, i.e., anticonvulsants, theophylline, digoxin, antidepressants.
- Consider electrocardiogram (ECG).
- Consider cervical spine x-rays for degenerative joint disease contributing to vertebral artery compression syndromes.
- **Consult with physician when considering the following tests:**
  - MRI: preferred when evaluating possible brainstem lesions.
  - Holter monitoring for possible cardiac arrhythmia.
  - Electronystagmography (ENG) to evaluate vestibular function.
  - Carotid and vertebral artery Dopplers.
  - Electroencephalography (EEG) to rule out seizure activity.
  - Cortrosyn stimulation study for adrenal insufficiency.

PREVENTION

- Discontinue nonessential medications; monitor drug levels.
- Refer for assessment and management of hearing problems.
- **See Protocol on Tinnitus.**
- Remove cerumen impaction if indicated. **See Protocol on Cerumen Impaction.**
- Correct vision problems.
- Maintain nutrition and hydration. **Dehydration and malnutrition can cause or exacerbate symptoms of dizziness in the elderly.**
- Consider referral for physical therapy (PT), falls and balance assessment, occupational therapy (OT) for home safety assessment. **See Protocol on Falls.**
- **See Protocol on Prevention and Health Maintenance.**

MANAGEMENT

Postural Dizziness Without Postural Hypotension

- Use support stockings.
- Recommend frequent contraction of leg muscles: rocking chair, walking.
- Maintain state of hydration: six to eight 8-oz glasses of water daily.
- Consider cardioselective beta-adrenergic blocking agent or sympathomimetic, i.e., Inderal (propranolol HCl) 40 mg bid or Sudafed (pseudoephedrine HCl) 30–60 mg bid.

✦ Consider Florinef (fludrocortisone acetate) 0.1 mg daily for volume expansion.

Benign Paroxysmal Positional Vertigo (BPPV)

✦ Viral labyrinthitis and head trauma (even in distant past) predispose.

✦ Course is generally gradual improvement over 4–6 weeks.

✦ Instruct patient to continue to move the head (refusing to move head slows recovery).

✦ Instruct on exercises to hasten recovery: falling or rolling on a bed several times in succession in a manner that provokes dizziness.

Labyrinthitis

✦ Single episode of vertigo with affected hearing; abrupt onset and gradual improvement over days.

✦ Consider Antivert (meclizine HCl) 12.5–25 mg tid, Phenergan (promethazine HCl) 12.5 mg tid, or Robinul (glycopyrrolate) 1–2 mg qid during acute phase. **Recovery is often slower in elderly. Monitor for excessive sedation with Phenergan.**

Vestibular Neuronitis

✦ Similar symptoms as labyrinthitis without hearing affected.

✦ Consider Antivert or Phenergan during acute phase. **Recovery is often slower in elderly.**

Meniere's Disease

✦ Recurrent episodes of vertigo associated with tinnitus and gradual onset of unilateral low-frequency hearing loss.

✦ Consider Antivert.

✦ Referral for hearing evaluation and treatment options.

Recurrent Vestibulopathy

✦ Recurrent episodes of vertigo without auditory symptoms.

✦ Consider Antivert.

Vertebrobasilar TIAs

✦ Episodic vertigo (rotatory dizziness) with an abrupt onset and lasting 20–60 min.

✦ May be associated with neurological symptoms: blurred vision, diplopia, limb numbness or weakness, or dysarthria.

✦ Initiate acetylsalicylic acid (ASA, aspirin) 81 mg daily.

✦ Consider anticoagulation therapy. Consult physician; consider other risk factors.

✦ Complete work-up or refer as needed to rule out embolic cardiac disease, epilepsy, thrombocytopenia, polycythemia, and thrombotic thrombocytopenia.

Cerebrovascular Accident (CVA)

✦ **See Protocol on Transient Ischemic Attack (TIA)/Cerebrovascular Accident (CVA).**

Cervical Etiology

✦ Vascular: temporary disruption of blood flow through one of the vertebral arteries. Occurs when turning head or looking up and an osteoarthritic spur pinches the vertebral artery. Presents as episodic vertigo provoked by specific positions of the neck.

✦ Proprioceptive: facet joints of the neck contain proprioceptive receptors that, when overstimulated, cause lightheadedness or vertigo.

✦ Consider referral to neurosurgery for further evaluation. Consult with physician.

Seizure Disorder

✦ **See Protocol on Seizures.**

Physical Deconditioning

✦ Recommend appropriate exercise program.

✦ Consider referral for home or outpatient PT.

✦ Consider assistive devices for safety.

✦ Consider subacute or rehabilitation referral for hospitalized patients.

Medication-Related Dizziness

✦ Review medications carefully; drugs that can cause or exacerbate dizziness include diuretics, calcium channel blockers, beta blockers, vasodilators, theophylline, antihistamines, tricyclic antidepressants, psychotropics, muscle relaxants, anticonvulsants, NSAIDs. **Antivert and Phenergan, commonly used for dizziness, can worsen dizziness through their anticholinergic effects.**

✦ Review patient's use of OTC medications such as cold preparations; decrease use of caffeine and EtOH.

Neurosensory Deficits

✦ Assess for multiple deficits for which the older patient cannot compensate, e.g., decreased vision, decreased hearing in a patient who has residual hemiparesis from a CVA and who is taking multiple antihypertensive agents.

- Identify and correct deficits when possible.
- Manage concomitant chronic diseases optimally.

Psychological Etiology

- Rare as a primary cause of dizziness in elderly.
- Assess for and treat underlying depression or anxiety.

KEY ISSUES

Patient/Caregiver Education

Patient/caregiver should be able to:

- Implement safety measures to prevent falls. **See Protocol on Falls.**
- Maintain a diary of episodes for review.
- Demonstrate maneuvers that may decrease dizziness.
- Discuss prescribed medication regimen.

Psychosocial Considerations

- Dizziness can greatly impair functional status, resulting in fear of falling and social isolation.
- Assess for underlying anxiety or depression.

Acute/Inpatient Setting

- Identify patients at risk for falling secondary to dizziness on admission; institute fall prevention protocols.

Extended Care Setting

- Implement fall prevention protocols.
- Assess new episodes of dizziness for previously undiagnosed problems. **Be alert to the fact that older patients with infection, electrolyte imbalances, or exacerbations of a chronic disease often present atypically.**

Home Setting

- Consider home safety assessment.
- If dizziness is episodic, consider having patient keep a diary of events to aid in diagnosis.

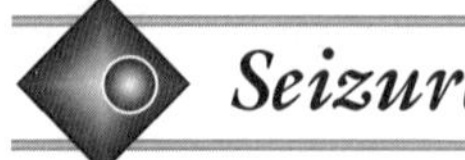

Seizures

HISTORY

✦ Onset, duration, timing of event? Number of events?

✦ Was the event witnessed? By whom?

✦ Describe event: presence of aura, loss of consciousness, staring, dizziness, confusion, lethargy, slurred speech, falls, loss of bladder, bowel, or salivary control, tongue biting, abnormal movements, vomiting, or aspiration? **Seizures may be focal or generalized, with or without motor involvement, with or without impairment of consciousness.**

✦ Postictal state? Symptoms: lethargy, somnolence, fever, confusion? Duration of symptoms? **Postictal state may be longer, more severe in the elderly.**

✦ History of known seizure disorder? Evaluation by neurologist? What did work-up entail? Results? Treatment recommendations?

✦ Recent fall? History of falls? Other trauma?

✦ History of CNS disorder, i.e., CVA, TIA, subdural hematoma, tumor, surgery, sleep disorder?

✦ History of cardiac problems, arrhythmias, syncope, carotid disease?

✦ History of diabetes mellitus, hypertension, renal problems, liver disease?

✦ History of anxiety, panic attacks, psychiatric disorder?

✦ EtOH use?

✦ Medications: prescription/OTC?

✦ Functional status?

✦ Social supports, caregiver?

PHYSICAL EXAMINATION

✦ Vital signs. Assess for orthostasis.

✦ General appearance, cognitive status, level of consciousness, breath odor for EtOH or ketones.

✦ Fundoscopic examination.

✦ Complete neurological examination: note any focal neurological deficits.

✦ Focused examination based on comorbid conditions or associated symptoms.

DIAGNOSTIC TESTS

✦ **See Protocol on Dizziness** for additional history, physical examination, and diagnostic tests if suspected dizziness vs. seizure.

✦ Consider electrolytes, BUN, drug/EtOH.

✦ Check anticonvulsant drug level if patient is on medication and continuing to have seizures.

✦ Monitor therapeutic drug level soon after beginning new anticonvulsant medication and at least every 6 months. Consider free phenytoin level in malnourished patient.

✦ Liver enzymes, CBC, and albumin level for baseline data prior to initiating anticonvulsant therapy

✦ Consider CT of the head to rule out structural brain lesion, i.e., stroke, tumor, subdural hematoma. Consult with physician.

✦ Consider lumbar puncture with cerebrospinal fluid analysis to rule out infectious process. Consult with physician.

✦ Consider EEG. Consult with physician. **Timing of study may not always coincide with seizure activity.**

✦ Consider referral to neurologist for further evaluation.

PREVENTION

✦ Recommend good oral hygiene; regular dental care. **Gingival hyperplasia is an adverse effect of Dilantin (phenytoin) and can predispose to gingivitis.**

✦ Assess for risk of falls and implement fall prevention strategies. **See Protocol on Falls.**

✦ Educate patient and family/caregivers on how to prevent injury during seizure activity, i.e., assist patient to a safe position with head turned to the side to prevent aspiration if vomiting occurs; avoid attempts to restrain patient; pad side rails and/or remove hard or sharp objects surrounding patient; stay with patient and provide supportive care.

✦ Anticonvulsant medications may be prescribed prophylactically for patients at high risk of seizure activity, i.e., new CVA, subdural hematoma, CNS lesion or tumor. Consider discontinuing prophylactic anticonvulsant therapy if no evidence of seizure activity for several months following acute events. Consult with physician.

✦ **See Protocol on Prevention and Health Maintenance.**

MANAGEMENT

✦ Support patient during seizure event to prevent injury or adverse complications, e.g., aspiration.

✦ Support patient during postictal state, i.e., assess need for IV fluids and medications; avoid oral feedings and medications if patient is somnolent and at higher risk of aspiration; consider need for hospitalization.

✦ Monitor medication regimen; review on each visit.

✦ Commonly used anticonvulsants include:

- ✧ Dilantin (phenytoin) 100–300 mg PO daily.
- ✧ Tegretol (carbamazepine) 200–400 mg PO daily.
- ✧ Phenobarbital 32–100 mg PO daily.
- ✧ Depakene (valproic acid) 15 mg/kg PO daily (maximum 60 mg/kg daily).
- ✧ Klonopin (clonazepam) start 0.5 mg PO tid, maximum 30 mg daily.
- ✧ Neurontin (gabapentin) 100–200 mg PO daily.

Begin with low dose and titrate to control seizures. May need combination of medications in some patients. Consult with physician on medication choice and dose.

✦ Check Dilantin level or other therapeutic drug levels when adjusting medication regimen. **Dilantin toxicity can occur when adding new medications to regimen, especially those that are highly protein bound, e.g., warfarin, antibiotics.**

✦ Address driving privileges. **Driving is contraindicated in patients with new or uncontrolled seizures.**

KEY ISSUES

Patient/Caregiver Education

Patient/caregiver should be able to:

✦ Verbalize understanding of medication regimen, interactions, and possible adverse effects.

✦ Verbalize signs and symptoms of impending seizure and act to maintain safety.

✦ Verbalize understanding of safety considerations for patient during seizures. **See Prevention.**

Economic Considerations

✦ Newer anticonvulsants are costly; may require formulary approvals.

✦ Loss of driving privileges may impair ability to continue to work when applicable.

✦ Seizure disorder may limit ability to live independently; assisted living arrangements can be costly and are primarily private pay. **See Chapter on Alternatives to Living Alone.**

Psychosocial Considerations

✦ Fear related to a seizure disorder may cause the patient to limit activities and result in social isolation. Loss of driving privileges is a significant threat to independence.

✦ Be alert to depression as a consequence of loss of independence.

✦ Consider referral for counseling if needed.

✦ Encourage patient to maintain normal activities when safe to do so.

Acute/Inpatient Setting

✦ Avoid oral feeding in postictal state; risk of aspiration is high. Provide for hydration and nutrition until sensorium has cleared.

✦ Anticonvulsants may be given IV if necessary. Loading doses may be recommended. Consult with physician.

✦ Initiate seizure precautions for patient with known seizure disorder.

✦ Implement fall assessment and prevention program.

Extended Care Setting

✦ Tube fed patients receiving Dilantin should have feeding held 1 hr pre- and post-dose to maximize absorption. Use of suspension may make administration easier but must be shaken well to prevent dose variation secondary to precipitant. Daily dose can usually be given in single night-time administration.

✦ Patient with protein malnutrition (low albumin or prealbumin) may require lower daily Dilantin dose. Consider drawing a free Dilantin level instead of bound Dilantin. **Dilantin is a highly protein bound drug.**

Home Setting

✦ Provide a safe environment for the patient with known seizure disorder. **See Protocol on Falls.**

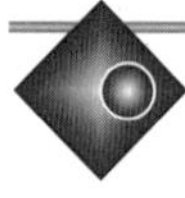

Transient Ischemic Attack (TIA)/ Cerebrovascular Accident (CVA)

HISTORY

✦ Race? **Higher incidence exists in African Americans—CVA occurs at younger age with worse outcomes.**

✦ Abrupt or gradual onset? Duration of symptoms?

✦ Associated signs/symptoms: Hypoglycemia, seizure? Headache, dizziness, loss of balance, syncope, fall? Any loss of vision; if so, which field(s)? Weakness (location)? Difficulty talking? Nausea/vomiting? Numbness, loss of sensation? Loss of consciousness? Incontinence? Rapid heartbeat? Change in behavior; memory loss?

✦ Past medical history/comorbid conditions: Previous TIA/CVA? **It is estimated that approximately one-third of patients will have a major CVA within 5 years after having a TIA.** Hypertension, hyperlipidemia, coronary artery disease (CAD), myocardial ischemia (MI) (note date), carotid stenosis, atrial fibrillation? **Approximately 50% of cardiogenic embolization results from nonvalvular atrial fibrillation.** Angina, mitral stenosis, prosthetic valve placement? Seizure disorder? Diabetes mellitus? Peripheral vascular disease (PVD), arteritis? Sickle cell anemia, polycythemia vera?

✦ History of head trauma?

✦ History of EtOH use, tobacco use (increases risk), use of illicit drugs (especially cocaine)?

✦ Family history of CVA, hypertension, CAD, diabetes mellitus, hyperlipidemia?

✦ Complete medication history including OTC diet pills?

✦ Functional status: change in ability to perform ADLs or inability to communicate?

✦ Cognitive status?

✦ Social situation, supports?

PHYSICAL EXAMINATION

✦ See Display 9-1.

✦ Vital signs. Assess for hypertension, orthostasis, irregular heart rate.

✦ Head: Auscultate for temporal bruits. Palpate scalp for indications of hemorrhage.

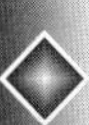

DISPLAY 9-1. *Normal Functions and Cognitive Skills Associated with Specific Areas of the Brain*

Frontal

Attention
Motivation
Emotional/impulse control
Control of social behavior
Personality
Judgment/insight
Decision making
Expressive language
Motor integration
Voluntary movement
Problem solving involved with executive IADLs

Temporal

Visual memory
Comprehension of verbal messages
Musical awareness
Sequencing skills
Receptive verbal and nonverbal language

Cerebellum

Posture/gait
Movements (**abnormally** there are awkward intentional movements)

Pons

Sensory perception
Cranial nerve function

Parietal

Temperature, pressure, tactile perception
Spatial relationship awareness
Academic skills such as reading, math
Voluntary movement

Occipital

Visual perception
Perception/recognition of written messages

Basal ganglia

Movements (**abnormally** there are awkward unintentional movements)

Midbrain

Visual and auditory reflexes

✦ Eyes: Assess visual fields for cuts; ask patient to cover one eye to assess cuts in each eye. Fundoscopic examination for arteriovenous crossings indicative of hypertension.

✦ Neurological: **Neurological examination likely to be normal in patient presenting with report of TIA symptoms unless currently experiencing TIA or has had previous CVA.** Assess level of consciousness, orientation, ability to speak and understand language. Perform mental status examination. Perform assessment of cranial nerves. Assess deep tendon reflexes; presence of Babinski's sign. Inspect for facial paresis. Assess motor function, sensory function, gait. Assess range of motion and muscle strength and coordination.

✦ Cardiovascular: Assess heart rate and rhythm. Assess peripheral pulses. Auscultate for temporal, carotid, and abdominal aortic bruits.

DIAGNOSTIC TESTS

✦ Serum electrolytes, glucose, and BUN for exclusion of metabolic disturbance as cause of neurological deficits and assessment for increased blood viscosity caused by dehydration.

✦ CBC to screen for infection.

✦ Platelet count, prothrombin time or international normalized ratio (INR), partial thromboplastin time.

✦ Serum thrombolytic factors: antiphospholipid antibodies (anticardiolipin elevation is an independent risk factor for CVA) and deficiencies in antithrombin III and protein C and protein S are associated with CVA.

✦ Fasting lipid panel (total cholesterol, low-density lipoprotein, high-density lipoprotein).

✦ Serological test for syphilis may be useful in or patients with atypical presentation.

✦ 12-Lead ECG to detect cardiac abnormality. Holter monitoring if cardiac arrhythmia is suspected.

✦ Echocardiogram to identify predisposing cardiac abnormalities. Transesophageal echocardiogram (TEE) is more expensive than transthoracic echocardiogram and requires intubation but can image the aortic arch and is more sensitive for identifying cardiac embolism.

✦ Carotid and vertebral artery ultrasound with Doppler to screen for occlusive disease.

✦ Transcranial ultrasound with Doppler provides information related to intracranial flow. Serial transcranial ultrasound is useful to detect and determine treatment for vasospasm after subarachnoid hemorrhage; to assess thrombolytic treatment; and to monitor for reocclusion after carotid endartectomy.

✦ Noncontrast CT to differentiate ischemia from hemorrhage and identify tumor, arteriovenous (AV) malformations, and subdural hematoma. In patients with ischemic CVA, CT scan usually normal until several hours after onset.

✦ Magnetic resonance angiography provides noninvasive imaging of cerebral vessels and is useful for patient selection for intra-arterial angiography. MRIs in the elderly with cardiovascular risk factors often show asymptomatic white matter lesions in multiple hemispheres. Clinical correlation by a neurologist is needed.

PREVENTION

✦ Inform families of patients at risk for CVA of the signs/symptoms of TIA/CVA and the importance of urgent evaluation and speedy treatment to improve outcomes.

✦ Control major risk factors for stroke:

✧ Elevated cholesterol. **See Protocol on Hyperlipidemia.**

✧ Hypertension. **See Protocol on Hypertension.**

✧ Atrial fibrillation. **See Protocol on Atrial Fibrillation** for anticoagulation recommendations for CVA prevention.

✧ Diabetes mellitus. **See Protocol on Diabetes Mellitus.**

✧ Smoking.

✦ Antiplatelet therapies for CVA prevention:

✧ For patients with history of previous TIA/CVA, consider aspirin 81 mg PO qd if no contraindications.

✧ Results remain unclear regarding the long-term efficacy of Ticlid (ticlopidine) 250 mg PO bid to reduce recurrent risk of thromboembolic CVA. In non-white populations, ticlopidine may be especially effective but serious side effects of neutropenia and thrombocytopenia mandate close monitoring. Ticlopidine therapy usually reserved for patients intolerant of aspirin or with ischemic symptoms while on aspirin therapy.

✧ Patients with recent history of MI, previous CVA, or established peripheral artery disease, may receive antiplatelet therapy with Plavix (clopidogrel bisulfate) 75 mg PO qd; contraindications: active bleeding, gastrointestinal (GI) ulcer, intracranial hemorrhage.

✦ Consider long-term anticoagulation with Coumadin (warfarin sodium) for patients with recurrent TIAs not responsive to previous regimens. **See Protocol on Atrial Fibrillation.**

✦ Consider Vitamin B_6 and Vitamin B_{12} therapy if elevated homocysteine levels.

✦ **See Protocol on Prevention and Health Maintenance.**

MANAGEMENT

✦ TIA and CVA both stem from etiology of insufficient blood flow to the brain. Cerebrovascular insufficiency may result from several pathologies. See Table 9-2.

✦ TIA results from temporary interference of blood flow to brain; duration is several minutes to several hours. Neurological deficits resolve within 24 hr. **TIA is a warning sign. Diagnostic testing and prevention are critical to avoid future ischemic events. See Prevention.**

✦ CVA presents with sudden loss of consciousness followed by neurological deficits and may be evolving or completed upon presentation. Severity and duration of deficits depends on location of affected arterial bed and size of infarct.

✦ **CVA is the third leading cause of death and a cause of significant disability in the elderly.**

✦ Most TIA/CVAs in the elderly are caused by ischemia rather than hemorrhage.

✦ On initial presentation of signs/symptoms of TIA/CVA, consult physician for appropriate diagnostic tests/management/referral. Acute CVA, especially evolving CVAs, may be appropriate for thrombolytic and anticoagulant therapy. **See Diagnostic Tests and Acute/Inpatient Setting.**

✦ Institute supportive management for functional consequences of established deficits:

✧ Refer to OT for assessment of safety hazard risks, ability to perform ADLs, and use of assistive devices.

✧ Refer to PT for assessment/therapy for prevention of contractures, pain from increased spasticity, loss of independence.

✧ Refer to speech therapy for diagnostics/management of language deficits, impaired swallowing. **Swallowing deficits increase risk for aspiration pneumonia.** Consider that failure to speak or comprehend may result from poor hearing. **See Protocol on Cerumen Impaction.**

✧ Control incontinence and fecal impaction. **See Protocols on Urinary Incontinence and Constipation.**

✧ Refer to social work services for referral to community resources.

✧ Refer to nutritionist. Many patients with CVA will require enteral feeding. **See Protocol on Management of the Enterally Fed Patient.**

KEY ISSUES

Patient/Caregiver Education

Patient/caregiver should be able to:

✦ Verbalize understanding of deficits and means for compensation (storing items for self-care on unaffected side, clothing affected side first).

TABLE 9-2. Differentiation of TIA/CVA Syndromes

Classification	Description/symptoms	Etiology
Hemorrhagic		
Subarachnoid hemorrhage	Sudden onset of headache; vomiting; decreased consciousness with or without focal neuro signs	Bleeding from aneurysm or AV malformations; drugs; amyloid angiopathy
Intracerebral hemorrhage	Headache (present in < 50% of cases) with co-existent focal deficits; vomiting. Generalized white matter changes on MRI with remote, small, clinically silent hemorrhages. Often co-exists with Alzheimer's disease	Chronic hypertension; amyloid angiopathy is common cause in the elderly; may be normotensive with neuro deficits. Anticoagulation or thrombolytic therapy; illicit drug use, OTC diet pills, decongestants
Ischemic		
Systemic hypoperfusion		Recent MI, cardiac dysrhythmias, shock, hypotension
Embolism	Abrupt onset of deficit and impaired consciousness. Suspected when CVA is in multiple vascular territories. Usually no history of prior TIAs	Valvular disease, atrial fibrillation, MI, atrial septal aneurysm, aortic arch lesion
Thrombosis	Symptoms depend on size and location of infarct. Sudden, gradual, or stepwise progression	Chronic hypertension, coagulopathies
Large artery (carotid, vertebral)	May be preceded by TIAs that suggest affected artery	Atherosclerosis of vertebral and carotid arteries
Small penetrating arteries (lacunar strokes)	Symptoms restricted to ataxic hemiparesis, pure motor, or pure sensory	Hypertension; diabetes mellitus

✦ Verbalize importance of maintaining safe environment (reducing clutter to avoid falls, using no-slip strips on floor areas, using adequate lighting).

✦ State understanding of prescribed diet and measures to prevent aspiration.

✦ State names of medications, possible side effects, prescribed doses and timing.

✦ Demonstrate proper use of assistive devices (walkers, canes, electric lift chairs, toilet/shower grab bars, raised toilet seats).

Psychosocial Considerations

✦ Distorted perception in patients with left hemiplegia may cause emotional insecurity. Educate caregivers to reinforce awareness of left side while assisting with ADLs.

✦ Be aware of potential for caregiver burden. Refer for hospice as needed.

✦ Post-stroke depression has been found to be associated with living in extended care settings, high pre-stroke EtOH intake, major functional impairment and divorced status.

✦ Refer for stroke support group if available.

Acute/Inpatient Setting

✦ Patients with new-onset CVA require IV fluids (normal saline) to promote perfusion and lowering of extremely elevated BP with adrenergic blocker (Normodyne, Trandate [labetalol HCl]). Be aware that lowering BP too aggressively may worsen evolving CVA.

✦ Surgery may be used for:

- ✧ Obliteration of aneurysm.
- ✧ Removal of hematomas in intracerebral hemorrhage.
- ✧ Dilation of vasospastic arteries.
- ✧ Treatment of AV malformations.

✦ Carotid endarterectomy has been shown to be superior to medical therapy for symptomatic, high-grade (70–99%) carotid artery stenosis. **Advanced age alone is not a contraindication to carotid surgery.**

✦ After CT exclusion of hemorrhagic etiology, patients with ischemic CVA may receive treatment with tissue plasminogen activator (t-PA) to improve outcomes. **Thrombolytic therapy must be initiated within 3 hr of onset of symptoms to be effective.**

✦ Acute anticoagulation is indicated to prevent recurrent cardiogenic embolism. Use of low-molecular weight heparin rather than regular heparin reduces the accompanying risk of hemorrhage.

✦ Acute inpatient rehabilitation should be encouraged.

✦ Before discharge, plan for appropriate level of care and housing.

Extended Care Setting

✦ Post-CVA patients may demonstrate emotional lability. Educate staff that use of restraints increases risk for falls and injury.

✦ Educate staff to position residents to avoid skin breakdown and aspiration and provide passive range of motion as indicated.

✦ Oral care and maintaining a sitting position after meals may also decrease aspiration risk.

✦ Advise staff of individual patient's impairments. Provide interventions to accommodate for deficits and encourage achievable independence.

Home Setting

✦ Refer to home health agency to address key issues: problems with performing ADLs, loss of identity, utilization of resources, and emotional support for patient/caregiver.

✦ Refer to OT for home safety assessment.

✦ Provide means of contact with community resources: companion services, senior centers, transportation services.

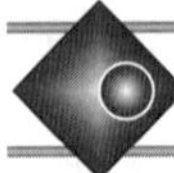

Parkinson's Disease (PD)

HISTORY

✦ Presence of primary symptoms: stiffness/rigidity, tremor, bradykinesia (delay in starting movement, slowness/poverty of movement, unpredictable/variable), postural instability (may be unable to maintain equilibrium or react to abrupt changes in position)? **Earliest symptoms are often nonspecific: weakness, fatigue, feel shaky, have difficulty getting out of a chair.**

✦ Secondary symptoms: speech difficulty (change in volume, pitch, phonation, articulation), changes in voluntary motor activity (difficulty walking, decreased arm swing, short/shuffling steps, difficulty turning, sudden/abrupt freezing spells), depression, sleep disturbances, sialorrhea, dysphagia, weight loss, constipation, shortness of breath, difficulty voiding, dizziness, postural hypotension, stooped posture, lower extremity edema, sexual dysfunction, seborrhea, excessive sweating? **Depression occurs in approximately half of patients with PD, may be an "agitated" depression and may occur early in the course of the disease preceding other symptoms.**

✦ Problems with memory or decision making? **PD without dementia usually begins in a person's 40s, 50s, or 60s and runs a long course responding well to medications. PD with dementia begins in older individuals and has a shorter, more severe course. Dementia resembles Alzheimer's disease; may be a variant called Lewy Body disease and may be associated with paranoia, delusions, and hallucinations.**

✦ Onset, duration, progression of symptoms? History of previous evaluations, examination by a neurologist?

✦ History of falls? Ability to perform ADLs?

✦ Presence of comorbid conditions?

✦ Medications? **Parkinson like symptoms (extrapyramidal) may be induced by certain medications, i.e., Thorazine (chlorpromazine), Haldol (haloperidol), Reglan (metoclopramide HCl).**

✦ Psychosocial assessment: patient's residence, social supports available, caregiver available? Caregiver stress? Use of/need for community resources, i.e., Meals on Wheels, respite care, home health services?

PHYSICAL EXAMINATION

✦ Vital signs with BP in three positions.

✦ General appearance: observe posture, gait, facial expression. **Face may lack expression and animation, "masked face."**

✦ HEENT: assess extraocular movements, accommodation; auscultate for carotid and temporal bruits; palpate for thyroid enlargement.

✦ Observe tremor, if present, at rest and with voluntary movement. **Characteristics of tremor: a to-and-fro resting tremor, begins in hand, rhythmic, "pill rolling," may only affect one side of the body especially early in disease. Common in 75% of patients.**

✦ Musculoskeletal examination: observe for rigidity of movement, assess for short-jerky "cogwheel" movements, range of motion, muscle tone and strength.

✦ Neurological examination: test cranial nerves, deep tendon reflexes, Romberg.

✦ Assess handwriting.

✦ Have patient perform a simple task, e.g., take off a coat.

✦ Ask patient to rise from a chair.

✦ Assess cognitive function; variety of screening instruments available.

✦ Assess for signs and symptoms of depression; variety of screening instruments available, such as the Beck depression screening.

DIAGNOSTIC TESTS

✦ There are no specific laboratory or radiological tests available. **PD is a clinical diagnosis.**

✦ Consider dementia work-up if patient is cognitively impaired. **See Protocol on Dementia.**

PREVENTION

✦ Address fall assessment and prevention. **See Protocol on Falls.**

✦ Maintain adequate nutrition and hydration.

✦ Adjust consistency of diet as needed, teach feeding techniques to prevent aspiration.

✦ Initiate and customize bowel regimen.

✦ Encourage appropriate exercise/activity/stretching program.

✦ Teach correct positioning to prevent contractures as mobility is decreased.

✦ **See Protocol on Prevention and Health Maintenance.**

MANAGEMENT

✦ Discuss advance directives with patient/caregiver. **See Chapter on Legal and Ethical Issues.**

✦ Discuss issues related to feeding options.

✦ Discuss issues related to appropriate level of care.

✦ Monitor weight, diet, changes in function, progression of symptoms.

✦ Consider adaptations for functional impairments.

✦ Consider OT and/or PT referrals for complete functional assessment and recommendations.

✦ Consider speech pathology referral for speech and swallowing assessment and recommendations.

✦ Consider evaluation by nutritionist for nutritional assessment, diet modifications, and recommendations. **A high-protein diet may limit effectiveness of levodopa.**

✦ Refer to social worker as needed for psychosocial assessment and discussion of community resources.

✦ Neurology referral for diagnosis and/or medication adjustment. Consult with physician.

✦ Consider neurosurgery referral for discussion of possible surgical interventions. Consult with physician.

✦ **Medication regimen for PD requires individualization to optimize effectiveness and minimize adverse effects.**

✦ Sinemet (carbidopa/levodopa) 25/100 tablets (½–1 tab) every 3–6 hr to maximum of 200 mg daily of carbidopa; Sinemet CR 50/200 tablets bid provides prolonged control. Initiate Sinemet CR with a 25% dose reduction of Sinemet. Sinemet is a CNS dopamine replacement; levodopa is converted to dopamine, carbidopa inhibits peripheral dopamine production to reduce side effects and increase CNS levodopa levels.

✧ Adjust timing of dosage if akinesia in morning or agitation at night. Side effects: dyskinesia, nausea, hallucinations, dizziness, choreiform movements. **Consult with physician as needed for medication side effects and associated CNS symptoms.**

✦ Eldepryl (selegiline HCl) 5 mg bid.

✧ An irreversible MAO inhibitor; use is controversial.

✧ **Contraindicated with selective serotonin reuptake inhibitor (SSRI) administration.**

✧ Side effects: dizziness, dysrhythmias, psychosis, hypotension.

✦ Parlodel (bromocriptine mesylate) 1.25–5 mg tid; Permax (pergolide mesylate) 0.05–1 mg tid.

✧ Dopamine receptor agonists; directly stimulate dopamine; mimic role of dopamine in brain; can be used alone or with levodopa.

✧ Side effects: nausea, headache, dizziness, hypotension, paranoia, hallucinations, confusion, edema.

✦ Consider antidepressants for associated symptoms. **The anticholinergic effects of tricyclics may improve motor symptoms, consider contraindications for tricyclics and other possible side effects.**

✦ Consider Clozaril (clozapine), Zyprexa (olanzipine), or seroquel (quetiapine fumarate) if psychosis complicates the clinical course of PD. **Monitor for blood dyscrasia with clozapine use. Consult with physician for individual dosing recommendations.**

✦ Treat symptoms related to dementia as appropriate. **See Chapter on Management of the Alzheimer's Patient.**

KEY ISSUES

Patient/Caregiver Education

Patient/caregiver should be able to:

✦ Describe the long-term course of PD and treatment plan.

✦ Describe management strategies to maintain function and prevent complications.

✦ Demonstrate correct transfer of positioning techniques.

✦ Describe medication regimen.

✦ Identify action/possible side effects of prescribed medications.

Economic Considerations

✦ Address economic issues related to appropriate level of care, e.g., assisted living or nursing home.

✦ Newer medications may require authorization through insurance/HMO.

Psychosocial Considerations

✦ Consider risk for depression and social isolation.

✦ Assess for caregiver stress.

✦ Consider support group for patient and family/caregiver.

✦ Consider counseling if indicated for adjustment to chronic disease.

✦ **See Protocols on Dementia and Depression; Chapter on Management of the Alzheimer's Patient.**

Acute/Inpatient Setting

✦ Avoid prolonged bedrest, immobility, restraints. **There is often a rapid deterioration when immobilized.**

✦ Refer to OT and PT for evaluation and maximization of function, prevention of functional decline, assessment of mobility and safety during hospitalization.

✦ Assess speech and swallowing ability; refer to speech pathology when appropriate. Consider video fluoroscopy for swallowing assessment. **See Protocol on Management of the Enterally Fed Patient** if patient is tube fed.

✦ Refer to social worker as needed for assessment of social supports and post-hospital needs.

✦ Observe for medication related complications, especially altered mental status.

✦ Assess condition of skin, risk for pressure ulcers, and initiate preventive measures.

✦ Refer for a nutritional assessment; maintain adequate nutrition and hydration.

✦ Reassess medication regimen and adjust as needed.

Extended Care Setting

✦ Maintain mobility: have patient out of bed for all meals, encourage participation in ADLs, recreational activities such as chair exercise.

✦ Maintain correct positioning for bed-to-chair patients to prevent contractures.

✦ Consider splinting if indicated to prevent contractures.

✦ Consult OT and PT as needed for recommendations for positioning, splinting, mobility, and function.

✦ Reassess need for assistive devices periodically.

✦ Maintain skin integrity; initiate preventive measures.

✦ Reassess nutritional status frequently.

Home Setting

✦ Address safety considerations.

✦ Assess for needed adaptive equipment or environmental changes to maintain function.

✦ Consider home health assessment with OT and PT for altered function.

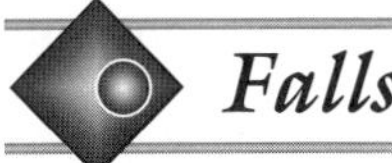

Falls

HISTORY

✦ First or recurrent fall? Was the fall witnessed? **Falls are often underreported by the elderly who fear loss of independence. The risk of accidental falls is increased when environmental hazards are combined with normal physiologic changes of aging and/or disease.**

✦ Slip? Trip?

✦ Location of fall? Time of day? During what activity? What clothing was worn? Footwear? Environmental hazards? If recurrent, are the circumstances the same or similar?

✦ Injury? **Lack of injury is common. Hip fractures increase after the age of 60. Complications of hip fractures can result in disability, loss of independence, and in some, death within a year of the fall. Falls account for approximately two-thirds of accidental deaths in the elderly.**

✦ Recent fracture? **Common fracture sites: hip, femur, humerus, ribs, wrist (Colle's fracture, especially in females), and lumbosacral spine. See Protocol on Hip Fracture.**

✦ Visual deficits? New lenses? Recent eye surgery? Cataracts? Difficulty with close/distant perception or adaptation to the dark? Recent CVA? **Diseases such as age-related macular degeneration, glaucoma, cataracts, and visual field cuts associated with a CVA can contribute to falls secondary to decreased proprioception. See Protocols on Age-Related Macular Degeneration, Glaucoma, Cataracts, and Transient Ischemic Attack (TIA)/ Cerebrovascular Accident (CVA).**

✦ Hearing deficits? Hearing aid(s)? **Vestibular senses often compensate in the presence of decreased visual proprioception and visual loss.**

✦ Tinnitus? **See Protocol on Tinnitus.** Dizziness? Vertigo? Syncope? **See Protocol on Dizziness.** Positionally related (especially upward or laterally)? **May suggest vascular insufficiency caused by carotid sinus or arterial compression.** Activity related? **Post-micturation syncope can lead to falls in elderly males. Post-prandial hypotension can result in falls.**

✦ Headaches following a fall? **Carry high level of suspicion for subdural hematoma.**

✦ General or localized weakness, paralysis, or contracture(s)? **Drop attacks are secondary to sudden weakness of lower extremities. There is usually no dizziness or syncope. May occur with rapid changes in position of the head.**

✦ Recent infection? Fever? Nausea, vomiting, or diarrhea?

✦ Incontinence? Nocturia? **Falls often result from hurried gait attempting to reach the bathroom or slips secondary to incontinence.**

✦ Tingling, numbness, or pain in hands, feet, legs?

✦ Difficulty with ambulation? Use of aid(s): walker, hemi-walker, straight or quad cane, scooter or wheelchair?

✦ Prolonged bedrest? If so, for what reason? **Complications of immobility greatly increase risk of fall.**

✦ Problems with memory? **Metabolic conditions may lead to cognitive changes. Confusion/cognitive impairment and wandering behavior associated with conditions such as multi-infarct dementia and Alzheimer's disease can lead to falls.**

✦ EtOH? Amount? **Alcohol usage often accounts for instability of gait, falls, and fractures and is under reported in the elderly. See Protocol on Substance Abuse.**

✦ Smoking?

✦ Medications? Polypharmacy? **Diuretics, antihypertensive agents, anxiolytic agents, hypnotics, antipsychotics, analgesics, and tricyclic antidepressants can increase risk of falls.**

✦ Functional status? Change in functional status since fall?

✦ Fear of recurrent falls? Effect on functional status/quality of life?

✦ History of: diabetes mellitus, anemia, hypothyroidism, TIA, CVA, normal pressure hydrocephalus, hypertension, heart disease, arrhythmias, psychiatric illness/depression, cancer, osteoporosis, chronic obstructive pulmonary disease (COPD), arthritis, cervical spondylosis, lumbar stenosis, peripheral vascular disease with or without amputation, vitamin B_{12} deficiency, Parkinson's, syphilis, myasthenia gravis, multiple sclerosis, Alzheimer's disease, seizure disorder or disorders of the feet? **See protocols on specific conditions. Severe osteoporosis and cancer with metastatic disease to the bone can cause a spontaneous (pathological) fracture, which results in a fall.**

✦ Refer to Displays 9-2, 9-3, and 9-4.

PHYSICAL EXAMINATION

✦ Vital signs; bilateral BP. **Hypothermia as well as febrile states increase risk of falls.** Orthostatic pulse and BP (absence of pulse increase and/or drop in SBP of 20 mm Hg from supine to standing). Weight.

✦ Skin: assess skin turgor (forehead, abdomen, or over sternum), assess for cyanosis, abrasions, lacerations, and ecchymosis. **Ecchymosis may not be apparent for 2–3 days following a fall.**

✦ HEENT: hearing and visual screening including visual proprioception. Check for nystagmus and associated vertigo. Otologic examination to rule

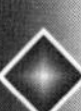

DISPLAY 9-2. *Epidemiology of Falls*

One-third of persons age 65+ will fall at least once a year.
Two-thirds of persons age 65+ in extended care will fall at least once a year.
Women aged 65–75 fall more frequently than men. After age 75, falls are similar in frequency.
Accidents are the fifth leading cause of death in the elderly; falls account for the greatest number of accidents in this age group.
Half of those who fall will fall repeatedly.
About 90% of those who fall have minor or no injuries.
About 5% of those who fall experience a fracture.
About 5% of those who fall experience other injuries that require medical attention.
Of those experiencing a fall requiring hospitalization, 50% will die within 1 year.
Of those experiencing a fall requiring medical attention, 25% will die within 1 year.
Some will develop functional decline related to injury, others become fearful and develop self-imposed immobilization and ADL dependence.
Approximately 40% of admissions to extended care are fall related.

out cerumen impaction or air/fluid levels in middle ear. Examine cervical spine for limitation in range of motion, presence of imbalance with motion. Auscultate carotids for bruit. Inspect and palpate thyroid for enlargement/nodule(s). Assess cranial nerves.

✦ Lungs: observe for hyperventilation; check oxygen saturation. Auscultate for crackles, decreased breath sounds (rule out congestive failure and pneumonia).

✦ Cardiac: auscultate for arrhythmia, murmur, gallop. Inspect jugular veins for distension.

✦ Extremities: Palpate femoral, popliteal, posterior tibial, and pedal pulses. Inspect amputation site and prosthesis if present. Inspect for misalignment, new onset of leg height variance, external rotation, or abduction suggestive of hip fracture. **See Protocol on Hip Fracture.** Inspect and palpate joints for acute inflammatory changes, pain, arthritic changes, abnormalities in range of motion and muscular strength/atrophy, and contractures. **Muscular strength that is especially important in fall prevention includes hip abduction, adduction, and extension; quadriceps and hamstrings (for extension and flexion of the knee); and ankle plantar and dorsiflexion.** Assess deep tendon reflexes and sensory paths to touch, vibration, pain, and sense of position. **Altered sense of vibration is the first sign of periph-**

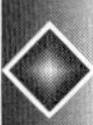

DISPLAY 9-3. *Fall Etiologies*

1. Extrinsic or environmental causes account for 1/3 of all falls.
2. Intrinsic or medical causes account for 2/3 of all falls.
   - Cardiovascular
   - Respiratory
   - Neurological
   - Orthopedic
   - Sensory
   - Cognitive impairment
   - Metabolic disorders such as hypoglycemia or hypoxia
   - Acute infections
   - Podiatric
   - Pharmacological

DISPLAY 9-4. *Risk Factors for Falls*

Gait impairment
Balance impairment
Cognitive decline
Depression
Incontinence
Polypharmacy
Medications: anticonvulsants, anxiolytics, antipsychotics, hypnotics, diuretics, antihistamines, tricyclic antidepressants, cardiac drugs, NSAIDs, antihypertensives
Sensory impairment
Previous fall
Use of assistive device for ambulation
Orthostasis
Number of chronic conditions
ADL dependence
Use of restraints

eral neuropathy. Assess for rigidity, spasticity, cogwheeling, and tremor. Assess for focal deficits. Inspect feet for dry, cracked, thickened soles; bunions; corns; calluses and poor nail hygiene. **Podiatric conditions are common causes/contributors to falls.**

✦ Palpate spine for tenderness.

✦ Assess patient's ability to get out of a chair; stand with eyes open, then closed; maintain balance during sternal nudge; ambulate (using appropriate adaptive aid if required); turn around; and sit down. Does the patient stop walking to speak? **A predictor of falls in the elderly.** Observe gait for sensory and cerebellar ataxia.

✦ Assess cognitive status using a standardized instrument. Consider dementia versus delirium. **See Protocols on Delirium and Dementia.**

✦ Assess for depression using a standardized instrument. Like dementia and delirium, depression causes lack of judgment and attention to safety. **See Protocol on Depression.**

✦ Assess baseline functional status (bathing, grooming, transferring, dressing, and continence). Observe for balance and difficulties in dressing. **Increased fall risk with dependent activities of daily living.**

✦ Assess wearing apparel and footwear for proper fit.

✦ Consider rectal examination and stool guaiac if suspected anemia.

DIAGNOSTIC TESTS

✦ Glucose, BUN, creatinine, calcium, and electrolytes.

✦ CBC.

✦ Thyroid profile.

✦ Therapeutic drug levels as appropriate (digoxin, phenytoin, lithium, valproic acid, etc.)

✦ Prothrombin time/INR if on coumadin.

✦ Consider urinalysis, culture and sensitivity.

✦ Consider prealbumin.

✦ Consider B_{12} and folate.

✦ Consider serological test for syphilis if suspicion is high for neurosyphilis.

✦ Consider baseline ECG, and as indicated by history and physical findings.

✦ X-ray suspected fracture site(s).

✦ Consider PA and lateral chest x-ray if pulmonary etiology is suspected.

✦ Consider Holter monitoring.

✦ Consider head CT/MRI with history of recurrent falls and head trauma or positive history/physical findings to rule out subdural hematoma/lesion, CVA/normal pressure hydrocephalus (NPH). Consult physician.

✦ Consider CT/MRI of cervical/lumbar spine as appropriate to rule out spondylosis/stenosis. Consult physician.

✦ Refer to ophthalmologist, audiologist if indicated.

✦ Consider referral to appropriate specialist, such as otolaryngologist, neurologist, cardiologist, podiatrist.

PREVENTION

- When addressing falls, prevention is the most important consideration.
- The goal of a preventive program is to reduce the risk of falls without creating functional limitation.
- Implementation of a fall prevention program begins with the identification of persons at risk of fall using a standardized assessment tool and a mechanism for communicating findings to care providers.
- The history and clinical findings guide an individualized fall prevention program.
- Any given fall usually has several underlying causes. Previous fall circumstances should be investigated.
- Prevention and management strategies overlap. **See Management.**
- Environmental risk factors to consider in the home:
  - Eliminate scatter rugs, buckled or loose carpeting.
  - Choose carpets with dense, short pile.
  - Avoid floor wax/buffing.
  - Redirect electrical/telephone cords.
  - Remove clutter.
  - Eliminate chairs that are unstable, too low, too soft, without arm rests, or on wheels.
  - Eliminate beds that are too high, too low. Patient should be able to sit safely on the side of the bed with both feet on the floor.
  - Apply protectors to furniture with sharp corners; consider placement of furniture for support, avoiding furniture as an obstacle.
  - Rearrange items in cabinets that are too high or too low.
  - Avoid ladders and step stools.
  - Avoid lighting that is too low or too bright, causing glare.
  - Provide accessible light switches to prevent walking in the dark to turn on a light.
  - Install night lighting; flashlight at bedside and other easily accessible areas in case of emergency.
  - Consider elevated commode seat/versa frame or grab bars if indicated; bedside commode/urinal use for nocturia/urge incontinence; grab bars in bathroom/bath tub or shower; and tub bench/transfer tub bench or shower chair/hand-held shower head.
  - Assure that shower or bath door is in good repair.
  - Provide slip-resistant surface in and outside the bath tub or shower.
  - Consider liquid instead of bar soaps; either, within easy access.
  - Apply contrasting tape or paint to stair edges inside and out.

- ✧ Install entryway handrails/ramps.
- ✧ Assure that outdoor walking surfaces are in good repair, well lit, and free of ice, snow, wet leaves, and loose gravel.
- ✧ Be alert for pets under foot.
- ✧ Be alert to items brought in or left by visitors, especially children.
- ✧ Assure that assistive devices (canes, walkers, wheelchairs, motorized scooters) are in good repair.
- ✧ Assure adaptive sensory aids such as corrective lenses and hearing aid(s) are appropriately cleaned and in good repair.

- ✦ Clothing:
  - ✧ Provide pants with legs of proper length. Consider use of suspenders.
  - ✧ Be alert to crepe-soled shoes. **May stick to floor covering if foot does not clear the floor during ambulation.**
  - ✧ Be alert to leather-soled shoes. **May be too slick.**
  - ✧ Proper shoe fit; low heel; be alert to imbalance secondary to wedged soles.
  - ✧ Avoid ambulation in hosiery or socks without shoes.
- ✦ **See Protocol on Prevention and Health Maintenance.**

MANAGEMENT

- ✦ Goal of acute fall management is the determination of injury followed by appropriate intervention.
- ✦ Adopt a multidisciplinary approach to fall evaluation and management.
- ✦ Treat/control underlying conditions when fall is related to an acute/chronic, stable condition (**see section on History**). **See Protocols on specific conditions.**
- ✦ Address polypharmacy. Initiate drug therapy at lowest possible dose, increasing slowly if needed. **See Chapter on Medication Issues.**
- ✦ For orthostatic hypotension: instruct patient to make changes in position slowly from supine to sitting, then standing, waiting several minutes between each change. Consider use of compression stockings. Avoid heavy meals. Consider sleeping with head of bed elevated at least 30°.
- ✦ For post-micturation syncope: encourage to sit while urinating.
- ✦ For balance and gait abnormalities: refer to PT and OT for evaluation, exercise treatment program, and assistive/adaptive devices.
- ✦ For recurrent falls: refer patient to PT to learn how to fall and get up safely.
- ✦ For weakness and impaired function: consider exercise/walking programs. For nonambulatory patients consider use of supervised rocking to increase muscle tone. Prevent immobilization.

✦ For drop attacks: consider evaluation for cervical collar. **Be alert to possible carotid compression with poorly fitted collar.**

✦ Consider referral to rehabilitation program to optimize function. Consult physician.

✦ For EtOH-related falls: suggest/refer willing candidate to substance abuse treatment program. **See Protocol on Substance Abuse.**

✦ Encourage use of mobile phone/telephone care lines/emergency call system.

✦ Suggest alternative living arrangement when level of function declines progressively and increased supervision is required.

✦ Consider sitting patient on nonskid mats with or without wedge cushions that position the patient backward in the chair. Consider recliners in nonambulating patients who are at risk of sliding or falling out of chairs. Refer to PT for training in wheelchair mobility if ambulation is no longer realistic.

✦ For falls associated with cognitive deficit and wandering, **see Chapter on Management of the Alzheimer's Patient** for behavioral management techniques.

KEY ISSUES

Patient/Caregiver Education

Patient/caregiver should be able to:

✦ Identify individualized risk factors.

✦ Verbalize understanding of prevention strategies as they apply.

✦ Demonstrate appropriate management skills.

Economic Considerations

✦ Home repairs/alterations may be costly. **Refer to social worker for community organizations/church groups willing to assist with minor home repairs at minimal cost.**

✦ Assistive devices are often not covered by insurance; financial limitations may prevent their use. **Refer to social worker for community organizations with "equipment closets" for temporary loan of equipment.**

Psychosocial Considerations

✦ Be alert to social withdrawal and further immobilization. **The psychological trauma of a fall is common. Fear of recurrent falls and loss of**

independence leads to further immobilization, increasing the risk of recurrent falls secondary to deconditioning.

✦ Consider referral to psychologist/psychiatrist if fear persists.

Acute/Inpatient Setting

✦ Identify patients at risk of falls/develop a multidisciplinary prevention program. **Falls within the hospital occur most commonly at the bedside during the transferring process.**

✦ Refer to PT/OT prior to patient becoming deconditioned.

✦ Prevent immobilization.

✦ Refer concerns of malnutrition, as a contributor to fall, to nutritionist.

✦ Place bedside table, telephone, grooming aids, glasses, hearing aid(s), medications, and dentures within easy access to patient.

✦ Assure that the nurse call light is available and patient demonstrates ability to use.

✦ Eliminate unnecessary tethers (IV, feeding tubes, Foley catheters, restraints).

✦ Initiate bladder and bowel training programs. Assure availability of urinal/bedside commode if indicated.

✦ Provide properly fitting nonskid footwear.

✦ Provide side rails/trapeze to increase bed mobility.

✦ Return bed to lowest position upon completion of patient care.

✦ Assure that the bed brakes are on and in good repair.

✦ Remove clutter, obstacles.

✦ Consider use of bed check monitors for cognitively impaired patient.

✦ Position cognitively impaired, agitated patient close to nurses' station, preferably within direct visualization.

✦ Assure that nightlights are in working order.

✦ Be alert to falls related to prepping procedures, fasting states, hypoglycemia, dehydration, and medications.

✦ Optimize pain management.

Extended Care Setting

✦ Initiate sensory deficit management including cleaning corrective lenses, cerumen management, and use of hearing aid(s) when indicated. **See Protocol on Cerumen Impaction.**

✦ Use contrasting colors to increase visibility. Avoid greens/blues.

✦ Implement orientation program.

✦ Consider implementation of a multidisciplinary falls consultant team.

✦ Refer foot disorders to a podiatrist.

✦ Provide adequate lighting.

✦ Avoid highly glossed floors with glare and flooring/carpeting with patterns that may lead to perceptual problems and abnormal gait in the resident with cognitive impairment.

✦ Educate all staff members to be alert for and clean up spills promptly.

✦ Assure that time-delayed doors are in working order to accommodate for slow-moving residents with assistive devices.

✦ Avoid restraints. **Physical restraints have been found to have a negative effect on quality of life and to contribute to functional decline, falls, injuries, and death.**

✦ Eliminate as many tethers as possible (such as IVs, tube feedings).

✦ Assure that side rails/bed brakes are in working order. Use recessed side rails.

✦ Provide nonslip flooring/skid-proof mats in bathing areas.

✦ Provide grab bars in bathrooms, elevated commode seats, and hand rails to assist in transfers.

✦ Assure that wheelchairs and assistive devices are in good repair.

✦ Implement fall risk identification and prevention program.

✦ Implement educational program for staff dealing with the resistive or combative cognitively impaired resident.

✦ In the presence of cognitive impairment, encourage involvement of significant other(s) in care. Reduce unnecessary stimulation (noise/activity).

✦ Implement bowel and bladder training programs.

✦ Place antiskid mat under hips on bedside to prevent slipping and a mat under feet at bedside to assist with transfers without sliding.

✦ Consider placement of the mattress on the floor to prevent recurrent falls from the bed, especially in the cognitively impaired.

✦ Consider "drug holidays."

Home Setting

✦ Consider home health PT/OT referral for safety check of environment and use of new adaptive equipment.

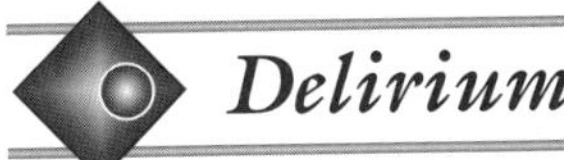

Delirium

HISTORY

✦ Description of current symptoms? **Sudden onset of cognitive impairment, disorientation, disturbances in attention, and perceptual disturbances suggest delirium. Agitation, change in sleep patterns, and/or irritability may be early signs of delirium. Hallucinations are more common with delirium than with dementia. Mental status may wax and wane.**

✦ Onset, duration, course of symptoms? **Delirium is an acute confusional state as opposed to a progressive memory impairment. Delirium may be superimposed upon a dementia and should be considered with an acute worsening of symptoms in patient with a diagnosed dementia.**

✦ Recent acute illness, infection, medication change, hospitalization or surgery?

✦ History of chronic diseases, i.e., diabetes mellitus, hypertension, cardiac disease, lung disease, liver disease, GI bleed, renal disease, TIAs, CVA, Parkinson's disease, dementia, depression, or cancer? **Delirium may be the result of an exacerbation of an underlying chronic disease. Patients with underlying dementia have an increased risk of delirium when stressed.**

✦ Review of systems? Note presence of fever, chills, or acute changes in any system, i.e., chest pain, dyspnea, dysuria, constipation, diarrhea, vomiting, recent falls, or neurological signs.

✦ Medications: prescription/OTC? **Common underlying cause of delirium. Any medication should be considered as potentially suspect (see Display 9-5).**

✦ EtOH use? Consider use of a questionnaire for alcoholism evaluation, such as the CAGE (JAMA 1984;252:1905–7) to assess.

✦ Baseline functional status? Change in functional status?

✦ Social situation, supports? Caregiver stress?

PHYSICAL EXAMINATION

✦ Vital signs, weight. Note orthostasis, change in weight from previous visits.

✦ Note facial expression, level of alertness, orientation, appearance, clothing, hygiene, ability to answer questions and follow commands.

✦ Focused physical examination based upon presenting symptoms and comorbid conditions.

✦ Cognitive assessment. **See Protocol on Dementia.**

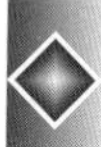

DISPLAY 9-5. ***Medications That May Cause Cognitive Impairment***

Antiarrhythmic agents	Antiparkinsonian agents
Antibiotics	Cardiotonic agents
Anticholinergic agents	Corticosteroids
Anticonvulsants	Histamine H2 receptor antagonists
Antidepressants	Immunosuppressive agents
Antiemetics	Muscle relaxants
Antihypertensive agents	Narcotic analgesics
Antimanic agents	NSAIDS
Antineoplastic agents	Radiocontrast agents
Antihistamine/decongestants	Sedatives

- Depression screening. **See Protocol on Depression.**
- Functional assessment. **See Protocol on Dementia.**

DIAGNOSTIC TESTS

- **See Protocol on Dementia.** Goal is to identify and treat underlying cause of delirium.
- Initial tests should focus on most common causes of delirium; check CBC, serum electrolytes, BUN, creatinine, urinalysis. Consider chest x-ray and assessment of oxygen saturation if respiratory symptoms. Proceed on to other tests as indicated. Assess status of comorbid conditions.
- Drug levels or screens if appropriate, i.e., anticonvulsants, digoxin, theophylline, ASA, antiarrhythmics, heavy metals, EtOH, benzodiazepines, valproic acid, illicit drugs.
- Consider computerized tomography (CT) of head to rule out CVA, subdural hematoma or other CNS lesion. Consult physician.

PREVENTION

- Maintain adequate hydration and nutrition in frail elderly at risk for delirium.
- Be alert to subtle changes in physical, cognitive, and functional status in frail and/or demented elderly at risk for delirium.
- Avoid medications that may cause or exacerbate delirium. **See Chapter on Medication Issues.** Review medications carefully at each visit.
- **See Protocol on Prevention and Health Maintenance.**

MANAGEMENT

✦ Delirium is a medical emergency. When possible, identify underlying cause. **Most common causes include fluid and electrolyte imbalances, infections, and medications. Refer if cause not readily determined.**

✦ Treat identified systemic abnormalities. Consult with physician.

✦ Stabilize underlying chronic diseases.

✦ Review medication regimen. Discontinue medications, when possible, which may cause or exacerbate delirium.

✦ Consider short-term symptom management. **See Chapter on Management of the Alzheimer's Patient, Table 19-2.**

KEY ISSUES

Patient/Caregiver Education

Patient/caregiver should be able to:

✦ Recognize acute changes in physical, functional, or cognitive status that may necessitate medical evaluation and intervention.

✦ Verbalize an understanding of the difference in dementia and delirium.

✦ Identify safety concerns with the patient and intervene appropriately to keep patient safe.

Economic Considerations

✦ Delirium can complicate or prolong co-existing illness, obscure underlying diagnosis, and result in or extend hospitalization.

Psychosocial Considerations

✦ Caregivers need support and education concerning delirium and its often unpredictable course.

✦ Delirium is frightening for patients. Reassurance, reorientation, attention to comfort, and provision of a safe environment are important considerations.

Acute/Inpatient Setting

✦ Be alert to delirium in the hospital setting; very common in the postoperative patient.

✦ Avoid medications that can cause or exacerbate delirium.

✦ Assess and manage pain effectively. **See Chapter on Pain Management.**

✦ Minimize tethers, i.e., IV lines, oxygen, catheters, side rails, restraints. Mobilize patient and maintain function.

✦ Promote an effective bowel regimen. **See Protocol on Constipation.**

✦ Provide consistent routine as much as possible, especially in patients with dementia.

✦ Provide prescribed sensory aids, i.e., corrective lenses, hearing aids, pocket talker.

✦ Avoid use of restraints when possible; place patient in room near nursing station, consider a sitter, use behavioral management techniques as alternatives to restraints. Follow restraint policy in terms of frequency of orders and appropriate documentation.

✦ Minimize use of Foley catheter. Increased incidence of urinary tract infection (UTI) with chronic Foley.

✦ Consider OT and PT consults to assess and maximize function during acute hospitalization.

✦ Consult pharmacist to review medications.

✦ Address safety issues related to wandering and falls. Implement fall prevention program. **See Protocol on Falls.**

✦ Approach patient in a calm manner, re-orienting him or her to your name and to what you are doing.

Extended Care Setting

✦ Be alert to signs of dehydration, malnutrition, and infection. **Common causes of delirium.**

✦ Avoid unnecessary medications; review medication regimen frequently.

✦ Avoid chronic Foley catheter use.

✦ Consider hospitalization of patient with acute delirium when etiology is not readily identified.

Home Setting

✦ Maintain adequate hydration and nutrition.

✦ Set up system for medication compliance if necessary.

✦ Address safety issues in the home environment.

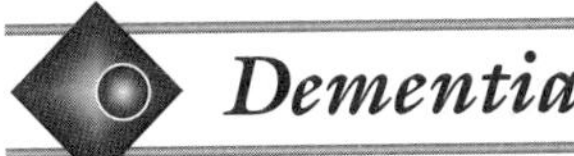

Dementia

HISTORY

✦ Description of current symptoms? **Family member or caregiver is often historian. Patient may deny symptoms. Be alert to early cognitive changes during routine evaluations. See Display 9-6.**

✦ Presence of aphasia, apraxia, agnosia, or disturbance of executive function? **See Display 9-7.**

✦ Onset (abrupt vs. gradual), duration, course (stepwise vs. continuous) of symptoms? **Family may overlook or compensate for symptoms for some time.**

✦ Behavioral problems: repetitive behaviors or speech, delusions, hallucinations (visual or auditory), paranoia, wandering, sleep disturbances, agitation, combativeness, lack of inhibitions, sexual aggressiveness?

✦ Safety concerns? **Ask about complex tasks, i.e., managing finances, paying bills, driving, cooking.**

✦ Previous medical/psychiatric evaluations? Previous dementia evaluation? When? What was family told?

✦ History of head trauma, especially if associated with loss of consciousness? **May be associated with increased incidence of dementia.**

✦ History and status of chronic diseases, i.e., diabetes mellitus, hypertension, cardiac disease, COPD, liver or renal disease, TIAs, CVA, Parkinson's disease, or cancer?

DISPLAY 9-6. *Warning Signs of Early Dementia*

- ✦ Difficulty learning and retaining new information.
- ✦ Repetitive conversation or behavior.
- ✦ Difficulty with short-term memory, i.e., misplaces objects, misses appointments, cannot recall recent discussions.
- ✦ Difficulty handling complex tasks that require multiple steps.
- ✦ Difficulty with problem solving in common situations.
- ✦ Difficulty driving; gets lost easily.
- ✦ Difficulty with word finding.
- ✦ Personality changes, i.e., more irritable, less self-directed, more suspicious.
- ✦ Changes in dress, appearance, hygiene, i.e., wears mismatched clothes, wears same outfit for several days, forgets to bathe.

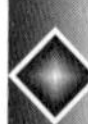

DISPLAY 9-7. *DSM-IV Criteria for Dementia*

- ✦ Multiple cognitive deficits including memory impairment and one or more of the following: aphasia, apraxia, agnosia, and/or disturbance of executive function.
- ✦ Must cause significant impairment in social or occupational function.
- ✦ Must represent a decline from previous function.
- ✦ Must *not* be due to a major depressive disorder or schizophrenia.

✦ History of Down's syndrome?

✦ Review of systems? **Especially note presence of sensory deficits, weight loss, anorexia, gait disturbances, or falls.**

✦ Recent acute illness or infection, i.e., pneumonia, UTI? Recent hospitalization or surgery?

✦ History of depression, mental illness, or mental retardation?

✦ EtOH use?

✦ Family history of dementia (especially early onset Alzheimer's disease), depression, mental illness?

✦ Current medications: prescription/OTC? **Wide range of medications can cause or exacerbate cognitive changes. Consider any medication potentially suspect.**

✦ Educational level? Primary language? Cultural background? Work history? Exposure to environmental toxins? **Patient with dementia may revert to native language. Consider use of an interpreter.**

✦ Functional abilities/limitations? Social withdrawal? Loss of interest in usual activities or hobbies?

✦ Social supports, living arrangement, caregiver(s)? Caregiver burden, level of understanding?

PHYSICAL EXAMINATION

✦ Complete physical examination on initial visit. **See Chapter on Management of the Alzheimer's Patient** for subsequent visits.

✦ Note facial expression, level of alertness, orientation, appearance, clothing, hygiene, and ability to answer questions and follow commands.

✦ Height, weight, vital signs. Note orthostasis.

✦ Assess skin: note presence and location of pressure ulcers, bruising, excoriations. Note skin turgor. Be alert for signs of possible elder abuse.

✦ HEENT: assess temporal arteries; assess eyes for visual acuity, presence of cataracts, retinopathy, glaucoma, macular degeneration; assess hearing and note presence of cerumen in ears; note condition of gums, teeth, dentures; palpate thyroid.

✦ Cardiovascular: note irregularities, abnormal heart sounds, presence of bruits, peripheral pulses.

✦ Respiratory: note respiratory rate, use of accessory muscles, breath sounds, adventitious sounds.

✦ Breasts: assess for nodules, drainage.

✦ Abdomen: note liver size, percuss for distended bladder, assess for abdominal aortic aneurysm.

✦ Rectal: assess sphincter tone, presence of stool, impaction, stool for guaiac.

✦ Neurological examination: note focal neurological changes or extrapyramidal signs. **Will have normal neurological examination with Alzheimer's disease.**

✦ Musculoskeletal: note gait, strength, range of motion. **Gait disturbances more common in extrapyramidal disorders, vascular dementia, and hydrocephalus.**

✦ Cognitive assessment. Use of a standardized tool is recommended, such as the modified Mini-Mental Status Examination (3MSE). Note impairment of language, word-finding, judgment, short-term memory throughout the interview. Clock drawing test may be useful. **Brief mental status tests are screening tools and are not diagnostic. There is risk of a false-positive result with patients with low educational levels and a false-negative result with patients with high educational levels. Tools are useful in establishing a baseline for monitoring cognitive impairment over time.**

✦ Depression screening. Use of standardized tool is recommended, such as the Beck depression screening or Geriatric Depression Scale.

✦ Functional assessment. Observe patient throughout examination, i.e., ability to undress/dress, rise from a chair, transfer to and from the examination table. Use of an informant-based standardized test, such as the Functional Activities Questionnaire (FAQ), may be useful.

DIAGNOSTIC TESTS

✦ Complete a dementia evaluation with focus on differentiating between treatable and untreatable etiologies.

✦ CBC, erythrocyte sedimentation rate (ESR), antinuclear antibodies, serum electrolytes, calcium, glucose, BUN, creatinine, albumin/prealbumin, liver function tests, thyroid-stimulating hormone (TSH), free T4, folate level, vitamin B_{12} level, syphilis serology, and urinalysis.

✦ Apolipoprotein E: not thought to be diagnostic alone, consider when patient meets clinical criteria of Alzheimer's disease.

✦ Consider specific laboratory tests based on history and physical examination, i.e., HIV antibodies, serum cortisol levels, hemoglobin Alc.

✦ Drug levels or screens if appropriate, i.e., anticonvulsants, digoxin, theophylline, ASA, antiarrhythmics, heavy metals, benzodiazepines, valproic acid, EtOH, illicit drugs.

✦ Consider oxygen saturation (O_2 sat or arterial blood gases) if history of respiratory problems Consider ECG to rule out silent MI, arrhythmias.

✦ CT of head (noncontrasted).

✦ Consider MRI if history suggests vascular dementia with brain stem involvement. Consult with physician.

✦ The role of single photon emission computed tomography (SPECT) and positron emission tomography (PET) is not fully established; generally only done in a research setting.

✦ Consider EEG if history suggestive of seizure disorder or in rapidly progressing dementia. Consult with physician. **See Protocol on Seizures.**

✦ Consider referral for lumbar puncture if history suggestive of metastatic disease, CNS infections, systemic lupus erythematosus, multiple sclerosis, hydrocephalus. Consult with physician.

✦ Consider referral for neuropsychological testing for comorbid mental health symptoms or to identify early dementia.

PREVENTION

✦ Address safety issues with patient and caregiver. **See Chapter on Management of the Alzheimer's Patient.**

✦ **See Protocol on Prevention and Health Maintenance.**

MANAGEMENT

✦ Early dementia may be difficult to detect especially in patients with high premorbid cognitive function. If dementia evaluation is normal, including mental status screening, reassure patient/family. Consider referral for neuropsychological testing especially if patient/family expresses extreme concern, or reassess in 6–12 months or if acute changes occur.

✦ If criteria for dementia are not met, consider diagnosis of depression, age-related cognitive changes, underlying mental illness, or delirium.

✦ If symptoms of depression, **see Protocol on Depression.**

✦ If evaluation suggests delirium, **see Protocol on Delirium.** Dementia can co-exist with delirium and/or depression.

✦ Refer as indicated to psychiatrist, psychologist, psychiatric clinical nurse specialist, licensed clinical social worker.

✦ Review diagnostic test results with physician and treat identified systemic abnormalities: Vitamin B_{12} deficiency (**see Protocol on Anemia**), hypothyroidism (**see Protocol on Hypothyroidism**), electrolyte disturbances (**see Protocol on Fluid and Electrolyte Abnormalities**), renal insufficiency (**see Protocol on Renal Failure**). See protocols for other conditions as appropriate.

✦ Refer as indicated for abnormal lesions on CT scan or MRI, i.e., CVA, subdural hematoma (SDH), abscess, primary CNS tumor, or brain metastasis.

✦ Review and adjust medication regimen as indicated. **Drug toxicity, drug–drug interactions, polypharmacy may contribute to symptoms. See Chapter on Medication Issues.**

✦ Treat underlying acute disease and stabilize chronic disease when present.

✦ Consider referral to geriatric psychiatry for troublesome behaviors if not responding to behavioral or pharmacological management.

✦ Consider referral for genetic testing and counseling if family requests.

✦ **Alzheimer's disease:** dementia with a gradual onset and progressive course not due to a CNS disease or systemic disease. No conclusive test available; remains a clinical diagnosis of exclusion. **See Chapter on Management of the Alzheimer's Patient.**

✦ **Vascular dementia:** dementia with focal neurological signs and symptoms or clinical and laboratory evidence of CV disease. Course is often a step-wise decline. Also called multi-infarct dementia. **See Chapter on Management of the Alzheimer's Patient** and **Protocol on Transient Ischemic Attack (TIA)/Cerebrovascular Accident (CVA).**

✦ **Lewy body dementia:** Alzheimer's like dementia characterized by marked visual hallucinations, mild Parkinsonian symptoms, delusions, fluctuating mental status, and neuroleptic sensitivity. Avoid neuroleptic medications that can worsen symptoms. **See Chapter on Management of the Alzheimer's Patient.**

✦ **Normal pressure hydrocephalus (NPH):** defined by the triad of dementia, gait dysfunction, and urinary incontinence. May be suggested by CT scan of head. Rare cause of dementia. Special neurological diagnostic studies required for confirmation. Consult with physician. **Longer the duration of symptoms, less likely to see improvement with shunting procedure.** Consider PT evaluation for recommendation for assistive devices.

✦ Consider less common causes of dementia: Pick's disease, Creutzfeldt–Jacob disease, Huntington's chorea, Wilson's disease, heavy metal toxicity, dementia pugilistica.

✦ **Patient may have a "mixed dementia," i.e., Alzheimer's disease and vascular dementia related to CVAs.**

KEY ISSUES

Patient/Caregiver Education

Patient/caregiver should be able to:

✦ Verbalize understanding of terms dementia, delirium, and depression.

✦ Verbalize understanding of the process of evaluation and diagnosis of dementia.

✦ Verbalize knowledge of community resources available.

✦ Recognize acute changes in physical, functional, or cognitive status that may represent new problems requiring medical evaluation and intervention.

✦ Identify behavioral strategies to effectively manage troublesome behaviors. **See Chapter on Management of the Alzheimer's Patient, Table 19-1.**

✦ Identify safety concerns with the patient and intervene appropriately to keep patient safe.

✦ Assist the patient in maintaining dignity and independence as long as possible.

Economic Considerations

✦ Ongoing dementia care is expensive, with care needs often not meeting the Medicare criteria for skilled home or facility care.

✦ Services such as respite care, adult day care, sitter services, transportation, and assisted living are generally not covered under Medicare.

✦ Pharmacological therapy is costly and often requires prior authorization under managed care plans; must document cognitive function with standardized mental status examination.

Psychosocial Considerations

✦ Caregiver stress is often significant and must be addressed as an important aspect of ongoing care in any setting.

✦ Be alert to signs of depression in both the patient with dementia and the caregiver(s).

✦ As dementia progresses, caregiver(s) will often begin grief process.

✦ Refer caregiver(s) as appropriate for counseling; support groups may be helpful.

Acute/Inpatient Setting

✦ There is a high incidence of delirium in the acute care setting; be alert to acute confusional states, even in the patient with dementia.

✦ Maintain a consistent routine as much as possible; contact family/caregiver or referring extended care facility to obtain information on routine, behavioral management strategies, bowel/bladder regimen, and baseline cognitive function.

✦ Address safety concerns related to falls and wandering. **See Protocol on Falls.**

✦ Avoid use of restraints when possible; place patient in room near nursing station, consider a sitter, use behavioral management strategies as alternatives to restraints. Follow restraint policy in terms of frequency of orders and appropriate documentation.

Extended Care Setting

✦ Implement fall prevention, wandering, and behavioral management programs. Educate nonlicensed staff on care of patients with dementia.

✦ Be alert to signs of dehydration, malnutrition, and infection. First sign may be a subtle worsening in mental status or an increase in behavioral problems, i.e., agitation, yelling.

✦ Provide stage-appropriate interventions to assist with ADLs and manage troublesome behaviors. **See Chapter on Management of the Alzheimer's Patient, Table 19-1.**

Home Setting

✦ Consider adult day care, inpatient/outpatient respite care, or support groups as modalities that may help maintain a patient in the home and decrease caregiver stress.

✦ Modify home environment as needed for safety, i.e., disconnect stove, lower temperature on water heater, remove harmful objects such as guns or knives, eliminate clutter.

Chapter 10

Endocrine System

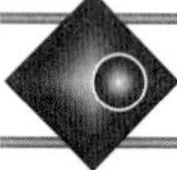

Diabetes Mellitus

HISTORY

✦ **Be aware that complications of diabetes mellitus (DM), i.e., retinopathy, nephropathy, impotence, gastroparesis, neuropathy, cardiovascular disease (CVD), peripheral vascular disease (PVD), balance/gait disturbances, are often presenting symptoms in the elderly rather than acute symptomatology.**

✦ Weight change? Polydipsia? Polyphagia? Anorexia? Early satiety?

✦ Polyuria (quantify)? Nocturia? Urinary incontinence? Dysuria?

✦ History of recurrent infections (bacterial and/or fungal)?

✦ Visual changes? **Especially note blurry vision.**

✦ Diarrhea?

✦ Any numbness, tingling, pain, or decreased sensation in extremities?

✦ Sexual dysfunction?

✦ Vaginal itching?

✦ Comorbid conditions? History of pancreatic disease, Cushing's disease, Grave's disease, hypothyroidism, hypertension, coronary artery disease (CAD)/angina, dyslipidemia, obesity, cerebrovascular accident (CVA), PVD, renal disease?

✦ History of gestational diabetes, delivery of infant > 9 pounds, or other complications of pregnancy?

✦ Medication review including OTC medications? **Note especially medications that can increase glucose levels, i.e., glucocorticoids, thiazide diuretics, furosemide, lithium, tricyclics, estrogen, beta-blockers, haloperidol, phenytoin, INH, nicotonic acid, levodopa.**

✦ Family history of diabetes, dyslipidemia, renal disease, or hypothyroidism?

✦ Race? **Hispanics, African Americans, Asian Americans, and Native Americans are at increased risk.**

✦ Diet history?

✦ Activity level (sedentary life-style increases risk)? Recent change?

✦ Functional status?

✦ Sensory or perceptual impairments?

✦ Economic status?

✦ Educational level? Literacy? Tobacco use? EtOH use?

✦ Living situation?

PHYSICAL EXAMINATION

✦ Height. Weight (> 20 pounds over ideal body weight increases risk). Vital signs: blood pressure (BP) in lying, sitting, standing positions to screen for autonomic dysfunction.

✦ Mental status examination. Depression screening, if indicated.

✦ Eyes: visual acuity, retinal examination for exudates, hemorrhages.

✦ Oral: caries, dry mucous membranes, gingival tenderness, signs of candidal infection.

✦ Neck: palpate thyroid, auscultate for bruits.

✦ Cardiovascular: assess heart sounds, palpate peripheral pulses, assess for signs of peripheral vascular disease.

✦ Skin: turgor, lesions, or ulcers; observe for signs of fungal or bacterial infection. **Careful examination of feet is critical.**

✦ Musculoskeletal: Assess for Duypyrtren's contractures; cheiroarthropathy; Charcot's joint.

✦ Abdomen: assess for organomegaly.

✦ Neurological: assess proprioception, vibratory sensation, sharp/dull, deep tendon reflexes.

✦ Genitourinary: palpate bladder for signs of urinary retention; females: assess for signs of vaginal candidiasis.

DIAGNOSTIC TESTS

✦ **Diabetes mellitus is diagnosed based on the following glucose levels:** Fasting plasma glucose (FPG) ≥ 126 on two occasions OR random plasma glucose ≥ 200 with symptoms of hyperglycemia OR plasma glucose ≥ 200 2 hr postprandial on two occasions even with FPG ≤ 126.

✦ **Impaired glucose tolerance** is indicated by FPG ≥ 126 AND 2-hr postprandial glucose ≥ 126 and < 200.

✦ Glucose tolerance testing (GTT) is not necessary for diagnosis when there is fasting hyperglycemia, and GTT is contraindicated in ill or inactive patients. Results may be affected by beta-blockers, diuretics, or nicotinic acid.

✦ **Glycosylated hemoglobin (HbA_{1c}). Normal 4.0–6.0.** Routine monitoring every 3 months. More frequent monitoring may be required when therapy is being adjusted to improve blood glucose (BG) control.

✧ HbA_{1c} ≅ average BG: 7.0 ≅ 150; 8.0 ≅ 180; 9.0 ≅ 210; 10.0 ≅ 240; 11.0 ≅ 270; 12.0 ≅ 300; 13.0 ≅ 330.

✦ **Electrolytes, blood urea nitrogen (BUN)** if suspected hyperglycemia or dehydration.

✦ **Serum creatinine.**

✦ **Urinalysis** for glucose, ketones, protein.

✦ Urine culture if symptomatic.

✦ **24-hr urine** to assess for microalbuminuria/albuminuria.

✦ Fasting lipid profile (total cholesterol, high-density lipoprotein [HDL], low-density lipoprotein [LDL], triglycerides). Triglycerides may be markedly elevated while hyperglycemia is present.

✦ Thyroid function tests.

✦ Liver function tests if indicated before beginning specific therapy.

✦ Electrocardiogram (ECG).

PREVENTION

✦ Given the results of the Diabetes Control and Complications Trial, the treatment goal for patients with Type 1 DM should be for tight control (HbA_{1c} of 7.2 and mean BG of 155) to prevent long-term complications. Results of the Kumaoto study indicate that similar control should be strived for in patients with Type 2 DM. However, intensive therapy with insulin or sulfonylureas increases the risk for hypoglycemia. Tight BG control may not be appropriate in elderly patients because atherosclerosis often co-exists with DM, posing increased risk for CVA or MI precipitated by hypoglycemia. Many patients with Type 2 DM are obese, and tight control with insulin or sulfonylureas contributes to weight gain. **Strive for the best BG control possible to prevent long-term complications without jeopardizing the elderly patient's safety and lifestyle.**

✦ **Smoking cessation** is of utmost importance.

✦ Annual dilated retinal examination especially important in patients with uncontrolled hyperglycemia.

✦ Daily foot examination for ulcers, lacerations. Wear protective foot covering at all times. **See Patient/Caregiver Education.**

✦ Emphasize importance of regular dental examinations and good oral hygiene.

✦ Correct the myth of "a touch of diabetes"; stress that potential complications from Type 2 DM are equivalent to those from Type 1 DM.

✦ Encourage weight loss/management in obese patients. Stress that even moderate weight loss can improve glucose tolerance significantly.

✦ **Control hypertension and hyperlipidemia. See Protocols on Hypertension and Hyperlipidemia.**

✦ The patient should carry identification that he or she has diabetes, **especially if taking insulin or oral hypoglycemic agents.**

✦ Emphasize critical need to check BG immediately before driving if on insulin or oral hypoglycemic agents.

✦ **See Protocol on Prevention and Health Maintenance.**

MANAGEMENT

✦ Consult physician if long-term complications exist, if refractory to treatment, or for emergent presentation. **See Acute/Inpatient Setting.**

✦ Goals are to safely maintain BG control as close to normal range as possible; monitor/prevent long-term complications; and maximize patient's quality of life.

✦ Individualize therapy based on etiology (Type 1/Type 2), presenting level of BG control, presence of long-term complications, co-existing illness, and risk factors.

✦ Refer to nutritionist if available or provide guidelines for daily food intake as follows: 10–20% protein; 20–30% fat; 50–60% carbohydrates. If weight loss is needed, institute moderate caloric restriction (500 calories less than average daily intake) coupled with regular exercise. Severe caloric restriction should be avoided in the elderly due to increased risk for nutritional deficiencies.

✦ After pre-exercise screening (exercise-stress ECG), begin 20-minute sessions (3 per week) of aerobic exercise.

✧ Instruct patient regarding the importance of appropriate warm-up and cool-down strategies

✧ Advise patient to check BG before exercise. Advise not to exercise if BG > 300. If BG < 140, carbohydrate intake will be necessary to prevent exercise-induced hypoglycemia (depending on intensity and duration of exercise). Refer to diabetes education clinic for more specific exercise guidelines.

✧ Isometric exercise should be avoided if retinopathy is present.

✦ Begin home blood glucose monitoring (HBGM). **See Patient/Caregiver Education.**

✦ Consider referral to diabetes education clinic/endocrinologist for deficits that complicate management.

✦ Consider use of blood glucose monitors, injection devices designed for patients with visual impairment/arthritis/musculoskeletal deficits.

Type I DM

✦ Caused by lack of insulin secretion by pancreas.

✦ Classic presentation includes symptoms of acute weight loss, polydipsia, polyuria, polyphagia, possible ketoacidosis. **See Acute/Inpatient Setting.**

✦ **New diagnosis in the elderly is uncommon.** May see elderly patient with life-long diagnosis of Type 1.

✦ Type 1 DM patients require insulin to sustain life. Basal insulin requirement is given as intermediate-acting insulin. Rapid-acting insulin provides meal coverage.

✦ Dosage is calculated based on body weight (usual 0.3–0.5 unit/kg; range 0.1–0.8 units/kg); 30–50% of daily dose is given as intermediate-acting (basal insulin) with the remainder in divided doses at meals to match carbohydrate intake. The ratio of insulin to carbohydrate intake varies among individuals; may begin with 1 unit insulin : 15g carbohydrates. Insulin doses must be adjusted based on HBGM results and level of activity.

✦ **Insulin preparations:** Human recombinant and DNA preparations are preferred for use in the elderly to reduce antigenicity.

✦ **Rapid-acting:**

✧ Regular—inject 30 minutes before eating

✧ Humalog (lispro)—inject Humalog when beginning to eat. Many elderly are erratic eaters which complicates choice of appropriate insulin dose with meals. Humalog, with its quick onset of action, is useful because it can be injected after a meal. Humalog also helps to reduce postprandial hyperglycemia quicker than Regular.

✦ **Intermediate-acting:**

✧ NPH, Lente, Ultrlente

Type 2 DM

✦ Caused by deficient β-cell function and insulin resistance.

✦ **Majority of patients over age 60 who present with new diagnosis have Type 2 DM.**

✦ Begin diet and exercise therapy to control BG.

✦ If use of diet/exercise does not control BG, pharmacological treatment usually begins with a single oral agent. If BG is uncontrolled with initial agent, (1) increase dose or (2) add second agent. May be necessary to proceed to combination of oral agent/insulin or insulin alone for control.

✦ **Oral agents:** Used as monotherapy or in combination with other oral agents or insulin as indicated. Selection of agent is dependent on patient profile.

✧ **Sulfonylureas: Glucotrol (glipizide) and Amaryl (glimepiride) are best choices because of lower incidence of severe hypoglycemia.** Begin Glucotrol (glipizide) 5 mg with breakfast, maximum dose 40 mg daily in divided doses before meals; also available as Glucotrol XL (sustained-release glipizide) 5 mg with breakfast, maximum dose 20 mg daily. Begin Amaryl (glimepiride) 2 mg with first main meal, in patients with impaired renal function or prior sensitivity to hypoglycemia agents—1 mg with first main meal; maximum dose 4 mg daily. Diabinese (chlorpropramide) is not recommended due to increased risk for hypoglycemia and subsequent myocardial infarction (MI) and CVA.

✧ **Biguanides:** Glucophage (metformin HCl) useful as adjunct to diet or in combination with sulfonylurea; may improve lipid profile; nausea/vomiting/diarrhea are potential side effects. Begin with 500 mg once daily and increase by 500 mg/day by 1-week intervals, take with meals, maximum dose 2,500 mg daily in 3 divided doses. **Contraindications:** renal dysfunction, creatinine > 1.5; liver dysfunction; heart disease; lung disease; history of EtOH abuse; acute or chronic metabolic acidosis or lactic acidosis. **Discontinue 48 hr prior to surgery or radiological tests.**

✧ **Alpha-glucosidase inhibitors:** Precose (acarbose) inhibits carbohydrate digestion; does not cause hypoglycemia but may potentiate hypoglycemia effect of sulfonylurea; does not cause weight gain; no effect on lipid profile; most frequent side effect is flatulence—improve tolerance with slow titration of dose. Begin with 25 mg with first bite of breakfast for 1–2 weeks; increase gradually to 25 mg tid with each meal, maximum dose 50 mg tid if weight < 60 kg, 100 mg tid if weight > 60 kg. **Contraindications:** liver impairment, irritable bowel syndrome, bowel obstruction, colostomy, bowel resection, history of cirrhosis or diabetic ketoacidosis.

✧ **Thiazolidinediones:** Rezulin (troglitazone) improves insulin sensitivity. Begin with 200 mg once daily, increase by 200-mg increments, maximum dose 600 mg once daily. If used in combination with insulin, insulin doses may require adjustment based on HBGM. **Contraindications:** hepatic dysfunction. Monitoring of liver function is required at initiation and throughout therapy. Patients should be aware of signs/symptoms of liver dysfunction.

✦ If poorly controlled with oral therapy, consider initiation of single morning dose of intermediate-acting insulin to control BG during day; if FBG remains elevated, add bed time dose; OR begin therapy with twice daily doses.

✦ Insulin dosage must be initiated based on weight (usual 0.3–0.5 units/kg, range 0.1–0.8 units/kg) and adjusted based on HBGM. Level of activity must also be considered in determining doses. Approximately 30–50% of total daily dose is given as intermediate-acting insulin (basal requirement). **Larger doses are usually required in Type 2 than in Type 1.**

✦ Add rapid-acting insulin with meals to control postprandial hyperglycemia. Dosages based on usual carbohydrate intake at meals.

✦ Both Regular and Humalog may be mixed in same syringe with NPH and Ultralente. Mixed doses of Regular or Humalog and Ultralente should be taken immediately.

✦ Frequency of follow-up is dependent on BG control, medication regimen changes, and existence of long-term complication.

KEY ISSUES

Patient/Caregiver Education

Patient/caregiver should be able to:

✦ Explain significance of HbA_{1c} results to self-management of DM.

✦ List potential long-term complications of uncontrolled hyperglycemia and discuss importance of good BG control.

✦ List dietary/exercise recommendations and their potential for improving BG control.

✦ Identify signs, symptoms, and alleviating strategies for hyperglycemia.

✦ Verbalize signs, symptoms, and treatment of hypoglycemia (if taking medications that can cause the condition). Caution not to overtreat hypoglycemia to prevent subsequent hyperglycemia.

✦ Demonstrate proper technique for HBGM including technique for obtaining sample, use of monitor, troubleshooting techniques when suspected false results, recording values. Identify importance of bringing results of HBGM to every clinic visit. Frequency and timing of HBGM varies with therapy, status of current control, and goals for BG control.

✦ Identify potential barriers to self-management and verbalize strategies for problem-solving.

✦ Verbalize medication regimen, doses, and potential side effects.

✦ When applicable, state proper technique for drawing up insulin, selection of site, injecting, storage of insulin, disposal of syringes, and transporting insulin for travel.

✦ Discuss importance of daily foot care and examination.

✦ Verbalize sick-day rules:

  ✧ If vomiting, diarrhea, elevated BG occur, call nurse practitioner (NP)/clinic.

  ✧ HBGM every 2–3 hours while ill.

✧ If BG > 240, check urine for ketones and report results to NP/clinic.

✧ If patient is not vomiting but solid foods cannot be tolerated, continue to take insulin and substitute fluids to fulfill usual carbohydrate intake. Continue to take oral agents except for those that require taking with food.

✧ Maintain hydration.

Economic Considerations

✦ Supplies and medications required for management are expensive. Consider cost of therapy. Assist patient with approval for nonformulary items.

✦ Insurors and Medicare are now required by federal legislation to reimburse for diabetes supplies and education.

✦ "Sugar-free" foods are usually more costly. Educate patients regarding lower-cost dietary alternatives.

Psychosocial Considerations

✦ Encourage verbalization of personal losses associated with diabetes mellitus, e.g., economic, body image, sexual relationships. Help patient to identify coping strategies.

Acute/Inpatient Setting

✦ Patients with Type 1 DM may present with symptoms of **diabetic ketoacidosis (DKA)** and should be **urgently admitted.** Usual presentation: BG > 300; pH < 7.3; serum bicarbonate < 15; positive serum ketones; increased creatinine; low, normal, or high potassium level; lethargy; dehydration; mental status changes; tachycardia; tachypnea, but often normotensive; polyuria; polydipsia; weakness; history of illness of short duration. **DKA is a less common presentation in elderly.**

✦ Most patients who present with **hyperosmolar hyperglycemia nonketotic coma** are elderly and have Type 2 DM with concomitant illness (infection, renal failure, MI, GI bleed, CVA). Usual presentation: BG 600–1,000+, serum osmolality ⩾320, elevated BUN, normal to mildly decreased serum bicarbonate (20–24), pH > 7.2, varying sodium and potassium levels (usually markedly decreased). **Requires urgent admission. Mortality high.**

✦ Obtain preadmission orders for adjustment of insulin therapy/oral agents prior to inpatient diagnostic testing (NPO status) or surgical procedures.

✦ Stress of acute illness often produces hyperglycemia that requires intensive management.

✦ Be aware that initiation of steroid therapy may induce hyperglycemia.

Extended Care Setting

✦ Educate staff regarding importance of HBGM, recognition and treatment of hypoglycemia and hyperglycemia, monitoring for signs of infection.

✦ **Safety (prevention of hypoglycemia-related injury) is critical issue.**

Home Setting

✦ Establish treatment plan for home setting and review periodically with patient and caregiver and/or home health staff.

✦ Be familiar with financial arrangements for services provided.

✦ Evaluate home environment for equipment needed if functional impairment, amputations, neuropathies exists.

✦ Consider home IV therapy for treatment of infections.

✦ Refer patients to podiatrist for foot care.

✦ Educate for proper insulin syringe/needle disposal.

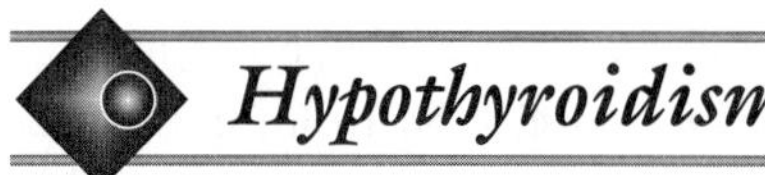

Hypothyroidism

HISTORY

✦ **Signs and symptoms of hypothyroidism in the elderly may be subtle and mistaken for normal changes of aging.**

✦ Common symptoms: fatigue; weakness; lethargy; depression; slowed intellectual functioning; memory impairment; weight gain; anorexia; decreased hearing ability; voice change; periorbital or peripheral edema; cold intolerance; dry skin; coarse hair or skin; constipation; muscular aches or cramping; paresthesia; ataxia.

✦ Age? Sex? **Hypothyroidism is more prevalent in the elderly and in females and is a progressive disorder.**

✦ History of hypercholesterolemia? Carpal tunnel syndrome?

✦ History of autoimmune disorders: Graves' disease, Addison's disease, Type 1 diabetes mellitus, myasthenia gravis, rheumatoid arthritis, pernicious anemia, systemic lupus erythematosus, scleroderma?

✦ History of treatment for **hyperthyroidism**: radioactive iodine therapy for Graves' disease or toxic nodular goiter? Neck irradiation for lymphoma or other malignancies? Subtotal thyroidectomy?

✦ Medications: **note especially antithyroid medications such as Tapazole (methimazole) and PTU (propylthiouracil).** Heparin, phenytoin, and salicylates may alter protein-binding of thyroid hormones. Estrogen, androgens, and glucocorticoids may affect levels of thyroid hormone-binding globulin (TBG).

✦ Diet history? Excess iodide intake can cause hypothyroidism but usually occurs in patients with underlying thyroid gland abnormality. Deficient iodide intake may be causative factor but is rarely seen in the United States.

PHYSICAL EXAMINATION

✦ Vital signs (increased BP or decreased heart rate, temperature); height; weight.

✦ Mental status examination. Depression screening. Assess affect, cognition.

✦ Eyes: assess for periorbital edema, lateral eyebrow loss.

✦ Ears: assess hearing ability.

✦ Hair: inspect for alopecia; assess texture.

✦ Oral: especially note size of tongue for possible enlargement.

✦ Neck: palpate thyroid for size, consistency, presence of goiter or nodules, assess swallowing and voice quality.

✦ Skin: observe for dryness, pallor, decreased perspiration, brittle nails.

✦ Cardiovascular: assess heart sounds for possible bradycardia; assess for peripheral edema. Severely ill patients may present with congestive heart failure or pericardial effusion.

✦ Respiratory: weakness of respiratory muscles; slow, shallow respirations; signs of airway obstruction?

✦ Abdomen: decreased bowel sounds, ascites, signs of bowel obstruction. Check for impaction if indicated.

✦ Neurological: Assess for slowed relaxation of deep tendon reflexes. Assess gait.

✦ Musculoskeletal: assess for presence of paresthesias, bradykinesia.

DIAGNOSTIC TESTS

✦ **Thyroid function tests: Thyroid-stimulating hormone (TSH)** triggers the release of **T_3 (triiodothyronine)** and **T_4 (thyroxine)** from the thyroid gland. T_4 is also converted in the periphery to T_3.

✧ **TSH radioimmunoassay** is the most sensitive test for hypothyroidism.

✧ **Circulating T_3 may be reduced with normal aging.** Also, T_3 levels may be normal, reduced, or elevated in hypothyroidism due to coexisting illness and, therefore, are not useful in establishing diagnosis.

✧ **Free T_4 and free T_4 index** provide an estimate of circulating T_4 unbound to other proteins and are reduced in primary hypothyroidism.

✦ **CBC:** Screen for co-existing normocytic or macrocytic anemia.

✦ **Serum electrolytes:** Screen for endocrine-related hyponatremia.

✦ **Lipid profile:** Presence of hypercholesterolemia, hypertriglyceridemia.

✦ **ECG:** May be affected by profound hypothyroidism. Be alert for low-voltage bradycardia.

PREVENTION

✦ Screening recommended for women over age 50.

✦ **See Protocol on Prevention and Health Maintenance.**

MANAGEMENT

Primary hypothyroidism is the most frequent cause of thyroid deficiency in the elderly. It may occur as result of an autoimmune disorder wherein the thyroid gland has failed (Hashimoto's thyroiditis); radioactive therapy for Graves' disease; lithium therapy; subtotal thyroidectomy; or inadequate or excessive iodide intake. Secondary and tertiary hypothyroidism (from hypopituitarism and hypothalamic dysfunction, respectively) are uncommon.

Primary Hypothyroidism

✦ Diagnosed by **low free T_4 or free T_4 index along with an elevated TSH level.**

✦ Consult physician or endocrinologist if goiter is present for possible ultrasound, thyroid scan, or needle biopsy.

✦ Consult physician before initiating therapy in patient with history of CAD, hypotension, or hyponatremia.

✦ Begin therapy with synthetic T_4 (levothyroxine, thyroxine, sodium L-thyroxine, Synthroid) in very low dose (12.5–25 μg PO qd) because **many elderly may have asymptomatic CAD that could be exacerbated by rapid thyroid replacement.**

✦ Avoid use of desiccated thyroid preparations (e.g., Euthroid), which may not be standardized. Symptoms of hyperthyroidism may be produced due to variability of biological activity. Convert patients from desiccated to non-desiccated formulations.

✦ Monitor TSH level after 4–8 weeks of therapy. Assess for signs of thyrotoxicity before increasing dosage. Increase dose slowly in small increments (by 25 μg every 4–8 weeks) continuing to monitor TSH until normalized. Low TSH level indicates overtreatment and dosage should be reduced until TSH normalizes.

✦ After establishment of equilibrium, monitor TSH every 6–12 months. Be aware that progressive loss of gland function may require increasing doses of thyroid hormone over time. Continue to be aware of effects of new medications on thyroid replacement.

Secondary and Tertiary Hypothyroidism

✦ Evidenced by low TSH levels and low free T_4 or free T_4 index.

✦ Consult physician or endocrinologist for further testing.

Subclinical Hypothyroidism

✦ Evidenced by elevated TSH level without symptoms of hypothyroidism and usually normal T_4 level.

✦ It is difficult to predict which patients will convert to overt hypothyroidism. Replacement in subclinical hypothyroidism may improve mental status, cardiac functioning, and lipid profiles. Risks of treatment include exacerbated cardiac disease and osteoporosis, but may be eliminated by careful monitoring of replacement. Decision to treat must be individualized. Consult physician.

Myxedema Coma

✦ Longstanding, untreated hypothyroidism may lead to myxedema coma in rare instances.

✦ Signs and symptoms include weakness, bradycardia, hypoventilation, hypothermia, and decreased mental status varying from stupor to coma.

✦ Occurs more frequently in elderly and may be precipitated by noncompliance with replacement therapy, stress of surgery, or concomitant illness such as infection, heart failure, GI bleed, MI, or stroke.

✦ Laboratory findings may include hypoglycemia and hyponatremia.

✦ Consult physician for immediate admission to ICU for passive rewarming, mechanical ventilation if necessary, IV fluids, IV levothyroxine, and corticosteroids.

KEY ISSUES

Patient/Caregiver Education

Patient/caregiver should be able to:

✦ List signs/symptoms of hypothyroidism.

✦ Verbalize correct dosage and frequency of replacement therapy.

✦ Verbalize understanding that taking daily supplements will probably be a life-long necessity.

✦ Identify signs of thyrotoxicity (**see Protocol on Hyperthyroidism**) and warning signals of exacerbated cardiac disease.

✦ Verbalize understanding that symptoms will gradually resolve with therapy.

✦ Identify interventions to alleviate current symptoms (high-fiber diet for constipation; warm dress for cold intolerance; frequent rest periods for fatigue).

Psychosocial Considerations

✦ Assess thyroid status of patients with neuropsychiatric manifestations.

✦ When converting to nondesiccated thyroid supplements, remember that demented patients on a longstanding dose of a specific number of tablets may have difficulty changing regimens to a different number of tablets. When possible, change to **same number of tablets** for new therapy.

✦ Patients and families should be instructed that symptoms will improve gradually with therapy.

Acute/Inpatient Setting

✦ Even though a patient is clinically euthyroid during acute or serious systemic illness, alterations in thyroid function tests (low T_4, normal TSH) may be present. This euthyroid sick syndrome often resolves as the patient improves. Monitoring of thyroid function until illness resolves is recommended.

Extended Care Setting

✦ Maintain periodic monitoring of residents on long-term replacement; requirements may change with aging.

Home Setting

✦ Monitor and assist with medication regimen to ensure compliance.

✦ Monitor for signs/symptoms of continued deficiency or thyrotoxicity from overreplacement.

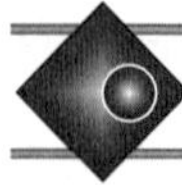

Hyperthyroidism

HISTORY

✦ **Age? 10–15% of those with hyperthyroidism are older than 60 years.**

✦ Classic symptoms include increased perspiration, palpitations, tachycardia, systolic hypertension, tremor, diarrhea, stare, lid lag, nervousness, insomnia, heat intolerance, increased hunger, proximal muscle weakness, hyperreflexia.

✦ **Symptoms may be atypical in the elderly:** coarse skin without diaphoresis; lack of tremor; elderly may report correction of constipation rather than diarrhea. Presentation may include anorexia, weight loss, failure to thrive, confusion, apathy, depression, or heart failure symptoms (apathetic hyperthyroidism).

✦ **60% of all elderly will present with new diagnosis or worsening of heart failure; atrial fibrillation; or new or worsening angina.**

✦ Past medical history/comorbidities: autoimmune disease (myasthenia gravis, pernicious anemia, Type 1 diabetes mellitus). Be alert for previous inappropriate thyroid replacement which may precipitate thyrotoxicity.

✦ Complete medication history—note especially exogenous thyroid hormone—**prolonged half-life of exogenous thyroid hormone increases risk of thyrotoxicity in the elderly;** nondessicated thyroid hormone formulations; amiodarone?

✦ Change in ability to perform activities of daily living (ADLs) due to myopathy?

PHYSICAL EXAMINATION

✦ Vital signs, weight, general appearance.

✦ Neurological: assess for mental status changes, depression, tremor, and hyperreflexia.

✦ Eyes: assess for periorbital and conjunctival edema, proptosis, lid retraction, and exophthalmos.

✦ Integument: assess skin temperature, texture, and presence of moisture; alopecia; excoriation from pruritus.

✦ Thyroid: auscultate for vascular bruit; palpate size and consistency; for presence of nodules and tenderness. **With normal aging, thyroid gland becomes more fibrotic and lies lower in the neck. Changes in gland size are less frequently seen in the elderly. Goiter may be substernal and difficult to palpate.**

✦ Cardiovascular: auscultate for tachyarrhythmia and presence of extra heart sounds.

✦ Extremities: assess proximal muscle mass and strength.

DIAGNOSTIC TESTS

✦ Thyroid function tests—diagnosis is confirmed by combination of elevated free T_4 index and undetectable TSH.

✧ In some cases, low TSH may be the only abnormal value.

✧ Lone elevation of total T_4 does not confirm hyperthyroidism.

✧ Elevated T_3 with normal T_4 is indicative of T_3 toxicosis and may be seen in the elderly.

✦ Increased uptake of radionuclide thyroid scans.

✦ Serum glucose level (hyperthyroidism increases insulin resistance).

✦ B_{12} level—may be decreased.

✦ Lipid profile—Cholesterol may be decreased by increased metabolism.

✦ Urine calcium level (increased level may result from increased bone resorption that may accompany hyperthyroidism).

PREVENTION

✦ Routine screening with TSH level should be considered in those > age 60 years; women > 40 years with one or more nonspecific complaints; and geriatric patients with atrial fibrillation.

✦ Effective treatment helps to prevent osteoporosis and decreases risk for fractures because hyperthyroidism increases bone turnover rate.

✦ **See Protocol on Prevention and Health Maintenance.**

MANAGEMENT

✦ The most common causes of hyperthyroidism in the elderly are Grave's disease and toxic multinodular goiter.

✦ Over-replacement of thyroid hormone may precipitate hyperthyroidism.

✦ Rare causes include:

✧ Subacute thyroiditis—usually preceded by a viral illness and produces mild signs and symptoms of hyperthyroidism.

✧ TSH-producing tumors—suspected when TSH is normal to high with an increased free T_4 index.

✧ Iodine-induced hyperthyroidism.

✦ 25% of patients > 60 years with atrial fibrillation have hyperthyroidism. Sinus rhythm may be restored on return to euthyroid state with antithyroid medications.

✦ In patients with concomitant diabetes, monitor for deterioration in blood glucose control.

Graves' Disease

✦ Autoimmune disorder that stimulates thyroid growth and overproduction of thyroid hormone.

✦ Diffuse goiter, exophthalmos, and pretibial myxedema may result but are rarely seen in the elderly.

✦ Elevated free T_4 or free T_4 index with decreased TSH are seen.

✦ Consult physician for management with antithyroid medications—PTU (propylthiouracil), Tapazole (methimazole), beta-blockers, or radioactive iodine treatment. Thyroidectomy may be indicated in persistent cases.

✦ Monitor for side effects of therapy: hypotension, bradycardia, hypothyroidism, agranulocytosis, skin rash, fever, toxic psychosis, myalgia, or arthralgia.

Toxic Multinodular Goiter

✦ Results from nodules that autonomously produce thyroid hormone.

✦ Multiple nodules may be found resulting in gland enlargement, asymmetry, and surface irregularity.

✦ May be accompanied by dyspnea or dysphagia.

✦ Consult physician for management with antithyroid medications, corticosteroids, beta-blockers, and radioactive iodine.

KEY ISSUES

Patient/Caregiver Education

Patient/caregiver should be able to:

✦ List dosages, timing, and side effects of medications.

Economic Considerations

✦ Thyroid testing should be performed judiciously. Frequent and repetitive testing is unnecessary as thyroid hormone levels may take 6–8 weeks to show changes.

Psychosocial Considerations

✦ Thyroid disease may mimic psychiatric disorders.

Acute/Inpatient Setting

✦ Severe illness (infection, MI, surgery, trauma) may precipitate **thyroid storm** (extreme thyrotoxicosis). Hospitalization is necessary for:

✧ Return to euthyroid state (PTU, iodine, beta-blockers, and corticosteroids).

✧ Heart rate control.

✧ Supportive care (rehydration with IV fluids and non-aspirin reduction of fever).

Extended Care Setting

✦ Periodic thyroid function tests may detect new onset thyroid disorders which develop insidiously.

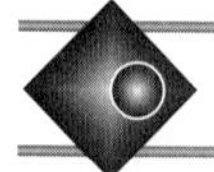

Hyperlipidemia

HISTORY

✦ **Age? The high incidence of CAD in the elderly suggests that even those who are asymptomatic may have significant atherosclerosis. CAD is the cause of death in more than 70% of individuals 75 and older.**

✦ **Gender?** Females older than age 55 years have greater total cholesterol, LDL, and HDL levels than males.

✦ Presence of risk factors for CAD: hypertension, diabetes mellitus, smoking, family history of CAD, sedentary life-style, obesity?

✦ Associated symptoms: angina, heart failure symptoms?

✦ Comorbidities: history of MI, TIA/CVA, peripheral vascular disease, pancreatitis?

✦ Medications: diuretics or beta-blockers (increase HDL, decrease LDL, and increase triglycerides); corticosteroids. Certain medications such as immunosuppressants, antifungals, and erythromycin may increase risk of rhabdomyolysis with concomitant hydroxymethylglutaryl coenzyme A (HMGCoA) reductase inhibitor ("statin") therapy for hyperlipidemia. **Multiple medication use increases risk of adverse effects from lipid-lowering agents.**

PHYSICAL EXAMINATION

✦ Vital signs.

✦ Neurological: assess mental status.

✦ Eyes: inspect eyelids for xanthomas (thickening or nodularity), iris for arcus senilus; fundoscopic examination for A/V nicking, papilledema, hemorrhages, or exudate.

✦ Cardiovascular: inspect for signs of peripheral vascular disease; auscultate for rate and rhythm and bruits; palpate peripheral pulses.

✦ Musculoskeletal: note presence of xanthomas at Achilles' tendon or extensor tendons of hands.

DIAGNOSTIC TESTS

✦ **Lipid profile: Controversy exists as to the panel that is most beneficial for therapeutic decision-making. Full lipid profile requires a fasting state to measure triglycerides. Screening with total cholesterol only may be misrepresentative, because elevated HDL contributes to total**

fraction and decreased HDL may go unnoticed; however, lone total cholesterol allows a nonfasting state prior to screen.

✦ Consider lipoprotein (a) [$Lp_{(a)}$] level when total cholesterol cannot explain the presence of CAD. $Lp_{(a)}$ is highly predictive of CAD in both men and women, but testing is expensive and no specific therapy exists at present for $Lp_{(a)}$ elevation.

✦ Baseline ECG.

✦ Serum glucose, liver function tests, creatinine, BUN, urinalysis, and TSH level to rule out underlying cause of hyperlipidemia. **See Management.**

PREVENTION

✦ Weight reduction if indicated.

✦ Regular, aerobic exercise.

✦ Maintain a diet low in saturated fats and cholesterol. Avoid overly aggressive restrictions in patients at risk for malnutrition.

✦ **See Protocol on Prevention and Health Maintenance.**

MANAGEMENT

✦ The National Cholesterol Education Panel (NCEP) guidelines include age as a major risk factor for CAD. Because the elderly have not been sufficiently included in clinical trials, it has not yet been shown that elevated cholesterol levels in older adults convey risk equivalent to that well-recognized in younger populations. **The power of total cholesterol levels to predict atherosclerotic cardiovascular risk declines after age 75; however, morbidity and mortality from CAD increase with aging.**

✦ **Decision to treat based on:**

✧ **Limitations of life-span:** Presence of significant comorbidity (cancer, CAD, malnutrition, depression) may justify decision not to treat.

✧ **Mental status/cognitive function:** patient's ability to maintain medication regimen.

✧ **Presence of comorbidities:** Dietary and pharmacological intervention may increase risk when patient has concomitant illness and takes multiple medications.

✧ **Patient's expectations of treatment:** Many community-dwelling elderly are concerned with their cholesterol levels and may be overzealous in lowering levels. Use average of two screenings before initiating treatment.

✦ Begin by treating underlying causes which may be responsible for hyperlipidemia:

TABLE 10-1. Goals of Treatment of Hypercholesterolemia in the Elderly

Patient	LDL goal	Use drug if LDL level
CAD patient	< 100 mg/dL	> 130 mg/dL
No CAD, ≥ 2 risk factors	< 130 mg/dL	> 160 mg/dL
No CAD, < 2 risk factors	< 160 mg/dL	> 190 mg/dL

LDL, low-density lipoprotein; CAD, coronary artery disease.

- ✧ Uncontrolled diabetes mellitus.
- ✧ Hypothyroidism.
- ✧ Renal failure or nephrotic syndrome.
- ✧ Obstructive liver disease.
- ✧ EtOH abuse.

✦ **Institute individualized management to achieve goals recommended by the NCEP.** See Table 10-1.

✦ An HDL level > 60 mg/dL is considered to be a beneficial (negative) risk factor.

✦ NECP recommends achieving an HDL level > 35 mg/dL.

✦ Triglycerides > 200 mg/dL are considered borderline and > 400 mg/dL are considered high.

✦ **Therapy begins with diet and exercise.**

✧ Refer for exercise treadmill test prior to exercise.

✧ Refer patients with known CAD to cardiac rehabilitation program.

✧ Refer to nutritionist for initiation of American Heart Association (AHA) Step 1 diet (daily totals: total fat $< 30\%$, saturated fat 10%, polyunsaturated fat 10%, monounsaturated fat 10%, cholesterol < 300 mg/day).

✧ If the Step 1 diet fails to control hyperlipidemia, the AHA Step 2 diet may be tried (saturated fat $< 7\%$, cholesterol < 200 mg/day).

✦ General dietary recommendations as follows:

✧ Maintain daily cholesterol intake equal to no more than one egg yolk/day.

✧ Eat less red meat and more poultry. Eat more soluble fibers (oat bran, barley).

✧ Use olive oil in cooking and avoid the use of coconut and palm oils. Excessive use of vegetable oil and complex carbohydrates to reduce total cholesterol may raise triglycerides and lower HDL.

✧ For the elderly, encourage meals with fish rather than fish oil tablets.

✦ If treatment goals are not achieved after 3–6 months of diet/exercise therapy, proceed to drug therapy. Consider initiation of estrogen replacement therapy in women > 65 years before initiating medications for hyperlipidemia, because estrogen decreases LDL, increases HDL, and decreases $Lp_{(a)}$.

✦ Pharmacological options for hyperlipidemia:

✧ Bile acid sequestrants: decrease LDL, increase triglycerides

✧ Questran Light (cholestyramine), available in 5-g packets or 210-g can, contains aspartame, or Questran (cholestyramine), available in 9-g packets or 378-g can; begin 1 packet or scoop mixed with fluid or food qd–bid; may increase to 2–4 packets or scoops tid; contains aspartame.

✧ Colestid (colestipol HCl), available in 5-g packets or 300-g bulk package; begin with 2 g qd–bid; may increase to 30 g/day; usual maintenance is 2–16 g/day.

✧ Common side effects include bloating, constipation, nausea, and flatulence. Consider concomitant Metamucil (**see Protocol on Constipation**). Be aware of potential for intestinal obstruction.

✧ Advise to take 1 hr before or 3 hr after other oral medications because these agents block absorption of many drugs (digoxin, propanolol, cyclosporine, vancomycin, warfarin, and numerous other medications).

✧ Deficiencies of iron, magnesium, zinc, and fat-soluble vitamins may be seen with long-term use.

✧ These agents may aggravate hypertriglyceridemia, and there is potential for pancreatitis with severe triglyceride elevations.

✧ Niacin (nicotinic acid): lowers LDL and triglycerides and increases HDL.

✧ Nicolar (nicotinic acid) usual initial dose 100 mg PO tid; geriatric dose: 50 mg PO tid; increase gradually to 1,000 mg PO tid.

✧ Potential side effects: glucose intolerance, liver function abnormalities, hyperuricemia, flushing, headache, and hypotension.

✧ Advise to take an aspirin 20–30 min prior to niacin to avoid flushing.

✧ Obtain baseline uric acid, serum glucose, and liver function tests before initiating therapy.

✦ **The elderly may be less tolerant of bile acid sequestrants or niacin than other agents.**

✧ Fibric acid derivatives: lower triglycerides and increase HDL.

✧ Lopid (gemfibrozil) 600 mg PO bid.

✧ Atromid-S (clofibrate) 1,000 mg PO bid.

✧ Potential side effects include gallstones and liver function abnormalities, but these agents are generally well tolerated.

✧ Tricor (fonofibrate) begin with 67 mg PO qd with food, may increase to 201 mg qd. This agent may also decrease LDL. Use is contraindicated in patients with hepatic or renal dysfunction or gallstone disease. Concomitant use with statins is contraindicated due to risk of rhabdomyolysis and acute renal failure. Potentiates anticoagulants; reduced dose is required.

✧ HMG-CoA reductase inhibitors (statins): lower LDL, raise HDL, and lower triglycerides.

✧ Mevacor (lovastatin) 20 mg PO every night; maximum 80 mg PO qd. Avoid combination with gemfibrozil to reduce increased risk of myositis.

✧ Pravachol (pravastatin sodium) 10 mg PO every night; maximum dose 40 mg/PO qd; usual maintenance 20 mg qd. Has been shown to reduce risk of first MI; reduces risk of TIA/CVA in patients with previous MI.

✧ Zocor (simvastatin) 10 mg PO every night; maximum dose 40 mg PO qd.

✧ Lescol (fluvastatin sodium) 20 mg PO every night; may increase up to 80 mg PO qd (in divided doses).

✧ Lipitor (atorvastatin) 10 mg PO qd, up to 80 mg PO qd. May decrease triglycerides by 50% at highest dose.

✧ Potential side effects include increases in serum transaminase and creatinine phosphokinase, myalgia, arthralgia, rash, fatigue, headache, and dizziness.

✧ Obtain baseline serum transaminase and creatinine phosphokinase. Monitor liver function tests at 6 and 12 weeks after initiation and after successive increases in dose. Discontinue if elevations occur.

KEY ISSUES

Patient/Caregiver Education

Patient/caregiver should be able to:

✦ Verbalize understanding of dietary/exercise recommendations.

✦ Verbalize timing, doses, and potential side effects of medications.

✦ **State the importance of continuing to take lipid-lowering medications even if no symptoms are felt.** It has been found that nearly half of older patients given prescriptions for antilipemic medications eventually discontinue their medications, and many never even have prescriptions filled despite adequate payment mechanisms.

Economic Considerations

✦ The direct medical costs for cardiovascular disease in the United States exceeds $100 billion.

✦ HMG-CoA reductase inhibitors are costly and not covered by many payment plans.

✦ Wide variation exists in costs for screening and medications. Check formularies/advise patients to check coverage.

Psychosocial Considerations

✦ Weigh the benefits of strict dietary curtailments versus the risk of deprivation of quality of life for frail elderly and those with significant comorbidity.

Acute/Inpatient Setting

✦ Utilize the acute care setting to educate patient/caregiver in risk factor reduction, diet, and medications.

Extended Care Setting

✦ Monitor patient for malnutrition and weight loss.

Home Setting

✦ Provide education and support for life-style/dietary changes to promote CAD risk reduction.

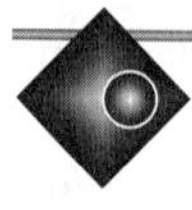

Fluid and Electrolyte Abnormalities

HISTORY

✦ **With increased age, these alterations in renal function are common:**

✧ **50% decrease in cortical blood flow.**

✧ **Markedly decreased renal mass and glomerular filtration.**

✧ **Reduced sodium concentration.**

✧ **Reduced urinary concentrating abilities.**

✧ **Thickening of tubular basement membranes with altered renal resorption/secretory function.**

✦ **Prediction of renal function is based on age:**

✧ **Creatinine clearance (CrCl)* (ml/min) =**

$$\frac{[140 - \text{age (yrs)}] \times \text{wt (kg)}}{72 \times \text{serum creatinine (mg/dL)}}$$

***May overestimate function when patient is cachectic.**

✦ **Multiply result by 0.85 for CrCl in females.**

✦ Associated signs/symptoms: mental status changes (disorientation, confusion, delirium, impaired concentration or memory, lethargy, agitation), depression, thirst, nausea, vomiting, anorexia, constipation, fever, edema, muscular weakness or cramping, paresthesia, bone pain, palpitations, dizziness, change in respiratory function, worsening of heart failure symptoms?

✦ Comorbid conditions: recent surgery, recent infection, renal insufficiency, malignancy, endocrine disorders (hyperthyroidism, hyperparathyroidism, diabetes mellitus, Cushing's syndrome, Paget's disease), sarcoidosis, heart failure, hypertension, arrhythmia, musculoskeletal disorder, GI bleeding, peptic ulcer disease, gastroesophageal reflux disease (GERD), tuberculosis?

✦ EtOH use?

✦ Medications: note diuretics, cardiac drugs?

✦ Diet history: note especially deficient calcium, Vitamin D intake, excessive salt use/restriction, salt substitutes.

PHYSICAL EXAMINATION

✦ Vital signs: Assess for signs of compromised fluid volume status (orthostatic hypotension, decreased weight). If possible, obtain baseline weight from caregiver.

✦ Neurological: Assess level of consciousness and cognitive status (mental status examination).

✦ Mouth: inspect for dry mucous membranes (volume deficit).

✦ Skin: Assessment of turgor at sternum area may be more reliable in the elderly than other sites.

✦ Cardiovascular: inspect for flat neck veins indicative of volume deficit; inspect for peripheral edema. Auscultate heart rate and rhythm. Auscultate for vascular bruits.

✦ Lungs: Note rate and quality of respirations, presence of adventitious sounds.

DIAGNOSTIC TESTS

✦ Serum electrolyte levels: sodium level reflects the body's water content or osmolality.

✦ BUN and creatinine to assess renal function. **Due to decreased muscle mass in the elderly, results may not accurately reflect fluid volume deficit or age-related changes in renal function. Calculation of creatinine clearance is recommended.**

✦ Hematocrit to detect hemoconcentration resulting from volume loss.

PREVENTION

✦ Encourage fluid intake to prevent dehydration.

✦ Conduct routine assessment of medication use to avoid use of those substances that may increase risk of electrolyte imbalance.

✦ Avoid drastic sodium-reduced diets to prevent volume depletion that may result in an acute reduction in renal function.

✦ Encourage regular at-home weights by patient or caregiver on same scale, at same time of day to monitor changes.

✦ **See Protocol on Prevention and Health Maintenance.**

MANAGEMENT

Hyponatremia/Hypernatremia

See Table 10-2.

Hypokalemia ($K^+ < 3.5$ mEq/liter)

✦ **Occurs most frequently due to diuretic use.**

TABLE 10-2. Sodium Balance

	Hyponatremia	Hypernatremia
Definition	Serum Na^+ < 135 mEq/liter	Serum Na^+ > 145 mEq/liter
Associated diagnoses/agents		
Renal (urine Na^+ > 20 mEq/liter)	Diuretics Osmotic agents Syndrome of inappropriate antidiuretic hormone Renal failure (acute, BUN/creatinine ratio > 20; chronic, BUN/creatinine ratio < 20)	Diuretics Osmotic agents Diabetes insipidus
Extrarenal (urine Na^+ < 10 mEq/liter)	Fluid loss Heart failure Cirrhosis	Free H_2O loss Dehydration Na^+ administration
Management		
Edematous states	Fluid restriction, diuretics	Free H_2O replacement
Volume loss states	Saline administration	

Calculate volume deficits using the following formula:

$$\text{Volume (liters)} = 0.6 \times \text{body weight (kg)} \times \left(1 - \frac{140}{[Na^+]\ \text{serum}}\right)$$

✦ Patients on digitalis are at highest risk for symptomatic hypokalemia.

✦ Other causes: vomiting, diarrhea, laxative use, high-dose sodium salt antibiotics such as penicillin, high-dose insulin, magnesium deficiency.

✦ Symptoms: weakness, cramping, altered mentation, arrhythmias.

✦ Management: oral or IV potassium.

Hyperkalemia ($K^+ > 5.0$ mEq/liter)

✦ **Occurs most frequently due to medication effects: angiotensin-converting enzyme (ACE) inhibitors, potassium-sparing diuretics, NSAIDs, potassium supplementation, and potassium-containing salt substitutes.**

✦ Common in elderly diabetics with hypertension (hyporenin/hyperaldosterone state).

✦ **$K^+ > 7.0$ is a medical emergency. Consult physician for cardiac monitoring, insulin/glucose administration, Kayexelate, and possible emergent hemodialysis.**

Other Mineral Derangements

CALCIUM

✦ **Hypocalcemia** ($Ca^+ < 8.8$ mg/dL with normal albumin)

✧ Symptoms include cramps, spasms, seizures.

✧ Rare except in malabsorption or following parathyroid surgery.

✧ Management depends on underlying etiology.

✦ **Hypercalcemia** ($Ca^+ > 10.5$ mg/dL with normal albumin)

✧ May cause weakness, altered mentation, nausea, vomiting, constipation.

✧ Seen in dehydration, metastatic cancer, hyperparathyroidism, and related to thiazide diuretic use.

✧ Management is determined by degree of severity and underlying cause.

MAGNESIUM

✦ **Hypomagnesemia** ($Mg^+ < 1.6$ mg/dL)

✧ Often seen in dehydration, related to diuretic use, or laxative abuse.

✧ May accompany hypokalemia.

✧ Symptoms may include muscular weakness, confusion, mental status changes.

✧ Replacement may be with oral preparations (magnesium oxide is best absorbed) or IV infusion depending on severity of deficit.

✦ **Hypermagnesemia** ($Mg^+ > 2.4$ mg/dL)

✧ Is rare and seen in association with excessive intake due to antacids or laxatives in the setting of renal disease. Magnesium is not removed by dialysis.

✧ Treatment is targeted to increase urinary loss of magnesium with normal saline infusion or loop diuretics.

PHOSPHORUS

✦ **Hypophospatemia** ($P^+ < 2$ mEq/liter)

✧ Seen in malnutrition and in critically ill individuals.

✧ Produces weakness and respiratory dysfunction.

✧ Mild hypophosphatemia (1.5–2.5 mg/dL) is managed with Phospho-soda 15–30 ml tid–qid or Neutra-Phos (250 mg elemental phosphorus) PO tid.

- **Hyperphosphatemia** ($P^+ > 4.5$ mEq/liter)
  - Often seen in renal failure.
  - Contributes to bone loss (renal osteodystrophy).
  - Management is with low phosphate diet and oral phosphate binders (aluminum hydroxide, calcium carbonate).

KEY ISSUES

Patient/Caregiver Education

Patient/caregiver should be able to:

- Promote adequate fluid intake.
- Verbalize medication doses and timing if indicated.
- Identify possible signs/symptoms of fluid and electrolyte abnormalities (change in weight, change in mental status).
- Verbalize that salt substitutes may induce electrolyte abnormality.
- Identify risk of overuse of magnesium-containing laxatives and antacids.

Economic Considerations

- Low socioeconomic status places individuals at higher risk for inadequate treatment of chronic renal failure.

Psychosocial Considerations

- Social isolation predisposes the elderly to dehydration, especially during periods of elevated heat index.

Acute/Inpatient Setting

- Monitor electrolytes and administer IV fluids carefully to elderly inpatients.
- Elderly patients admitted with an acute problem and co-existing dehydration have substantially increased risk of mortality as compared with elderly patients admitted without dehydration.

Extended Care Setting

- Promote adequate dietary and fluid intake.

✦ Dehydration is a geriatric syndrome frequently seen in frail, institutionalized elders and often associated with acute infections.

✦ Be alert to fluid and electrolyte abnormalities as a common cause of acute confusion in the elderly.

Home Setting

✦ Monitor electrolytes, adjust free water in individuals receiving enteral alimentation.

✦ Monitor electrolytes in individuals with edematous states, taking diuretics, with fluid/nutritional intake deficits, and with chronic renal failure, heart failure and diabetes.

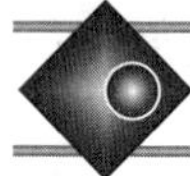

Osteoporosis

HISTORY

✦ **Osteoporosis progresses without symptoms until a fracture occurs; note risk factors on history with any elderly patient.**

✦ Demographics? **Whites and Asians are at highest risk; affects 70% of females over age 45 years.**

✦ Postmenopausal or history of hysterectomy with oophorectomy? **Women lose between 1–4% of bone mass per year during the first 10 years after menopause (age-related or surgical).**

✦ Hormone replacement therapy (HRT)? Duration? Tolerance?

✦ History of fractures? Location? **Fractures most associated with osteoporosis are spine, hip, and wrist.**

✦ Excessive loss of height with aging? **Normal aging is consistent with a 2-inch loss in height between age 20 and 70.**

✦ History of falls? Fall risk? Fear of falling?

✦ History of osteoarthritis or rheumatoid arthritis? Associated impaired mobility? Use of assistive devices?

✦ History of Cushing's syndrome, hyperthyroidism, hyperparathyroidism, hepatic disease, renal disease, multiple myeloma, hypogonadism, or lymphoma?

✦ History of malnutrition, vitamin deficiencies, sun avoidance (vitamin D deficiency), osteomalacia?

✦ Family history of osteoporosis-related fractures, breast cancer?

✦ Medications? **Chronic corticosteroids, heparin, antiepileptics, and thyroid medications increase risk of osteoporosis. Psychotropics, pain medications, and benzodiazepines increase risk of falls.**

✦ Smoking and EtOH history?

✦ Diet history: 24-hr recall, calcium intake?

✦ Exercise/activity level? Weight-bearing exercise?

✦ Functional status? Recent change in functional status?

PHYSICAL EXAMINATION

✦ Weight and height.

✦ Vital signs; check for orthostatic hypotension.

✦ Observe stature, presence of kyphosis. **Small-boned, thin women have highest risk of osteoporosis.**

✦ Musculoskeletal examination: note factors that increase fall risk; assess gait and balance, ability to rise unaided from a chair.

✦ Neurological examination: note factors that increase fall risk.

✦ Pelvic examination and Pap smear. Perform when initiating HRT and annually thereafter; not indicated if history of hysterectomy.

DIAGNOSTIC TESTS

✦ Bone mineral densitometry (BMD) or dual energy x-ray absorptiometry (DEXA) scan. Treatment is recommended when values are 2 or more standard deviations below peak bone mass. **Most precise measurements are taken at the lumbar spine and hip.**

✦ Screening: focus on patients with spinal deformity, loss of height, fractures of forearm or vertebrae, premature menopause, contraindications to postmenopausal HRT, or on chronic corticosteroid therapy.

✦ Consider laboratory tests based on the individualized clinical assessment: CBC with erythrocyte sedimentation rate, renal and liver function tests, serum albumin or prealbumin (for nutritional assessment), calcium (increased in hyperparathyroidism), phosphate (low in osteomalacia), alkaline phosphatase (increased with osteomalacia), thyroid function tests (to exclude hyperthyroidism).

✦ Consider specific x-rays if a fracture is suspected.

PREVENTION

✦ Consider HRT for perimenopausal or postmenopausal women. **See Chapter on Management of the Postmenopausal Woman** for discussion of use of HRT.

✦ Consider Evista (raloxifene HCl) 60 mg daily as alternative to HRT in postmenopausal woman. Reduces bone resorption. A selective estrogen receptor modulator that does not affect breast and uterine tissue.

✦ Dietary elemental calcium: for postmenopausal women recommend 1,500 mg daily (approximately four 8-oz glasses of milk daily or calcium carbonate 500 mg tid taken with meals). Encourage adequate fluid intake if using calcium supplements; do not take at same time as iron supplement.

✦ Vitamin D: 600–800 IU per day in a multivitamin or in combination with calcium.

✦ Weight-bearing exercise at least 3 times weekly. Stress proper body mechanics.

✦ Fall risk assessment and prevention program. **See Protocol on Falls.**

✦ Education/referral for smoking cessation.

✦ Limit EtOH intake.

✦ Adequate/balanced caloric nutritional intake.

✦ **See Protocol on Prevention and Health Maintenance.**

MANAGEMENT

✦ For high risk patients or those with osteoporosis, review risks and benefits of pharmacological treatment.

✦ Consider Bisphosphonates: Fosamax (alendronate sodium) 10 mg daily.

✧ Action: prevents bone resorption; may contribute to increased bone density.

✧ Common side effects: esophagitis.

✧ Patient education: take with 8 oz water on awakening in a.m. at least ½ hour before any food, drink, medications. Remain upright for 30 minutes.

✦ Consider calcitonin: Miacalcin (calcitonin salmon) 200 IU per day intranasally, alternating nostrils daily or Calcimar, Osteocalcin, or Salmonine 100 IU of salmon preparation subcutaneously 3 times weekly at bedtime (to minimize possible nausea and facial flushing). Due to the possibility of systemic allergic reactions, skin testing prior to treatment is recommended.

✧ Action: prevents bone resorption; effective in short-term management of bone pain.

✧ Side effects: nausea, GI symptoms, flushing, and nasal irritation.

✧ Patient education: patient or family/caregiver must be taught medication administration technique.

KEY ISSUES

Patient/Caregiver Education

Patient/caregiver should be able to:

✦ Describe risk factors and potential consequences of osteoporosis.

✦ Describe key strategies in preventing osteoporosis.

✦ Explain indications, potential side effects, and correct administration of medications.

✦ Identify environmental hazards associated with high risk for falling; modify the environment as appropriate.

✦ Demonstrate correct use of assistive devices for gait and balance.

✦ Demonstrate safe practices in transfers and ambulation.

Economic Considerations

✦ Consider expense of medications to treat osteoporosis, especially for older individuals on fixed income; some health plans require BMD before approving Fosamax or calcitonin.

✦ Consider expense of BMD screening and questionable reimbursement.

Psychosocial Considerations

✦ Evaluate for depression or social isolation resulting from fear of falling, changes in self-concept secondary to changes in stature, decreased ability to perform ADLs, potential loss of independence.

Acute/Inpatient Setting

✦ Implement fall risk assessment and prevention program. **See Protocol on Falls.**

✦ Consider referral to physical therapist (PT) to assess gait and safety, and to prevent functional decline while hospitalized.

✦ Consider referral to occupational therapist (OT) to assess and maximize function and to recommend needed adaptations.

✦ Avoid bedrest/immobility for prolonged periods; mobilize as soon as possible to prevent functional decline.

✦ Avoid/eliminate tethers when possible: IV, oxygen, Foley catheter, continuous tube feeding, and restraints that contribute to immobilization.

Extended Care Setting

✦ Implement fall risk assessment and prevention program. **See Protocol on Falls.**

✦ For ambulatory residents, offer weight-bearing exercise programs, encourage walking.

Home Setting

✦ Perform home safety assessment to identify and correct potential fall hazards.

✦ Consider home OT and PT evaluations.

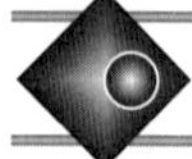

Erectile Dysfunction

HISTORY

✦ Onset of problem? Sudden or gradual?

✦ Continuous or intermittent occurrence?

✦ Any remaining ability to have erections? If so, duration? When do erections occur? Early morning erections? Nocturnal erections? Partial erection or erection lost during intercourse? Does erection ability vary with different partners? Erection on visual stimulation but not with partner(s)?

✦ Pain on erection?

✦ Characteristics of ejaculation? Ejaculation with soft penis? Does semen (fluid) come out of penis?

✦ Change in sensitivity of penis? Change in shape of penis?

✦ Change in libido?

✦ Engage in foreplay? Duration of foreplay?

✦ Frequency of intercourse prior to problem?

✦ Change in beard growth or frequency of shaving? **Suggests androgen deficiency.**

✦ Buttock pain? **Buttock claudication suggests aortic bifurcation narrowing that is a remedial cause of erectile dysfunction.**

✦ **Patient's perception of what may be causing problem?**

✦ Past medical history for conditions associated with erectile dysfunction: atherosclerosis and CVD, decreased HDL, tobacco use, EtOH use, recreational drug use, CVA, multiple sclerosis, temporal lobe epilepsy, depression, Parkinson's disease, musculoskeletal disabilities, Cushing's syndrome, hypothalamic–pituitary disease, cirrhosis, renal failure, Addison's disease, hyperthyroidism, hypothyroidism, diabetes mellitus, morbid obesity, systemic disease or cancer, incontinence, traumatic or surgical injury (radical prostatectomy, renal transplant, transurethral prostatectomy)?

✦ Marital status?

✦ Sexual preference?

✦ Number of partners? Extramarital experiences?

✦ Profile of current partner: age, health status and effect on sexual function, interest in sex, quality of relationship, communication patterns, desired duration of foreplay, partner's desire for treatment of problem?

✦ Medications: note especially those which may be associated with erectile dysfunction: antihypertensives, hormonal agents, antipsychotics, anticonvulsants, muscle relaxers, anorectic agents, EtOH, nicotine, antidepressants, narcotics, tranquilizers, digoxin, cimetidine.

✦ Current EtOH intake, current tobacco use?

✦ Living arrangements: especially note setting that might compromise privacy or decrease ability to seek partner.

✦ Psychosocial stressors?

PHYSICAL EXAMINATION

✦ Vital signs (BP in three positions to screen for autonomic disturbance), height, weight.

✦ Neurological: affect, cognition, gait. Loss of sensation in distal extremities, particularly with co-existing diabetes mellitus. Deep tendon reflexes in lower extremities.

✦ Eyes: cuts in temporal visual fields may suggest impotence caused by pituitary tumor.

✦ Integument: hair pattern, texture, pigmentation, evidence of vascular disease.

✦ Breasts: Assess for gynecomastia.

✦ Cardiovascular: palpate strength of all pulses to assess for PVD, including penile pulse.

✦ Penis: size, discharge, consistency (soft testes occur in primary hypogonadism after puberty); palpate shaft for fibrosis; inspect for hypospadias. Bulbocavernous reflex is not a very sensitive test.

✦ Scrotum: size of testes, consistency, masses. Assess for varicocele and hydrocele.

✦ Rectal: sphincter tone (if adequate, indicates intact innervation of pelvic floor).

✦ Prostate: size, texture, tenderness, masses.

DIAGNOSTIC TESTS

✦ CBC to screen for anemia or macrocytosis suggestive of nutritional deficiencies.

✦ Serum electrolytes, glucose, BUN, creatinine.

✦ Thyroid function tests.

✦ Liver function tests.

✦ Testosterone (serum and bioavailable). Due to variability, necessary to take three morning samples 15–60 min apart (may pool samples to reduce cost). If decreased, measure follicle-stimulating hormone (FSH) and leutinizing hormone (LH) levels (both increase **gradually** with aging). If FSH or LH ↓, consider hyperprolactinemia (prolactin level) or hypopituitarism. **Hyperprolactinemia secondary to pituitary lesion is uncommon.** If LH ↑ and FSH ↑, suggests primary hypogonadism.

✦ Consider zinc level in patients with uremia, diabetes, sickle cell disease, patients on dialysis, and patients taking diuretics.

✦ Consider at-home snap gauge test to assess for nocturnal penile tumescence (NPT) to differentiate organic from psychogenic dysfunction. **Because rapid eye movement (REM) sleep (when NPT occurs) lessens with aging, test may produce false-positive results and is not useful in patients with depression, sleep apnea, or if taking impotence-causing medications.**

PREVENTION

✦ Thorough sexual history is part of a complete patient evaluation. **Impotence is present in 25% of men over age 65 years.**

✦ To prevent erectile dysfunction caused by performance anxiety (fear of failure), counsel regarding **normal changes associated with aging:**

- ✧ Erection may be less firm.
- ✧ Takes longer to achieve an erection.
- ✧ Ejaculation may be less forceful.
- ✧ Volume of semen ejaculated may be reduced.
- ✧ Refractory period between ejaculations may be prolonged.
- ✧ More direct penile stimulation may be necessary for erection.
- ✧ If partner is postmenopausal female, the relaxed vagina may not provide required stimulation to maintain erection.

✦ Explain that the belief that the elderly do not engage in sex is a **myth of ageism.**

✦ To prevent vasculogenic impotence, stress importance of smoking cessation and reduction of other cardiovascular disease risks.

✦ Encourage intimacy rather than intercourse as sexual fulfillment goal.

✦ Suggest use of EtOH after rather than before sexual activity.

✦ For elders with joint pain, encourage use of comfort measures: warm bath, analgesic 30 min prior to sexual activity, use of pillows, and alternate positions for intercourse.

✦ For elders with chronic obstructive pulmonary disease (COPD), suggest use of inhaler prior to sexual activity.

✦ **See Protocol on Prevention and Health Maintenance.**

MANAGEMENT

Exclude physiological causes of impotence before treating as psychogenic unless there is a frankly evident stressor that can be identified from history. Psychogenic impotence is more common in younger men than in older.

Physiological Impotence

✦ If serum or bioavailable testosterone, LH, FSH, or prolactin levels are abnormal, consult physician and refer to endocrinologist for further treatment. **Be aware that testosterone replacement in the elderly with normal levels does not increase sexual functioning except for possible placebo effect. Administration may cause water retention, which can worsen hypertension or congestive heart failure; stimulate prostatic growth; produce gynecomastia and polycythemia.**

✦ If thyroid function test abnormal, treat as indicated. **See Protocols on Hyperthyroidism or Hypothyroidism.**

✦ Consult physician if patient requests therapy with Viagra (sildenafil citrate). This oral medication has been shown to be effective in treating erectile dysfunction but has serious potential side effects. Concomitant use of Viagra with nitrates causes severe, prolonged hypotension with risk of death, and ventricular tachycardia may occur when Viagra is used by patients with cardiac disease.

✦ If zinc level is decreased, administer zinc supplementation.

✦ If concomitant illness (e.g., hypertension, diabetes), implement management strategies to control.

✦ If NPT is not present on snap gauge test, consider vascular abnormality. Refer to urologist for assessment of penile-brachial systolic blood pressure index and further diagnostics and treatment including injection therapy, vacuum constriction devices, penile prostheses, or vascular reconstructive surgery.

✦ If NPT is present on snap gauge test, consider psychogenic cause.

Psychogenic Impotence

✦ May result from performance anxiety or other psychosocial stressors.

✦ Assess for depression with geriatric depressing screening tool. Begin antidepressant therapy if indicated. **See Protocol on Depression.**

✦ Initiate preventive and educational strategies.

✦ Refer to psychotherapist or sex therapist.

✦ Consult physician and consider referral to urologist for temporary penile injection therapy to aid patient in overcoming fear of failure.

✦ Refer to Impotents Anonymous, a self-help group for patients and their partners. National headquarters: 119 South Ruth St., Maryville, TN 37801; (615) 983-6064.

Iatrogenic Impotence

✦ Determine if dysfunction coincided with beginning of new medication (especially sedatives, antihypertensives, analgesics, antidepressants).

✦ Substitute another medication or discontinue as appropriate.

✦ Be aware that some elderly may welcome medication-induced impotence (or impotence from any other etiology) as a reason for no longer feeling obligated to engage in sexual activity. Respect the individual's desires.

✦ Consult physician. If medication substitution or discontinuation is impossible, support patient and partner by suggesting other means of intimacy and refer to support group.

KEY ISSUES

Patient/Caregiver Education

Patient/caregiver should be able to:

✦ Identify that prevalence of erectile dysfunction increases with age but **impotence is not a normal change of aging.**

✦ Verbalize the importance of:

✧ Alternate means of sexual fulfillment, e.g., touching, kissing, dancing.

✧ Positive aspect of increased time before ejaculation—longer intercourse before ejaculation may increase partner's pleasure.

✦ Verbalize that not all counselors have expertise regarding sexuality and geriatrics. Identify that although religious counselors may be helpful, some offer only an orthodox point-of-view.

✦ Explain that female partners may need topical estrogen or lubrication to increase comfort if partner regains erectile ability.

Economic Considerations

✦ Many treatment options for erectile dysfunction are expensive and not covered by insurance plans.

✦ Free counseling may be available through family agencies. Be aware of the qualifications of counselors before making referrals.

✦ Because of the sensitive nature of the problem to some elderly patients, they may request a quick technological solution rather than divulge information to health care providers. Creation of a trusting atmosphere is essential to prevent unwarranted, costly testing and procedures.

Psychosocial Considerations

✦ Because elderly females far outnumber elderly males, the newly widowed male may be placed unwillingly in a situation with a new partner after his wife's death. Stress to perform may cause transient erectile dysfunction until the elderly male has finished grieving for his spouse.

✦ The partner of a demented patient may be concerned by inappropriate sexual behaviors exhibited by the patient. The patient's inability to remember his/her partner's name or recent intercourse may offend the partner. The partner may feel like an onlooker because of lack of intimacy. In late Alzheimer's, patient may not have adequate cognitive function to perform, leaving the spouse with no partner. **See Chapter on Management of the Alzheimer's Patient.**

✦ Offer treatment to the elderly with or without current partner. In some senior citizen communities, a man may be unable to get a date if there is gossip that he has an erectile dysfunction.

✦ Consider the sex-role stereotype as defined by the patient's culture. Men who have lost the traditional role of financial provider (due to extended illness or loss of employment) may experience erectile dysfunction.

Acute/Inpatient Setting

✦ Collaborate with physician to give post-MI patients instructions for intercourse prior to discharge. Instruct to take anti-anginal medications prior to sexual activity.

✦ Instruct patients with COPD, arthritis, or exertional angina to use different sexual positions that will decrease exercise and movement requirements.

✦ Assess knowledge of prostatectomy patients regarding possible lack of ejaculate after surgery. Instruct patients that lack may be due to retrograde ejaculation, which is physiologically harmless.

Extended Care Setting

✦ Assess potential causes of residents' erectile dysfunction:

- ✧ Anxiety related to lack of privacy.

✧ Fear of reprimand by staff for engaging in sexual activity.

✧ Threat to adult children that parent may face expulsion from facility for engaging in sexual activity.

✦ Initiate staff education related to needs of the elderly for sexual fulfillment.

✦ Consider home visits (for residents who are capable) as opportunity for intimacy in stress-free environment.

Home Setting

✦ Identify elders who live with family members or other caregiver. Assess for caregiver bias against sexuality in the elderly, which may impair privacy, independence, and ability to contact potential partners.

✦ Explain sexual needs of the elderly to caregivers.

✦ Encourage dialysis patients to plan for times off dialysis and times of least fatigue for sexual activity.

Chapter 11

Hematologic System

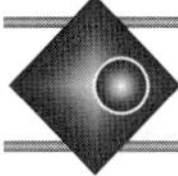

Anemia

HISTORY

✦ Associated or presenting symptoms: Weakness, fatigue, shortness of breath, lightheadedness? **Be aware that elderly may present with symptoms of irritability, confusion, and inappropriate behavior.** Weight loss? Nosebleeds? Sore tongue? Palpitations, syncope, increase in number of anginal episodes, orthopnea, edema? Change in bowel habits; black, tarry, or red-streaked stool; constipation; diarrhea; hemorrhoids? Abdominal discomfort, heartburn, reflux?

✦ **Duration of symptoms?**

✦ Recent fever, infection?

✦ Comorbid conditions/past medical history: Alcohol (EtOH) use, history of colon cancer, polyps, Crohn's disease, inflammatory bowel disease, peptic ulcer disease, hiatal hernia, gastroesophageal reflux disease (GERD), pancreatic insufficiency, gastric surgery, B_{12} deficiency, pernicious anemia, arthritis, congestive heart failure (CHF), coronary artery disease (CAD), diabetes mellitus, renal insufficiency/dialysis, frequent phlebotomies?

✦ Ethnicity: African Americans at risk for sickle cell disease or thalassemia; East Asians and those of Mediterranean descent at risk for thalassemia.

✦ Medications: especially NSAIDs, aspirin, glucocorticoids, or OTC aspirin-like compounds? Note especially antacids, which may interfere with iron absorption. Medications with potential to interfere with B_{12} absorption: aminosalicyclic acid, biguanides, colchicine, neomycin, omeprazole? Medications with potential to interfere with folic acid metabolism: sulfasalazine, methotrexate, pyrimethamine, phenytoin, antituberculosis drugs?

✦ First-degree relative with colon cancer?

✦ Diet history? Vegetarian diet? History of pica (eating ice, clay, or raw potatoes)? **Increased fiber in diet may cause available iron to be unabsorbable.**

✦ Functional status: inability to walk without fatigue?

✦ Social supports/caregiver?

PHYSICAL EXAMINATION

✦ Vital signs. Assess for postural hypotension. Assess for fever as sign of underlying infection.

✦ Neurological: Assess mental status. Assess proprioception and vibratory sensation (alterations may indicate malnutrition or B_{12} deficiency).

✦ Skin: Note pallor. Inspect for koilonychia (spoon nails), brittle nails.

✦ Oral: Inspect for caries, gum inflammation (possible bleeding/infectious sites). Assess for glossitis, angular chelitis (sign of vitamin and iron deficiency).

✦ Eyes: Inspect color of sclera: paleness, **blue tint may be sign of iron deficiency in the elderly.** Pale conjunctiva may also be evident.

✦ Cardiac: Assess for tachycardia, systolic murmur.

✦ Lungs: Increased respiratory rate.

✦ Abdomen: Palpate for mild splenomegaly which may indicate iron deficiency.

✦ Rectal: Stool for guaiac.

DIAGNOSTIC TESTS

✦ CBC with differential:

✧ Hemoglobin (Hgb) level is screen for anemia. Criteria for diagnosis of anemia: males: Hgb < 14 g/dl; females Hgb < 12 g/dl.

✧ Hematocrit measures RBC concentration. Hgb and hematocrit levels are more useful if compared with patient's previous levels. Both are influenced by age and gender and may not provide additional critical information if diagnosis of anemia has already been derived from RBC count and analysis of blood smear.

✧ Mean corpuscular volume (MCV) differentiates microcytosis from macrocytosis.

✧ Red cell distribution width (RDW) measures variation in red blood cell size. Neither RDW nor MCV provide definitive diagnosis because life-span of red blood cells is 120 days and only about 1% are replaced daily.

✦ Reticulocyte count represents new RBC production from marrow. Count is usually low in vitamin B_{12}, folate, and iron deficiency; high in anemia caused by blood loss or hemolysis. Reticulocyte production index (RPI) is a calculated value that assesses RBC production correcting for increased erythropoietin and degree of anemia. See Figure 11-1.

✦ Serum iron level; normal range at most labs 50–200 μg/dL. Used in conjunction with ferritin and transferrin to differentiate iron deficiency from other anemias.

✦ Total iron-binding capacity (TIBC) reflects total amount of transferrin available in the blood; normal at most laboratories 200–450 μg/dL.

✦ Transferrin saturation (calculated by dividing serum iron by the TIBC); not valid if TIBC $<$ 250 μg/dL.

✦ Serum ferritin level to differentiate between iron deficiency and anemia of chronic disease. Correlates with total body iron stores. May be elevated in states of inflammation, hepatocellular damage, or malignancy.

✦ Microscopic analysis of blood smear, currently less frequently used, but reveals:

✧ Uniformity or variance in RBC size.

✧ Presence of sickle cells—confirms diagnosis of sickle cell anemia.

✧ Presence of target cells—deformities seen in iron deficiency, thalassemia.

✧ Hypersegmentation of nuclei of neutrophils—suggestive of vitamin B_{12} or folate deficiency.

✧ Presence of elliptocyte cells—deformities suggestive of thalassemia minor and iron deficiency.

✦ Blood urea nitrogen (BUN) and creatinine to monitor for kidney disease, which may inhibit normal production of erythropoietin.

✦ Albumin or prealbumin level. **Protein malnutrition may cause anemia.**

PREVENTION

✦ **See Protocol on Prevention and Health Maintenance.**

MANAGEMENT

✦ Differentiate type of anemia through analysis of laboratory findings and examination of peripheral smear if available.

✦ See Table 11-1 and Figure 11-1.

Iron Deficiency

✦ **Most common type of anemia seen in elderly population. Contributing factors: reduced absorption and increased iron turnover due**

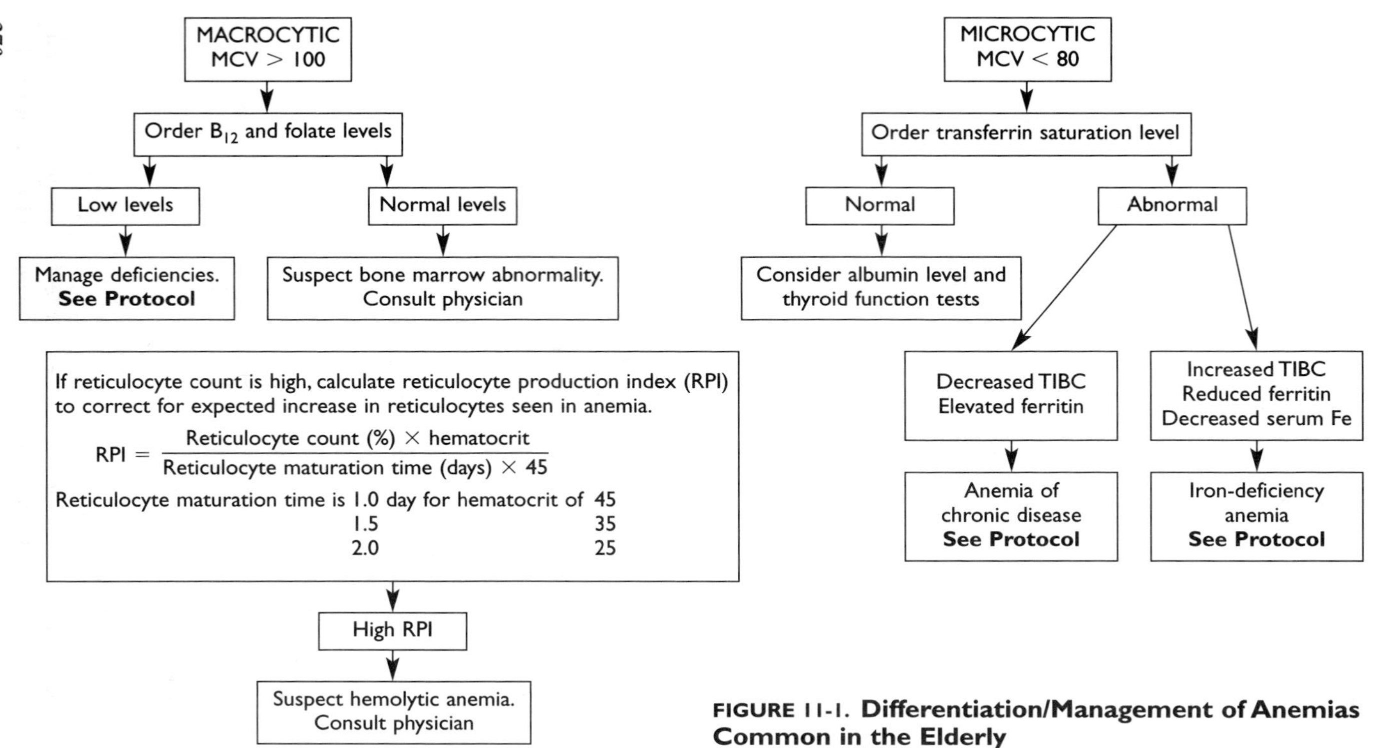
MACROCYTIC
MCV > 100
Order B_{12} and folate levels
Low levels
Manage deficiencies.
See Protocol
Normal levels
Suspect bone marrow abnormality.
Consult physician
If reticulocyte count is high, calculate reticulocyte production index (RPI) to correct for expected increase in reticulocytes seen in anemia.
$RPI = \frac{\text{Reticulocyte count (\%)} \times \text{hematocrit}}{\text{Reticulocyte maturation time (days)} \times 45}$
Reticulocyte maturation time is 1.0 day for hematocrit of 45
1.5 35
2.0 25
High RPI
Suspect hemolytic anemia.
Consult physician
MICROCYTIC
MCV < 80
Order transferrin saturation level
Normal
Consider albumin level and thyroid function tests
Abnormal
Decreased TIBC
Elevated ferritin
Anemia of chronic disease
See Protocol
Increased TIBC
Reduced ferritin
Decreased serum Fe
Iron-deficiency anemia
See Protocol

FIGURE 11-1. Differentiation/Management of Anemias Common in the Elderly

TABLE 11-1. Laboratory Findings in Anemias Common in the Elderly

	Types of anemia		
	Macrocytic (MCV > 100)	Microcytic (MCV < 80)	
Laboratory findings	B_{12} and folate deficiency	Iron deficiency	Anemia of chronic disease
Iron	High	Low	Low
TIBC	Normal	High	Normal or low
Ferritin	High	Low	Normal or high
Transferrin	—	Low	Normal
Reticulocyte count	Low	Low	Normal or low
Transferrin saturation	—	Low	Normal or low

to age-related atrophy of gastric mucosa; reduced absorption caused by decreased gastric acidity; medications; adherence to high-fiber diet; chronic blood loss.

✦ Females are at greater risk until after menopause when their risk becomes equal to that in men.

✦ **Primary cause of iron deficiency in the elderly is gastrointestinal (GI) blood loss. Cause of blood loss should be investigated prior to treatment of iron deficiency. See Protocol on GI Bleeding. Poor dietary iron intake should not be assumed.**

✦ May be caused by high-fiber diet that renders iron unabsorbable.

✦ It is necessary to discontinue iron supplementation 1 week prior to checking serum ferritin level to diagnose iron deficiency.

✦ Dietary treatment is of little value because there is low bioavailability of dietary iron.

✦ Supplemental iron therapy:

✧ Standard dose: 60 mg Fe tid between meals to maximize absorption.

✧ Feosol (ferrous sulfate) 200 mg capsule, 1–2 capsules qd.

✧ Fergon (ferrous gluconate) 300 mg qd.

✧ Nonenteric-coated preparations are preferred because enteric coating may prevent release of iron into gastric environment.

✧ **Consider concomitant oral ascorbic acid therapy to facilitate absorption of iron because elderly may be deficient in ascorbic acid.**

✧ Treatment should be continued for 6 months after resolution of anemia to replenish iron stores in the liver, bone marrow, and other sites.

✦ 2–3 weeks required for normalization of serum ferritin level.

✦ Possible GI side effects from oral iron supplementation: nausea, vomiting, constipation, abdominal cramping, epigastric distress. Intensity of side effects is dose related. Most likely cause of poor therapeutic response is noncompliance. Consider reducing dose to bid or qd schedule taken with meals to alleviate side effects.

✦ Indiscriminate iron supplementation should be avoided to prevent iron overload in patients homozygous for hereditary hemochromatosis (1 in every 250 of northern European heritage).

✦ Parenteral iron therapy is reserved for cases of malabsorption, intolerance to oral iron preparations, or iron loss greater than the maximum oral replacement. **See Acute/Inpatient Setting.**

Anemia of Chronic Disease

✦ Caused by ineffective iron utilization in protein/calorie malnutrition, failure to thrive, dementia, chronic inflammatory states (pressure ulcers, osteomyelitis, tuberculosis), and cancers.

✦ Symptoms and physical findings are usually less marked than in iron-deficiency anemia.

✦ Management includes treatment of underlying disorder and malnutrition. Iron supplementation is usually not effective.

Vitamin B_{12} Deficiency

✦ Serum B_{12} level < 100 pg/mL is diagnostic, < 300 pg/mL is highly suggestive.

✦ Results in progressive decrease in RBCs. Characterized by muscular weakness, GI and neural disturbances. **Be aware that initial presentation may resemble symptoms of dementia. Accurate diagnosis is critical because anemia of vitamin B_{12} deficiency may be fatal ultimately, if untreated.**

✦ Most common cause of B_{12} deficiency is gastric malabsorption rather than dietary inadequacy of vitamin B_{12}. Found in gastrectomy or gastric cancer patients and also pernicious anemia, an autoimmune disorder that causes lack of intrinsic factor. **Incidence of pernicious anemia increases with aging and is also associated with thyroid disease.**

✦ If B_{12} deficiency suspected based on laboratory analysis, check antibodies to intrinsic factor, a specific test for pernicious anemia but positive in only about 60% of cases. Consider also homocysteine level (elevated in B_{12} and folic acid deficiency) and methylmalonic acid level (specific for B_{12}, elevation confirms B_{12} deficiency).

✦ The Schilling test for B_{12} absorption is indicated to further evaluate low B_{12} levels. Oral intrinsic factor corrects malabsorption of radiolabeled oral

B_{12} in pernicious anemia but not in ileal disease or bacterial overgrowth of small bowel. Consult physician.

✦ Consider empiric B_{12} supplementation for patients in whom evaluation for malabsorption would be difficult to obtain (incontinent elderly, extended care residents).

✦ Supplemental vitamin B_{12} therapy:

✧ Various regimens exist for replacement of vitamin B_{12}. Due to high water solubility of cyanocobalamin, lower dose is now recommended.

✧ Cyanocobalamin 100 mcg IM/deep SQ daily for 7 days followed by 100 mcg IM/deep SQ monthly for life; or

✧ Cyanocobalamin 1,000 mcg IM/deep SQ q week for 4 to 6 weeks followed by 1,000 mcg IM/deep SQ monthly for life.

✧ Maintenance therapy can be given as 1 mg PO q month because 1% will be absorbed even in patients with malabsorption.

✧ Follow-up laboratory studies: CBC, B_{12} level, reticulocyte count, serum potassium to monitor for hypokalemia secondary to rapid mucosal replacement from B_{12} therapy.

Folate Deficiency

✦ Diagnostic criteria: macrocytic, megaloblastic state with RBC folate level < 150 ng/dL.

✦ **More common in the elderly who are institutionalized, disabled, or mentally ill. Also seen in alcoholism.**

✦ Results from dietary insufficiency (inadequate fruit and vegetable intake); impaired absorption from small bowel resection or chronic illness; iatrogenesis (phenytoin, trimethoprim).

✦ Patients with cancer and rheumatoid arthritis have increased requirements for folate.

✦ Replacement with oral folate, 1–2 mg qd, and iron.

✦ **It is important to ensure that patients receiving folate therapy are not B_{12} deficient to avoid worsening of neurological complications. Consider concurrent folate and B_{12} until serum B_{12} normalizes.**

KEY ISSUES

Patient/Caregiver Education

Patient/caregiver should be able to:

✦ Verbalize supplementation regimen; doses, timing, possible side effects.

✦ Administer monthly B_{12} maintenance injections if indicated.

✦ Monitor medication compliance.

Economic Considerations

✦ Combination tablets of oral iron may contain substances that slightly increase absorption of iron, but additional expense is probably not justified.

✦ Controlled-release preparations of iron supplements (Feosol spansule) decrease GI side effects but are more costly.

Psychosocial Considerations

✦ If indicated, refer for EtOH abuse counseling. **See Protocol on Substance Abuse.**

✦ Anemia may cause fatigue/weakness suggestive of depression or dementia.

Acute/Inpatient Setting

✦ Transfusion required for hematocrit < 25 or in setting of hypoxia, CHF, and preoperatively.

✦ Transfusions may be given in infusion areas/emergency department to avoid hospitalization.

Extended Care Setting

✦ Screen for anemia—common with NSAIDs, aspirin usage, malnutrition, and weight loss.

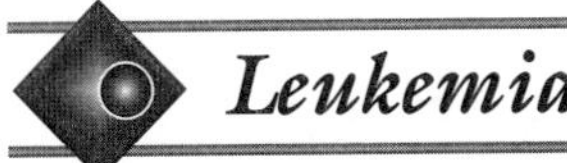

Leukemia

HISTORY

✦ Onset and duration of symptoms? **Signs and symptoms of leukemia may mimic other conditions often seen in the elderly. Leukemia is the cancerous production of one or more types of blood-forming cells, usually the leukocytes. The abnormal cells in the peripheral blood accumulate in the bone marrow. Leukemia is seen more in adults than children; age of onset is between 50 and 60 years, with most cases occurring at age 60 and older.**

✦ Leukemia is either acute or chronic and myelogenous or lymphocytic (see Display 11-1). Onset, progression, and cell maturity differentiates acute and chronic leukemia. Chronic forms of leukemia are different than chronic phases of acute forms. The four major types of leukemia are:

✧ Acute myelogenous leukemia (from myeloid stem cell)—AML (also referred to as acute nonlymphocytic leukemia—ANLL.

✧ Acute lymphocytic leukemia—ALL (from lymphoid stem cell).

✧ Chronic myelocytic leukemia—CML.

✧ Chronic lymphocytic leukemia—CLL. **Leukemia of the elderly.**

✦ Fever? Recent or recurrent infections?

✦ Heat intolerance? Night sweats? **Especially seen in chronic myelogenous leukemia (CML).**

✦ Visual changes? **Retinal hemorrhages can occur.**

✦ Headache? Change in mental status?

✦ Tachycardia? Dyspnea? Edema?

✦ Nausea/vomiting? Anorexia? Weight loss?

✦ Abdominal discomfort? **Left upper quadrant discomfort/fullness is common.**

✦ Bony pain? **Seen in CML.**

✦ Sternal pain? **Seen in CLL.**

✦ Fatigue, malaise, weakness? **Secondary to anemia.**

✦ Decline in functional status? Effect on quality of life?

✦ Bruising? Bleeding? Nosebleeds?

✦ Pruritus? **See Protocol on Pruritus.**

✦ Gout? **Especially in CML.**

✦ History of Down's syndrome, multiple myeloma, ovarian cancer, or Hodgkin's? **May increase risk of acute leukemia.**

DISPLAY 11-1. *Types of Chronic Leukemia*

Chronic Leukemias

Chronic Myelogenous Leukemia (CML)

Characteristics: Philadelphia chromosome + high WBC/polys

Clinical presentation: Frequent infections. May progress to blast crisis

Prognosis: 3–4 years

Treatment: Chemotherapy; bone marrow transplant (BMT) if < 60 years of age

Chronic Lymphocytic Leukemia (CLL)

Characteristics: High WBC/lymphocytes; splenomegaly; lymphadenopathy; anemia; hypogammaglobulinemia

Clinical presentation: Frequent infections. May progress to lymphoma

Prognosis: 10 years

Treatment: Chemotherapy

Myelodysplastic Syndromes (MDS)

Characteristics: Decreased RBC, WBC, or platelet counts

Clinical presentation: May transform to leukemia

Prognosis: 1–5 years

Treatment: Supportive; BMT if < 60 years of age

Monoclonal Gammopathies

Waldenstrom's Macroglobulinemia

Characteristics: Elevated total protein and calcium; renal failure; splenomegaly; anemia; monoclonal IgM proteinemia

Clinical presentation: Frequent infections

Prognosis: 2–10 years

Treatment: Chemotherapy; BMT if < 60 years of age

Multiple Myeloma

Characteristics: Elevated total protein and calcium; renal failure; splenomegaly; anemia; monoclonal IgG, IgA; proteinuria

Clinical presentation: Frequent infections; pain in rib cage and back

Prognosis: 2–5 years

Treatment: Chemotherapy; adjunct radiation therapy for pain control; BMT if < 60 years of age

PHYSICAL EXAMINATION

- Vital signs. Weight. **Note fever, hypotension or orthostasis.**
- Assess eye grounds for evidence of hemorrhage.
- Assess for tenderness over sinuses, nasal secretions. **Sinusitis may be presenting infection.**
- Assess skin and mucus membranes for pallor, ecchymosis, purpura, and petechiae, oral plaques and ulcerations, groin and perineal areas for rash with satellite lesions.
- Assess for lymphadenopathy.
- Palpate abdomen noting tenderness, hepatomegaly, and splenomegaly.
- Assess for peripheral edema.

DIAGNOSTIC TESTS

- CBC and differential. **Note anemia, lymphocytes, neutropenia, thrombocytopenia, blasts, and normal, low, or extremely high WBC. Abnormal leukocytes and myeloblasts occur with AML, abnormal lymphoblasts with ALL, abnormal granulocytes and Philadelphia chromosome with CML, and abnormally high lymphocytes in CLL. Mild pancytopenia may be only abnormality early in disease process.**
- Erythrocyte sedimentation rate.
- BUN, creatinine, electrolytes. **Hypo- and hypernatremia have been seen.** Hyperkalemia may occur secondary to high WBC and platelet counts. **A plasma potassium can clarify possible pseudohyperkalemia.**
- Calcium, phosphorus, albumin, prealbumin. **Hypercalcemia may be present.**
- Leukocyte alkaline phosphatase. **Zero or decreased in CML.**
- Uric acid and B_{12} levels. **Often elevated, especially in CML.**
- Lactic dehydrogenase (LDH).
- Urine for urinalysis, culture and sensitivity (to rule out hematuria and infection secondary to leukemia).
- Stool for guaiac.
- X-ray chest and areas of bony pain.
- Consider CT scans and MRI. **Consult physician.**
- Refer to hematologist for bone marrow biopsy if indicated. **Diagnosis of CLL can be made on peripheral smear; bone marrow is not required.**

PREVENTION

- ✦ Avoidance of excess radiation, benzenes, alkylating agents, chloramphenicol, and phenybutazone. **Thought to increase risk of acute leukemia.**
- ✦ No known prevention for chronic leukemias.
- ✦ Considered high risk for infection—encourage influenza and pneumococcal vaccination. **See Protocol on Prevention and Health Maintenance.**

MANAGEMENT

- ✦ **The elderly have a decreased rate of response to treatment, remission, and cure.**
- ✦ **Counsel regarding advance directives. See Chapter on Legal and Ethical Issues.**
- ✦ Without treatment: life expectancy for acute forms of leukemia is a few months; chronic forms, 5 years or longer.
- ✦ With treatment, acute leukemias may have longer survival time than chronic leukemias.
- ✦ Treatment for acute leukemias is chemotherapy. Bone marrow transplantation (BMT) is not considered in most centers if >60 years of age.
- ✦ Treatment for chronic leukemias also includes chemotherapy and BMT for selected CML patients. Goal of treatment is a normal leukocyte count, timely treatment of infections, and control of bleeding and anemia.
- ✦ Comorbidities or debilitations often prevent or complicate intense chemotherapy.
- ✦ Potential risks of hypertension, congestive heart failure, diabetes mellitus, peptic ulcer disease, osteoporosis, and visual and mental status changes must be considered when management with corticosteroids is indicated.

AML/ANLL

- ✦ Aggressive chemotherapy includes induction therapy with Ara-C (cytosine arabinoside) and daunorubicin followed by post-remission consolidation. Chemotherapy is indicated in the elder who is otherwise healthy. For those not considered a candidate for chemotherapy, palliative therapy consists of Hydrea (hydroxyurea) or etoposide.
- ✦ Approximately 40–50% of elderly > 60 years achieve remission.

ALL

- ✦ No cure in the elderly.

- ✦ Incidence increases with age.
- ✦ Less common than AML/ANLL.
- ✦ Bone marrow aspirate is negative for Auer rods.
- ✦ Induction chemotherapy with daunorubicin, vincristine, and prednisone.
- ✦ Treatment is palliative to control symptoms.

CML

✦ Only cure is allogeneic BMT. Procedure is not presently done if ≥60 years of age.

✦ Palliative treatment goal is to maintain WBC in the range of 10,000–20,000. Hydrea (hydroxyurea) 1–3 g daily. Alpha interferon has been added with good results; however, may be accompanied by flu-like symptoms, which can be managed with acetaminophen.

CLL

✦ No cure in the elderly.

✦ Initial treatment with alkylating agents such as Leukeran (chlorambucil) or Cytoxan (cyclophosphamide). Prednisone is often given with the alkylating agent.

✦ Requires close monitoring for development of autoimmune hemolytic anemia.

KEY ISSUES

Patient/Caregiver Education

Patient and caregiver should be able to:

✦ Verbalize understanding of disease process.

✦ Identify signs and symptoms that necessitate consult to medical provider.

✦ Verbalize understanding of management interventions.

✦ Verbalize the need for and ability to follow through with adequate nutrition/hydration, especially during chemotherapy.

✦ Demonstrate appropriate use of analgesics, antiemetics, antipruritic, and bowel management agents.

Economic Considerations

✦ Some treatment modalities may not be covered by insurance carrier/HMO.

- Medications are costly.
- Disease process is chronic and requires close monitoring.

Psychosocial Considerations

- Be alert to fear and depression related to chronicity and/or uncertainty of prognosis.
- Alternative housing may be required as functional status declines.
- Consider community resources to assist with transportation and nutritional support.

Acute/Inpatient Setting

- Be alert to pain management, bowel management, antiemetic concerns, and nutritional needs associated with aggressive chemotherapy.
- Consider anxiolytic and/or antidepressant use.
- PT/OT referrals to maintain baseline function.

Extended Care Setting

- Referral may be required for blood transfusions.
- Continue PT/OT to prevent functional decline.
- Evaluate for protective devices for prevention of skin breakdown due to pressure, shear, and trauma.

Home Health

- Assess ability to self-medicate, especially if using injectable agents such as alpha interferon.
- Consider OT referral for energy conservation techniques.

Chapter 12

Psychiatric Disorders

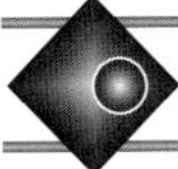

Depression

HISTORY

✦ **Most common psychiatric disorder in elderly but often underdiagnosed. Be alert to subtle signs and symptoms during evaluation for any problem. Depression may be a feeling, a mood, a syndrome, or a psychiatric disorder.**

✦ Onset, duration, course of symptoms?

✦ Memory impairment? **Approximately 20% of older, depressed patients demonstrate cognitive deficits, i.e., depressive pseudodementia or dementia syndrome of depression. See Protocols on Delirium and Dementia.**

✦ Depressed mood or loss of interest or pleasure? **A core feature for major and minor depression by DSM-IV criteria.**

✦ Presence of secondary features (**DSM-IV criteria**):

- ✧ Weight change,
- ✧ Sleep disturbances,
- ✧ Psychomotor agitation or retardation,
- ✧ Fatigue or loss of energy,
- ✧ Feelings of worthlessness, excessive or inappropriate guilt,
- ✧ Decreased ability to think or concentrate; indecisiveness, and/or recurrent thoughts of death, recurrent suicidal ideation with/without a specific plan, or suicide attempt.

✦ **Suicide is more likely in older single, divorced, or widowed males with positive family history.**

✦ Symptoms related to anxiety, i.e., palpitations, dyspnea, dizziness? **Patient with multiple complaints, somatized complaints, vague complaints, complaints of chronic pain, frequent visits and phone calls, or lack of motivation in a rehabilitation setting should be evaluated for possible depression.**

✦ Recent bereavement or loss? **Consider loss of function or loss of independence, i.e., recent cerebrovascular accident (CVA) or giving up driving; major change in lifestyle, i.e., retirement or relocation; death of spouse, sibling, child, friend, pet.**

✦ History of dementia, depression, mental illness? Hospitalized for depression? Received counseling, electroconvulsive therapy (ECT)?

✦ Medications? Trials of antidepressants? Results?

✦ Alcohol (EtOH) use? Consider use of a screening tool such as the CAGE questionnaire (*JAMA* 1984;252:1905–1907) to assess EtOH use.

✦ Comorbid conditions? **Depression may be associated with debilitating chronic disease(s).**

✦ Functional status? Baseline? Any recent change?

✦ Educational background? Work history? Cultural background? Spiritual beliefs? Coping strategies?

✦ Social situation, supports?

PHYSICAL EXAMINATION

✦ Weight, vital signs.

✦ General appearance, facial expression, level of alertness, orientation, clothing, hygiene, ability to answer questions and follow commands.

✦ Focused physical examination based on symptoms and comorbid conditions.

✦ Cognitive assessment. **See Protocol on Dementia.**

✦ Depression screening. Use of a standardized tool is recommended such as the Beck Depression Screening or the Geriatric Depression Scale (GDS).

✦ Functional assessment. **See Protocol on Dementia.**

DIAGNOSTIC TESTS

✦ **See Protocols on Dementia and Delirium.**

✦ **See protocols on appropriate comorbid condition(s).**

PREVENTION

✦ Assess coping mechanisms and teach healthy strategies for coping with stressful life events.

✦ **See Protocol on Prevention and Health Maintenance.**

MANAGEMENT

✦ **See Chapter on Special Issues** for management of the suicidal patient.

✦ Frequency of follow-up appointments will depend on the severity of the depression. Maintain telephone contact between appointments.

✦ Review medications and discontinue potentially offending medications when possible, i.e., antihypertensives, analgesics, antiparkinsonism drugs, antimicrobials, cardiovascular medications, hypoglycemic agents, psychotropic agents, and steroids.

✦ Refer to mental health professional(s) for further evaluation and/or counseling.

✦ Consider referral to support groups when appropriate for caregiver issues and stress.

✦ Consider trial of an antidepressant:

✧ **Selective serotonin reuptake inhibitors (SSRIs): Recommended as initial agents for elderly patients due to low side effect profile.**

✧ Celexa (citalopram Hbr): 20 mg daily; added benefit of avoiding weight loss often associated with other SSRIs;

✧ Effexor (velafaxine): 25–150 mg daily in divided doses.

✧ Paxil (paroxetine HCl): 10–20 mg daily in morning, maximum dose 40 mg daily.

✧ Prozac (fluoxetine HCl): 10–20 mg daily, maximum dose 40 mg daily.

✧ Serzone (nefazodone HCl): 50 mg bid, maximum dose 300–600 mg daily in divided doses.

✧ Zoloft (sertraline HCl): 25–50 mg daily in morning with food, maximum dose 200 mg.

✧ Tetracyclic:

✧ Remeron (mirtazapine): 15–30 mg daily; begin with ¼ to ½ of a 15 mg tablet and increase gradually as tolerated. Unrelated to the SSRIs, TCAs, and MAOIs; has added benefit of stimulating appetite.

✧ **Tricyclic antidepressants: Have varying anticholinergic effects; relatively contraindicated in patients with cardiac arrhythmias or other cardiovascular disease. Use cautiously in patients with increased intraocular pressure, urinary retention, seizure disorders (may lower seizure threshold), hyperthyroidism, or impaired renal or hepatic function. Discontinue as long as possible prior to elective surgery.**

✧ Asendin (amoxapine): 25 mg daily–tid, maximum dose 100 mg daily.

✧ Aventyl or Pamelor (nortriptyline HCl): 10–150 mg daily in divided doses.

✧ Elavil (amitriptyline HCl): 25–50 mg at bed time, maximum dose 300 mg daily, **has significant anticholinergic effects, may cause dry mouth, urinary retention, confusion. Avoid in the elderly.**

✧ Norpramin (desipramine HCl): 25–50 mg at bed time, maximum dose 200 mg daily.

✧ Sinequan (doxepin HCl): 25 mg daily–tid, maximum 150 mg daily, **may be useful in depression associated with anxiety and sleep disturbances.**

✧ **Heterocyclics:**

✧ Desyrel (trazadone HCl): 25–200 mg daily in divided doses, may be useful in depression associated with anxiety and with vascular dementia.

✧ Wellbutrin (bupropion HCl): 25–150 mg daily–tid, contraindicated in patients with history of seizures.

✧ **Monamine oxidase inhibitors: Caution: tyramine-rich foods must be avoided. Potential for drug–drug interactions is great. Consult with psychiatrist.**

✧ Nardil (phenelzine sulfate): 15 mg daily–tid, maximum dose 60–90 mg daily.

✧ Parnate (tranylcypromine sulfate): 10–30 mg daily in divided dose, maximum 60 mg daily.

✧ **Psychostimulants: May be added to antidepressant therapy initially to prompt an earlier response. Controlled substance. Consult with physician.**

✧ Ritalin (methylphenidate HCl): 5–30 mg daily.

✦ Increase dosage of antidepressants at intervals of not less than 1 week.

✦ Educate patient/family that medication effects may not be seen for 2–6 weeks.

✦ Reassess need for continued antidepressant use after several months; may be required long term.

✦ Refer patient with vegetative symptoms; may consider ECT. Address nutritional concerns; may need feeding tube.

KEY ISSUES

Patient/Caregiver Education

Patient/caregiver should be able to:

✦ Verbalize understanding of the role of antidepressants as a treatment modality; recognize that maximum effectiveness does not occur immediately; may take several weeks to notice any change in mood.

✦ Verbalize need to take medications exactly as directed.

✦ Verbalize need to continue medications as directed.

Economic Considerations

✦ SSRI medications are more costly, may require formulary approval.

✦ Ongoing counseling may be expensive; may be limited by coverage under insurance plan.

Psychosocial Considerations

✦ The role of caregiver is associated with a high incidence of depression and increased health problems. Be alert to depression in caregiver(s) of elderly patients.

Acute/Inpatient Setting

✦ Be alert to possible depression in patient who exhibits poor motivation, anorexia, lack of cooperation, or chronic pain. Patient who has suffered recent acute illness and loss in function is at increased risk.

✦ Be alert to depression vs. delirium in acute confusional state. **See Protocol on Delirium.**

✦ 50% of acute stroke patients experience depression.

Extended Care Setting

✦ Be alert to signs and symptoms of depression in poorly motivated patient in rehabilitative setting.

✦ Be alert to possible depression in patient transitioning to extended care setting from independent living.

Home Setting

✦ Reassess need for continued antidepressant after several months.

✦ Suicide risk requires supervision of medications.

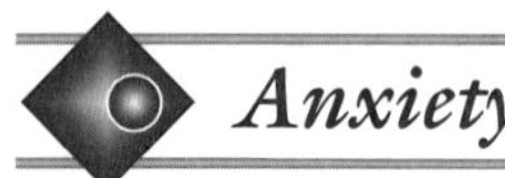

Anxiety

HISTORY

✦ Description of symptoms? **Symptoms of anxiety in the elderly may mimic manifestations of physical illness, i.e., cardiovascular, endocrine, or neurological conditions. May range from mild apprehension to a disabling emotional disorder.**

✦ Decreased concentration, attention, or memory?

✦ Subjective feelings of tension, feeling "keyed up," or irritable?

✦ Expressions of fear over loss of independence, physical health/ability, social isolation, financial security? **Fear may be based on real concerns.**

✦ Difficulty falling asleep or other sleep disturbance?

✦ Alteration in appetite?

✦ GI symptoms: nausea, heartburn, indigestion, constipation, diarrhea?

✦ Cardiovascular symptoms: chest pain, increased heart rate, palpitations, dyspnea?

✦ Musculoskeletal symptoms: trembling, muscle tension, or aches?

✦ Neurological symptoms: dizziness or complaints of "feeling faint"?

✦ Autonomic symptoms: dry mouth, sweating, flushes?

✦ Chronic pain?

✦ Onset, course, and duration of symptoms?

✦ Medications? **Caffeine, OTC cold or diet preparations, antidepressants with stimulating properties can cause or exacerbate anxiety.**

✦ History of dementia, depression, other mental illnesses, comorbid conditions? **Anxiety and depression often co-exist. Common illnesses can present with concomitant anxiety, i.e., cardiovascular disease, respiratory disease, endocrine disorders, neurological disorders, vitamin B_{12} deficiency.**

✦ EtOH use? Consider use of a tool such as the CAGE to assess.

✦ Tobacco use?

✦ History of or risk of falls? **Benzodiazepines are associated with an increased risk of falls in the elderly.** **See Protocol on Falls.**

✦ Functional status? Impact of anxiety on ability to perform activities of daily living (ADLs) and instrumental ADLs (IADLs)?

✦ Social situation/support?

PHYSICAL EXAMINATION

✦ Weight, vital signs. Note change in weight. Note hypertension, tachycardia, dyspnea, or tachypnea.

✦ General appearance, facial expression, level of alertness, orientation, clothing, hygiene, ability to answer questions and follow commands.

✦ Note presence of tremors, sweating, wringing hands, pacing, restlessness, inability to sit still.

✦ Focused physical examination based on symptoms and comorbid conditions.

✦ Cognitive assessment. **See Protocol on Dementia.**

✦ Depression screening. **See Protocol on Depression.**

✦ Functional assessment. **See Protocol on Dementia.**

DIAGNOSTIC TESTS

✦ **See Protocols on Dementia and Delirium** for recommendations on diagnostic evaluation if associated with cognitive changes.

✦ **See protocols on appropriate comorbid conditions.**

PREVENTION

✦ Assess coping mechanisms and teach healthy strategies for coping with stressful life events.

✦ Educate on fall prevention strategies. **See Protocol on Falls.**

✦ **See Protocol on Prevention and Health Maintenance.**

MANAGEMENT

✦ **Extreme states of anxiety, i.e., panic, obsessive-compulsive disorder, and phobias, are less common in the elderly.**

✦ **Decision to treat anxiety is based on impact symptoms are having on social, emotional, or cognitive function, or on a co-existing physical illness. Potential toxicity of treatment must be considered. Treatment usually limited to symptom relief.**

✦ Consider social work referral for complete psychosocial assessment, education, and counseling on available resources.

✦ Consider referral to a mental health professional(s) for psychotherapy, cognitive-behavioral therapy, relaxation training, or possible admission to a psychiatric unit for detoxification and drug withdrawal.

✦ Avoid or limit EtOH and caffeine.

✦ Consider antidepressant if anxiety is associated with depression. **See Protocol on Depression.**

✦ Consider behavioral management, counseling, reassurance techniques before initiating drug therapy.

✦ Consider benzodiazepines for symptom relief. **Use with caution in the elderly.** Highly protein-bound, therefore may cause increased sedation in elderly with low albumin. Elimination half-life is prolonged secondary to slower hepatic metabolism, therefore increased potential for toxicity especially with longer-acting benzodiazepines. There is also an increased sensitivity to CNS effects of benzodiazepines with age. Comorbidity, polypharmacy further increase toxicity risk. Most common side effects are sedation, ataxia, dysarthria, decreased coordination, and psychomotor and cognitive impairment.

✧ **Benzodiazepines with short or intermediate half-life:**

✧ Serax (oxazepam): 15–45 mg daily in three divided doses.

✧ Ativan (lorazepam): 0.5 mg initially, range 0.5–1 mg bid–tid.

✧ Xanax (alprazolam): 0.25–2 mg daily in divided doses.

✧ **Benzodiazepines with long half-life: May see toxic effects in elderly days to weeks after discontinuing drug. Advantage: Can be prescribed in once daily or every other day dosing.**

✧ Librium (chlordiazepoxide HCl): 5–25 mg daily, maximum 100 mg daily in divided doses; can cause increased drowsiness, apathy, and ataxia.

✧ Valium (diazepam): 2 mg daily initially, gradually increase as needed and tolerated; **half-life of 75–90 hr.**

✧ Discuss ability to drive; benzodiazepines often cause psychomotor impairment which can increase risk with driving. Consider driving evaluation through OT if available.

✧ Be alert to increased toxicity risk with increasing age; patient can develop toxicity over time on same dose secondary to increasing age.

✧ Be alert that side effects of benzodiazepines may be mistaken for age-related memory impairment.

✧ Avoid use of benzodiazepines in patients with dementia or with history/high risk of falls.

✧ Taper slowly over weeks to discontinue if patient has been on benzodiazepines long term. **Long term use should be limited secondary to development of physiological dependence and withdrawal. In general,**

the higher the dose, the shorter the time required to produce dependence.

✧ Be alert to withdrawal symptoms, i.e., a rebound increase in anxiety, restlessness, insomnia, cognitive disturbance when benzodiazepines are discontinued abruptly, especially with short half-life agents.

✦ Non-benzodiazepine medications:

✧ **Barbiturates and propanediols:** Potentially hazardous for elderly. Use is not recommended.

✧ **Buspirone:** May be useful as anxiolytic; has been used for agitation in patients with dementia.

✧ **Beta-blockers:** Reduce autonomic symptoms associated with anxiety; little clinical data on effectiveness in anxiety.

✧ **Antidepressants:** Useful with mixed depression/anxiety.

✧ **Antihistamines:** May be useful short-term; can cause confusion and oversedation.

✧ Benadryl (diphenhydramine HCl): 25–50 mg daily—bid.

✧ Atarax (hydroxyzine HCl): 50–100 mg tid–qid.

✧ **Neuroleptics:** Useful for severe agitation with dementia; usefulness in treatment of anxiety has not been demonstrated.

KEY ISSUES

Patient/Caregiver Education

Patient/caregiver should be able to:

✦ Verbalize appropriate nonpharmacological strategies recommended for stress reduction.

✦ Verbalize understanding of medication regimen, benefits/risks of prescribed medications, need to take medications exactly as directed.

Economic Considerations

✦ Behavioral health treatment modalities may not be covered under insurance; may require prior authorization.

Psychosocial Considerations

✦ Elderly experience many losses over time; be alert to concomitant depression in older patient with symptoms of anxiety.

Acute/Inpatient Setting

✦ Anxiety may coexist with acute/chronic medical problems or may mimic medical conditions. Assess and manage underlying problems.

✦ Be alert to withdrawal symptoms with long-term use of benzodiazepines. Taper slowly.

✦ Intravenous benzodiazepines available if needed.

✦ Use benzodiazepines with caution in combination with hypnotics, sedatives, analgesics, or narcotics.

✦ Be alert to malignant neuroleptic syndrome related to use of neuroleptic medications.

Extended Care Setting

✦ Health Care Financing Administration (HCFA) guidelines, Omnibus Reconciliation Act (OBRA) 1987, restrict use of benzodiazepines and neuroleptics in nursing homes; must have clear indications and/or attempt to discontinue.

Home Setting

✦ Anxiolytics, especially long-acting agents, are associated with increased risk of falls. Be alert in individuals living alone. Consider emergency notification system.

✦ Compliance and dependency may be difficult to monitor in individuals living alone.

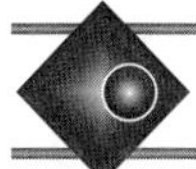

Substance Abuse in the Elderly

It is estimated that 17% of the over-60 population is affected by substance abuse. Alcohol, prescription analgesics, anxiolytics, sedatives, hypnotics, and tobacco are the most commonly abused or misused substances, while illegal or recreational drugs are used to a lesser extent. More is known about tobacco (nicotine) abuse, which will be discussed separately. Little research has been done in this area in the over-80 population.

Research findings vary depending on the environment studied (community/primary care/acute inpatient/nursing home/veterans's facilities). More complex problems in the form of housing, education, legal issues, and psychiatric and medical comorbidities are found among abusers/misusers in the veteran population and public programs. There are multiple concerns. The chemically dependent patient requires an increased rate of health care and may require premature institutionalization. The elderly have more hospitalizations for alcoholism and its consequences than for acute myocardial infarctions. The cost of treating substance abuse is $200 million, whereas the cost of treating the consequences of substance abuse is >$30 billion. Insurance and HMO coverage is often restricted or denied.

Alcohol consumption in the elderly is often done secretly and is commonly associated with rationalization, blame, manipulation, denial, shame, and embarrassment. Commonly, more than one substance is abused; chemical substance abuse often co-exists with tobacco abuse. Alcohol abuse is more prevalent among men and prescriptive drug abuse is more prevalent among women. A high level of suspicion should be maintained while routinely screening for alcohol/drug/tobacco abuse or misuse in all patients. Substance abuse is frequently a missed diagnosis. See Display 12-1.

AGING AND THE EFFECTS OF SUBSTANCE ABUSE/MISUSE

A number of normal physiological changes of aging alter the effects substances can have on the elderly. A decline in the lean body mass, an increase in body fat, and a decrease in the body water to fat ratio, increases the blood levels of the abused/misused substance. There is a decrease in the number of brain cells especially in the basal ganglion, hippocampus, and reticular activating system. Because EtOH is water-soluble the elderly are more susceptible to the effects of a higher blood/brain level at lower quantities of intake. Altered mental status, behavioral changes and susceptibility to falls are consequences of increased CNS sensitivity. Withdrawal also carries a higher incidence of complications in the elderly.

Changes in thermoregulation, combined with the vasodilating effects of EtOH, increase the risk of hypothermia. This risk is a concern out of doors

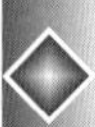

DISPLAY 12-1. *Terminology*

Substance: A chemical, medication, or drug; prescribed or OTC; legal or illegal. As referred to here, is a psychoactive agent that has an effect on the CNS.

Misuse: Use of a prescription or OTC drug, alone or in combination, for a purpose other than its intention.

Abuse: The deliberate use of a substance to alter mood or awareness that has adverse affects on the user.

Dependence: The preoccupation of obtaining and using a substance; the development of tolerance; signs and symptoms of withdrawal; and an inability to discontinue its use.

as well as during clinical procedures. Reduction of up to one-half the hepatic blood flow may alter the metabolism of the substance. Other changes in liver metabolism affect drug–drug interactions and associated consequences. A decline in glomerular filtration may impair excretion.

History

The clinical history may provide multiple positive findings, many of which can also be attributed to other conditions commonly seen in the elderly. See Display 12-2.

Multiple risk factors have been identified. See Display 12-3. In addition, the duration of substance use is a concern. Two-thirds of the elderly alcohol abusers have had an early onset (prior to the age of 50–60 years) and usually have a positive family history for alcoholism. At any age, especially in males, alcoholism in a first-degree relative markedly increases this risk. The remaining one-third has had a late onset of substance abuse (after the age of 50–60 years). Family history is less of a factor in the latter group, but psychosocial issues may prompt the abusive behavior. Substance abuse often co-exists with psychiatric conditions, referred to as dual diagnosis. This co-existence is seen especially with schizophrenia and affective disorders, but may occur with dementia or delirium. Mood-altering effects can be attained with decreased quantities and frequency than during younger years. The pattern of substance abuse should be noted. Be alert to the need of daily use, alcohol/drug-consuming friends, and the use of medications prescribed for significant other(s) and friends. The functional assessment further defines impairments that have occurred since the onset of abuse. A high level of suspicion should be maintained when there are treatment failures of comorbid conditions such as diabetes mellitus, hypertension, and/or infection. There are often multiple health care providers ordering multiple medications and

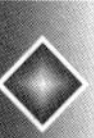

DISPLAY 12-2. ***Clinical Presentation of Substance Abuse by History***

Fatigue
Irritability
Chest pain
Constipation
Impotence
Paranoia
Social withdrawal
Loss of energy
Weight loss
Heartburn
Diarrhea
Falls/accidents
Hallucinations
Social isolation
Motivational decline
Cough/fever (due to aspiration)
Nausea/vomiting
Incontinence
Tremors ("the shakes")
Disruptive behaviors
Depression/suicidal ideation

Cognitive change:
  Acute memory change = decreased attention
  Chronic memory change = confabulation

Self-neglect suggested by poor hygiene and grooming; clothing with holes secondary to unsafe smoking practices

interventions. The history may reveal discontinuation of services by the patient when medications were not prescribed.

Further assessment includes a history of the consequences of abuse, such as the effects on relationships, marriage(s), and legal problems. Standardized tests such as the CAGE questionnaire for alcoholism or the Michigan Alcoholism Screening Test—Geriatric Version (MAST-G) provide valuable screening information. A score of 2 "yes" answers on the CAGE is considered positive for alcohol abuse. The consequences of alcoholism are numerous, many debilitating. See Display 12-4.

It is also helpful to interview the significant other(s) when possible. The informant can provide information on personality changes associated with abuse, living and safety conditions, and the effect of substance usage on

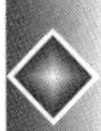

DISPLAY 12-3. ***Risk Factors of Substance Abuse***

Family history
Change in living situation
Anxiety
Loss of finances
Loss of independence
Psychiatric disorder
Loss of home
Caregiver burden
Recent change in health status
Retirement
Death of significant other(s)
Abusive relationship

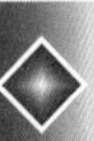

DISPLAY 12-4. *Consequences Associated with Alcoholism*

Hypothermia
Electrolyte imbalance and dehydration
Premature signs of progressive aging
Oropharyngeal squamous cell carcinomas
Stomatitis
Parotid gland enlargement
Cardiomegaly/cardiomyopathy
Tachycardia
Atrial fibrillation
Hypertension
Esophageal varices
Esophageal malignancy
Gastritis
Gastric malignancies
Pancreatitis
Fatty metamorphosis of the liver
Cirrhosis
Anemia (macrocytic)—due to vitamin B_{12} deficiency, iron/folate deficiency
Hemolytic anemias
Thrombocytopenia
Acute mental status changes of Wernicke's encephalopathy
Chronic, progressive mental status changes (dementia, confabulation, apathy) of Korsakoff's syndrome
Early onset peripheral neuropathy with/without diabetes mellitus
Malnutrition:
- Protein–calorie
- Thiamine deficiency
- Vitamin D deficiency

Hypomagnesemia, hypophosphatemia, hypocalcemia

family/social relationships. Codependent relationships are common. Denial in the significant other is also common, especially prior to the establishment of a trusting relationship with the health care provider. Homeless elderly are often the victims of theft and assault.

Physical Examination

There may be multiple positive findings on physical examination. See Display 12-5.

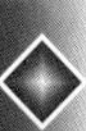

DISPLAY 12-5. *Substance Abuse and Potential Positive Findings on Physical Examination*

General: Poor hygiene/grooming; agitation and/or mental status impairment

Vital signs: Secondary hypertension; hypotension (especially orthostatic); hypothermia; weight loss; cachexia

Head, eyes, ears, nose, throat (HEENT): Diplopia; nystagmus; slow pupil reaction; horizontal/vertical gaze palsy; odor of EtOH; and oral lesions. Lymphadenopathy

Chest: Decreased breath sounds, wheezing, rhonchi, crackles in the presence of aspiration or tobacco abuse; gynecomastia*; spider angioma*

Cardiovascular: Cardiac murmurs associated with cardiomyopathy, tachycardia, atrial fibrillation

Abdomen: Ascites; hepatomegaly

Extremities and integument: Asterixis, needle marks, ecchymosis/lacerations; icterus; edema; Dupuytren's contractures; palmar erythema*; clubbing of fingernails; skin tears and pressure ulcers

Neurological: Positive focal signs associated with head injury; hyperactive deep tendon reflexes (following EtOH ingestion); muscle wasting and diminished strength; diminished peripheral sensation to touch, vibration, and position. Cerebellar ataxia; wide-based gait; impaired sitting balance; truncal ataxia

Genital: Testicular atrophy*

Rectal examination: Guaiac positive stool

***Gynecomastia, spider angioma, palmar erythema, and testicular atrophy are secondary to an increased ratio of free estrogen to testosterone.**

Diagnostic Tests

The patient may present alert, but ill, or comatose with ketoacidosis, an increased anion gap, or a low arterial blood pH. Hypoglycemia may be present secondary to malnutrition and the inhibition of hepatic gluconeogenesis. Liver failure may exist, although liver function studies may be within normal limits. Chronic alcohol use can be suspected when the rise in AST (SGOT) is more than twice the ALT (SGPT). The gamma-glutamyl transferase (GGT), alkaline phosphatase, and bilirubin may be elevated as well. Increased GGT is indicative of recent heavy EtOH use. A prolonged prothrombin time (PT) and low albumin may be indicative of end-stage liver disease. The progression of the PT is often a measure of progressive hepatic decline. Radiological examination of the chest often demonstrates multiple old rib fractures, which are suggestive of falls related to alcohol when not accounted for by history of other etiology. A screening for tuberculosis is also advisable in this high-risk group. Screening should include a two-step purified protein derivative (PPD) with controls. **See Protocol on Tuberculosis.** Refer to Display 12-6 for suggested diagnostic work-up.

Management

Identification and recognition is the first step in management. Often the presentation is post-operative delirium or agitation and the onset of seizures. Treatment outcomes demonstrate that the elderly do as well as, if not better than, younger treatment program participants. Often, several attempts to enter a treatment program have failed and commonly the patient has enrolled in several treatment programs before there is continued abstinence. Mini-intervention techniques are often successful when the interdisciplinary team, patient, and significant other(s) are involved. Late-onset alcohol abusers seem to respond to pressures to discontinue the offending substance.

Formal treatment programs of mixed ages may not be as therapeutic secondary to comorbid conditions, sensory deficits, and or functional impairments. An age-specific rehabilitation program with less emphasis on confrontation and an increased focus on socialization, self-esteem, reminiscence, and support is encouraged. In addition, psychotherapy, exercise, and relaxation techniques are important program components. The goal of any treatment intervention is total abstinence of the offending substance and to decrease the number of potentially abusive substances. Involvement of the significant other(s) and participation in an Al-Anon program should also be encouraged.

Detoxification programs require hospitalization because the severity and duration of withdrawal increases with age. Seizures can occur up to 2 weeks after the last drink of alcohol. Delirium tremens (DTs) presents with disorientation, agitation, perceptual problems (especially visual and at times auditory hallucinations), and tremors. DTs can lead to death. The elderly are at increased risk due to comorbidities and multi-organ reserve deficits. Supportive therapy includes sedation, maintenance of electrolyte balance and hydration, and/or thiamine and folate administration. Benzodiazepines are used to prevent DTs but can precipitate delirium in the elderly. Shorter-acting benzodiazepines such as lorazepam or oxazepam can be substituted, but the risk of recurrent withdrawal symptoms is increased. Short-term benzodiazepines are also associated with increased sedation, cerebellar ataxia, and periods of amnesia. The use of Antabuse (disulfiram) is not encouraged in the elderly due to the risk of oversedation, delirium, and psychosis. There is also a strong cross-addiction of benzodiazepines and alco-

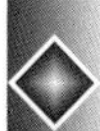

DISPLAY 12-6. *Diagnostic Considerations*

CBC
Folate, B_{12}
Blood urea nitrogen (BUN), creatinine, electrolytes, glucose
Consider arterial blood gas
Liver function studies
Prothrombin time may be prolonged
Albumin/prealbumin to assess nutritional status
Ammonia level if hepatic encephalopathy is suspected
Consider CPK level to rule out rhabdomyolysis, especially if the patient has been found on the floor/ground after being down for some time
Free T_4 and thyroid-stimulating hormone (TSH)
Consider serum amylase, lipase
Consider drug/EtOH screening
Consider electrocardiogram in the presence of arrhythmia
Consider echocardiogram if cardiomyopathy is suspected
Consider two-step purified protein derivative (PPD)
Chest x-ray
Consider referral to gastroenterologist for further work up; consult physician
Consider pulmonary function tests with tobacco abuse; consult physician

hol. Detoxification programs for prescription or illegal drug abuse also require hospitalization secondary to the severity and duration of withdrawal.

Outpatient services for continued support are found at Veterans' facilities, Alcoholics Anonymous, Narcotics Anonymous, mental health clinics, Senior centers, and some churches. Home health social workers should be considered to help evaluate available resources to aid in chronic supportive care, including nutritional support; psychiatric home health nurses are available through selected home health agencies. Occupational and physical therapy referrals are encouraged to assess for safety of function within the environment (including the kitchen), adaptive equipment needs, and ability to perform money management. Comorbid conditions require ongoing simultaneous monitoring and treatment. Patients should be advised to select one pharmacy to prevent multiple prescribers ordering multiple prescriptions. Health care providers, caregivers, and patients alike must be alert to alcohol-containing cough and cold preparations, mouth washes, and certain food items.

Substance abuse in an extended care facility is often missed. Staff must be educated to be alert to patients drinking alcohol-containing mouthwashes and aftershave, especially in the patient experiencing dementia. Well-meaning significant other(s) may supply anxiety or pain medications, alcohol or alcohol-containing products, and/or tobacco products with the thought of providing quality to remaining life. Implementation of Alcoholics Anonymous, Narcotics Anonymous, or Al-Anon meetings, and a smoking cessation program should be considered for the facility residents and their families. When these programs are not feasible, transportation to and from community support groups should be arranged.

TOBACCO (NICOTINE) ABUSE

Tobacco is the most commonly used OTC drug. Between 16% and 20% of smokers are in the 65-to-74 year age group, whereas 8% to 9% are 75 years or older. In the rural South, older women use snuff whereas older men use both snuff and chewing tobacco. The use of tobacco increases the risk of pulmonary and cardiovascular diseases as well as cancer of the lip, mouth, pharynx, larynx, esophagus, lung, stomach, and bladder. Osteoporosis and cataracts have been associated with a history of smoking. **See Protocols on Osteoporosis and Cataracts.** Dental health and denture maintenance are also affected by the use of tobacco products. Smoking is a major cause of fires and burns in the elderly.

Nicotine is more addictive than alcohol. The addiction has physical, psychological, and habitual components. Longevity and, potentially, the quality of life can be increased with the discontinuation of tobacco. Recognition and awareness of the impact of tobacco use on the current health condition(s) are the first steps in management.

Management

Counseling from the health care provider has been very effective and may include contracting for a cessation date. Self-help literature is available through agencies such as the American Lung Association and the American Cancer Society. Community-based smoking cessation programs are available and provide social support. Commonly, abrupt cessation is successful.

Switching to lower tar and nicotine products is not advised since withdrawal symptoms can be prolonged. Withdrawal symptoms may be atypical and include arthralgia, lethargy, and indigestion. Typically withdrawal rarely lasts more than 2–3 weeks. If the patient is depressed, treatment for depression should be initiated prior to entry into a smoking cessation program. **See Protocol on Depression.**

The antidepressant Zyban (bupropion HCl) has been effective in treating addiction related to smoking. Zyban is contraindicated in patients with a history of seizure disorder and must be used with caution in renal, hepatic, and cardiovascular disease.

Nicotine substitutes are available as gum, patches, and inhalants. These replacement products can be expensive and are not covered by insurance. They should be avoided in patients who are not motivated or who continue to smoke. The products are contraindicated for persons with unstable cardiovascular or endocrine disorders, hypertension, advanced renal or liver disease, or gastric ulcers. Serious adverse effects, including stroke and myocardial infarctions, have been documented with high doses of nicotine replacement.

When used, nicotine gum should be chewed intermittently throughout the day and is not meant to be chewed continuously. Dentition may prohibit the use of gum in the elderly. Both the gum and patches are prescribed based on the number of cigarettes smoked per day. In some persons, long-term use of the gum (12–14 months) has been required to continue abstinence. The patches are tapered every 4–8 weeks. Nicotine patches are advised for approximately 3 months, not to exceed 6 months. An educational and/or behavioral modification program is advised in conjunction with nicotine replacement therapy.

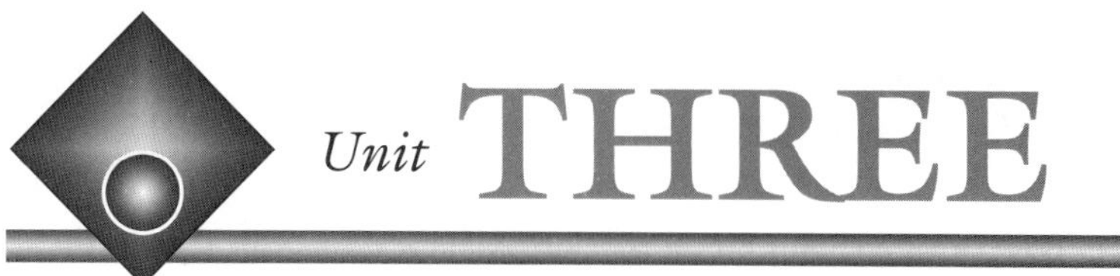

Management Issues in Geriatrics

Chapter 13

The Frail Elderly

The majority of the elderly population in the United States live independently and remain active in the community, requiring minimal or no assistance in their ability to perform tasks necessary for daily living. As the numbers of seniors increase, however, many more are presenting as the oldest old (age > 75 years) with multiple chronic illnesses. Often, elderly patients are seen with complaints that are not readily attributable to a specific diagnosis or disease process but, rather, could be caused by a number of co-existing etiologies (see Display 13-1). Anorexia, unexplained weight loss, and decreased cognitive or physical functioning comprise a syndrome of **failure to thrive** that is often compounded by malnutrition and sensory deficits. The frail elderly may be found living at home, in an extended care setting, or on admission to an acute-care facility. Assessment and management of the frail elderly require a systematic, interdisciplinary team approach.

SENSORY DEFICITS

Age-related losses in the sensorium contribute to inability to perform basic tasks of daily living in some elderly (see Display 13-2). Quality of life may be diminished by these age-related losses, which become more severe when accompanied by pathological deficits. Sensory deficits predispose to injuries, such as hip fracture, that have potential to seriously limit independence.

DECLINE IN FUNCTIONAL LEVEL

Decreased functional level can be precipitated by psychosocial and physical losses that cause decline in appetite and general well-being. Elderly individuals are at increased risk for frailty in the presence of acute and chronic illnesses that cause decline in functional ability (see Display 13-3). Failure to accomplish the developmental tasks of aging may result in depression, grieving, or apathy (see Display 13-4).

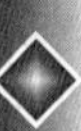

DISPLAY 13-1. ***Causes of Failure to Thrive in the Elderly***

- Physical illness
  - Malignancy
  - Chronic obstructive pulmonary disease
  - End-stage renal disease
  - Cerebrovascular accident
  - Gastrointestinal disease (peptic ulcer, inflammatory bowel disease)
  - Diabetes mellitus
  - Hip fracture
  - Cardiac disease (heart failure, myocardial infarction)
  - Musculoskeletal disorders (arthritis)
  - Chronic infection (recurrent urinary tract infections, tuberculosis)
  - Malnutrition
- Sensory deficits
- Medication use/polypharmacy
- Dementia
- Decline in psychosocial functioning
  - Poverty
  - Elder abuse/neglect
  - Loss of social contacts/isolation
  - Institutionalization
  - Depression
- Alcoholism

MALNUTRITION

Alterations in the Gastrointestinal System

Even though tooth loss is not a normal change of aging, many elderly are edentulous. Ill-fitting dentures impair eating ability and contribute significantly to malnutrition. Strength of chewing is reduced. Dry mouth may also contribute to eating difficulties. The presence of two or more oral problems increases the risk of malnutrition by >80%. Constipation is a frequent problem in the elderly that can alter nutritional status. **See Protocol on Constipation.** Absorption of Vitamin B_{12}, folate, iron, calcium, and other micronutrients and minerals is impaired by the decrease in hydrochloric acid, pepsin, and intrinsic factors seen most frequently in the elderly with atrophic gastritis. Decreased absorption is also possible with

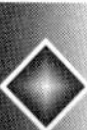

DISPLAY 13-2. *Age-Related Sensory Losses*

Presbycusis (loss of ability to hear high-frequency sounds)
Presbyopia (inability to focus on near objects/farsightedness)
Diminished perception
Narrowing of visual fields
Decreased sense of smell
Changes in taste sensation
Reduced tactile sensation
Reduction in pain signals
Decreased awareness of position in space (alteration in proprioception)

many of the medications frequently used by the elderly. **See Chapter on Medication Issues.**

Protein–Calorie Malnutrition

Calorie requirements diminish with aging while protein needs remain relatively constant throughout the life-span and may increase during illness. Reasons for lower caloric intake in the elderly include age-related decrease in lean body mass, reduction in physical activity, and decrease in appetite. This decline in caloric intake will lead to weight loss and may result in deficiencies unless accompanied by an increase in the nutrient density of foods eaten. Limited income, dentition problems, and changes in taste may cause the elder to make nonprotein food choices. The active, community-dwelling elderly generally remain guarded from protein deficiency by dietary intake. At increased risk for malnutrition are older individuals who have chronic diseases and who live in extended-care facilities, are homebound, poor, or have dementia. There is a 10% prevalence of protein–calorie malnutrition in com-

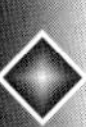

DISPLAY 13-3. *Limitations that Contribute to Frailty*

Limited mobility
Inability to prepare food
Lack of transportation to shop and obtain food
Inability to eat caused by motor dysfunction, cognitive impairment, or musculoskeletal impairments
Chronic, disabling pain

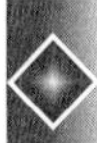

DISPLAY 13-4. ***Developmental Tasks of the Elderly***

Adapting to role losses (widowhood, retirement)
Adjusting to change in living situation (dependent status—living with adult children, living alone, or institutionalization)
Dealing with loss of significant others (spouse, peer group) and avoiding isolation
Dealing with reduced or fixed income
Adapting to increased physical and emotional dependence
Accepting approaching death

munity-dwelling elderly, increasing to 30–60% prevalence among institutionalized elderly. Signs and symptoms of protein–calorie malnutrition are nonspecific but are often detected during laboratory screening for acute illness or discovered on hospital admission. Pressure ulcers, burns, tissue loss, and infection increase protein requirements. Older individuals are less efficient in utilizing protein intake.

Malnutrition in the elderly may take the form of marasmus (calorie deficiency), kwashiorkor (protein deficiency), or a combination of both conditions. Patients with marasmus often present in the primary care setting with gradual weight and energy loss, wasting, anorexia, and irritability. Serum protein levels are usually normal. Kwashiorkor occurs acutely and is precipitated by increased metabolic demands from severe illness or injury. Hypoalbuminemia will be found. Weight is preserved, and edema is present. Kwashiorkor with serum albumin < 3.5 g/dL is associated with increased mortality and morbidity in hospitalized elders. Protein–calorie malnutrition should be aggressively sought and managed in the elderly to prevent its potentially fatal consequences of compromised immunity, poor healing, and reduced functional status.

ASSESSMENT

Most elders followed in a primary care clinic are evaluated over time with assessment focused on changes as clues to developing frailty.

History

- Associated signs/symptoms: change in weight over time, anorexia, early satiety, dyspepsia, dysphagia, nausea, vomiting, diarrhea, constipation, pain. **Any unintentional weight loss is a risk factor for malnutrition.** Screen for alcohol abuse.
- Comorbidity (see Display 13-1).

✦ Medications: note especially drugs that may cause anorexia or alter gastrointestinal motility: digoxin (even within therapeutic range), laxatives, antibiotics, pain relievers, narcotics, benzodiazepines, beta-blockers, diuretics, selective serotonin reuptake inhibitors (SSRIs), anticholinergics, and OTC preparations such as antihistamines. Note number of medications patient is taking.

✦ Diet history: note dietary restrictions (low-salt, low-cholesterol). Use screening tool to determine nutritional risk.

✦ Functional level/living situation: determine if patient provides all self-care or if there is a caregiver. Use screening tools to assess ability to perform activities of daily living (ADLs/IADLs) and caregiver burden. The concerns of the patient and caregiver may differ. Determine use of corrective lenses, hearing aids, assistive devices for bathing, dressing, eating, cooking. Living alone can decrease the desire to prepare or eat meals.

Diagnostic Tests

✦ CBC to assess for anemia caused by nutritional deficiency.

✦ Serum albumin or prealbumin. Albumin has a half-life of 18–21 days and is a better predictor of long-term nutritional status. Prealbumin has a half-life of 3–5 days and is a better assessment of acute changes and repletion efforts (level should increase 1 mg/dL per day).

✦ Serum cholesterol level <160 mg/dL indicates poor nutritional status.

✦ Consider thyroid function tests, B_{12} level, and creatinine/blood urea nitrogen. Customize diagnostic work-up based on acute presentation and comorbidities.

✦ Consider tuberculin skin test.

✦ Consider swallowing study.

Physical Examination

✦ **Weight:** Evaluate using age-adjusted tables. Poor nutritional status/ malnutrition is indicated by any of the following:

✧ $<80\%$ ideal body weight [50 kg + (2.3 kg × inches over 5 ft)]; in women [45.5 kg + (2.3 kg × inches over 5 ft),

✧ 10% loss in body weight over the past 6 months,

✧ 5% weight loss in the past month,

✧ body mass index [wt (kg)/ht^2 (m)] < 22–24. Measure mid-arm circumference and skin-fold thickness for comparison with standardized tables.

✦ **Head:** Inspect for temporal wasting.

✦ **Mouth:** Inspect teeth and gums; note signs of ill-fitting dentures or poor oral hygiene. Inspect for signs of Vitamin B_{12} deficiency (glossitis, cheilosis, angular stomatitis). Observe swallowing.

✦ **Skin:** Inspect for edema (hypoalbuminemia), wounds, or pressure sores.

✦ **Heart:** auscultate for S_3 (congestive heart failure).

✦ **Lungs:** auscultate for adventitious sounds (chronic obstructive pulmonary disease [COPD]).

✦ **Abdomen:** palpate for hepatomegaly or masses.

✦ **Rectal:** assess for large amount of stool in rectal vault or impaction (constipation) and obtain sample for guaiac testing.

✦ **Neurological:** Assess gait and balance. Perform mental status examination. Assess for depression.

✦ **Musculoskeletal:** Assess muscle strength and mass. Assess mobility.

✦ **Functional:** Assess ability to rise from a sitting position and to reach for objects.

Management

The frail elderly require coordinated management by the interdisciplinary team. The physician should be consulted for findings suggestive of severe illness and for further diagnostic work-up as indicated. Underlying physical morbidity should be treated to the extent desired by the patient or appointed decision-maker.

Medications without a definite indication or shown efficacy should be discontinued (**see Chapter on Medication Issues**). If needed, nutrient supplements and pain control should be provided. Patients/caregivers should be educated to increase palatability of food with herbal seasoning. Encourage meal-preparation and eating with others. Monitor serum protein, prealbumin and cholesterol levels, and CBC over time to assess efficacy of interventions.

At-risk patients should receive referral to:

✦ Nutritionist for calculation of daily protein/calorie needs and planning for interventions (food choices, dietary supplements, or enteral feeding as indicated). **See Protocol on Management of the Enterally Fed Patient.** Severe dietary restrictions should be avoided in the elderly.

✦ Social work service to aid in obtaining resources (transportation, Meals on Wheels, adult daycare) and financial assistance.

✦ Physical/occupational therapy for detailed assessment of functional ability, strengthening exercise, need for assistive devices, and home evaluation.

✦ Dental service for evaluation of dentition needs.

✦ Optometrist/ophthalmologist for visual evaluation/correction.

✦ Geriatric team meeting (physician, nurse practitioner, nutritionist, social worker, physical therapist, occupational therapist, pharmacist) involving the patient and family/caregiver for discussion of possible interventions and advance directives.

Chapter 14

Pressure Ulcers

Pressure ulcers are common; most occur in patients older than 65 years of age. Reports of incidence and prevalence vary. Although there is an increased number of pressure ulcers in extended care facilities, many are acquired prior to admission. Likewise, the pressure ulcers seen among the medical-surgical patients often have their onset perioperatively or while the patient is in an intensive care setting. Accompanying the aging process are a number of changes that increase the risk of pressure ulcer development and delays in healing. See Display 14-1.

The cost of ulcer treatment continues to rise. Pressure ulcer development delays the rehabilitation process, increases the length of stay, and may not be covered under diagnosis-related groups (DRG) reimbursement. Complications of localized infection, sepsis, and osteomyelitis not only increase the financial burden but also carry the risk of increased mortality in the elderly. The discomfort and stress associated with the development and treatment of a pressure ulcer are often overlooked.

Treatment of pressure ulcers is at least 2.5 times as costly as prevention. Preventive strategies encouraged by the Agency for Health Care Policy and Research (AHCPR) have been shown to be cost effective. Much has been published regarding the treatment and prevention of pressure ulcers. The products associated with assessment, prevention, and treatment are ever changing and research continues to provide new treatment options. The formation of a pressure ulcer is multifactorial, and prevention and treatment require the expertise of an interdisciplinary team. The wound, ostomy, continence specialist is an invaluable resource to the interdisciplinary team in geriatrics.

PREVENTION

Pressure ulcer prevention begins with the identification of persons at risk using a standardized screening/assessment tool, and a mechanism for communicating findings to care providers. The patient's history and clinical findings are used to develop an individualized program of prevention. Numerous medical conditions increase the risk of pressure ulcer development. The elderly often experience more than one of these conditions concurrently. See Display 14-2.

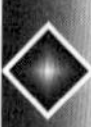

DISPLAY 14-1. *Normal Changes of the Aging Skin*

Number of Pacini's and Meissner's corpuscles are reduced, resulting in altered perception of pressure and pain.
Epidermis is thinner.
Epidermal cell proliferation is decreased.
Stratum corneum turnover is delayed.
Changes in the microcirculation reduce local tissue blood supply. There is an alteration in thermoregulation and a reduction in the ability to handle waste products.
Dermal and epidermal junction is flattened, resulting in separation of the two layers.
T-cell activation is decreased, delaying local inflammatory response.
Slower epithelialization and contraction result in a longer healing process.
Elasticity decreases and tensile strength is lower due to a decrease in dermal collagen production.
Subcutaneous fat is lost.
Number and activity of eccrine glands decrease, resulting in increased dryness.

There are a number of risk screening/assessment tools. The AHCPR recommends use of the Braden or the Norton scale. Assessment should be done on admission to a health care facility (i.e., hospital, subacute care, rehabilitation, extended care, adult day health) or home health. Reassessment for risk should be done routinely per the facility's protocol and when there is a change, either decline or improvement, in the physical or mental status of the patient.

There are four major etiological factors in the formation of pressure ulcers: pressure, shear, friction, and maceration. Pressure is the most critical factor.

✦ **Pressure** leads to ischemia when the capillary closure pressure exceeds 32 mm Hg for a prolonged or recurrent period of time. Ischemia causes death of the cell and tissue necrosis. The amount of time and intensity of pressure are key in the formation of a pressure ulcer. The ulcer can occur during shorter periods of time with increased intensity of pressure or prolonged periods of time with less intense pressure.

✦ **Shear** occurs when two layers of tissue slide in opposite directions, causing twisting or bending of the blood vessels and tearing of the tissue. This action also results in cell death followed by tissue necrosis.

✦ **Friction** results in the loss of epithelial cells.

✦ **Maceration** is caused by excessive moisture. This excess may be due to drooling, incontinence, ostomy output, wound drainage, diaphoresis, or soaks used for local wound care.

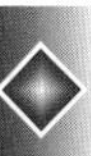

DISPLAY 14-2. *Conditions Associated With Increased Risk of Pressure Ulcer Development*

Immobility	Trauma
Obesity	End-stage renal/hepatic disease
Delirium	Altered sensory perception
Malignancy	Peripheral vascular disease
Diabetes mellitus	Cachexia
Arthritis	Depression
EtOH/drug abuse	Anemia
Chronic steroid use	Edema
Parkinson's	Cerebrovascular accident
Urinary/fecal incontinence	Tobacco use
Malnutrition	Generalized weakness
Dementia	Spinal cord injury
Infections	Multiple sclerosis
Autoimmune conditions	Xerosis

Conditions requiring a critical care setting
Perioperative conditions, especially orthopedic procedures

Friction and maceration affect the superficial layers of skin, whereas pressure and shear affect the deeper tissues and work their way to the outermost layers. Shear may present clinically with minimal change to visual inspection; however, the injury increases progressively through the tissue to muscle and bone. This effect is commonly referred to as the "iceberg" phenomenon.

Pressure ulcers can occur anywhere on the body where pressure results in ischemia. There are potentially a variety of sources, many of which are not readily considered (see Display 14-3). Sites of pressure ulcers are frequently associated with specific positions of the body (see Display 14-4). Interventions of prevention and management overlap as supported by the AHCPR guidelines. Strategies are suggested in Display 14-5.

ASSESSMENT

When a pressure ulcer is identified, a thorough history and physical examination should be completed. Assessment of a pressure ulcer in isolation of this holistic approach is of little value in developing an individualized plan of management. A number of factors, including laboratory determinations, must be considered (see Display 14-6).

Essential documentation includes "staging" and a description of the pressure ulcer and the intact surrounding tissue (see Display 14-7). The

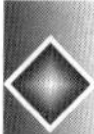

DISPLAY 14-3. *Frequently Overlooked Sources of Pressure*

Oxygen tubing and nasal prongs
IV tubing
Catheters, stabilizing and anchoring devices, catheter clamps
Ill-fitting condom catheters
Nasogastric tubes
Endotracheal tubes
Tracheostomy tubes
Ostomy appliances
Percutaneous endoscopic gastrostomy (PEG) tubes and bumpers
Wrinkled bed linens and underpads
Items found in patient's bed:
- Needle caps
- Medication cups
- Prong closures for elastic wraps
- Grooming aids
- Pens/pencils
- Hearing aids/dentures
- Food, especially crumbs

Braces, prostheses, splints, slings
Ambulatory aids, especially walkers, canes, crutches
Ill-fitting corrective shoes, worn seams or soles
Items found in patient's shoe:
- BB pellets
- Tacks
- Nails
- Gravel

Ill-fitting corrective lenses, dentures, or hearing aids
Helmets/halos used during surgical procedure
Restraints
Overlapping digits associated with advanced arthritis
Contractures
Excessive padding placed on specialty support surfaces

universal staging system was introduced by the National Pressure Ulcer Advisory Panel (NPUAP) in 1989 and was later adopted by the AHCPR. The staging system (see Display 14-8) can be found in both sets of the AHCPR Clinical Practice Guidelines for Pressure Ulcers. This detailed assessment is the basis of reference when evaluating the effectiveness of treatment interventions. Instant photo documentation has provided additional qualitative documentation, especially if done in a serial manner by

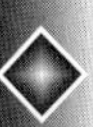

DISPLAY 14-4. *Potential Pressure Points by Body Position*

Sitting in bed

Sacrum
Coccyx
Scrotum
Ischial tuberosity
Heel

Sitting in wheelchair

Sacrum
Coccyx
Scrotum
Ischial tuberosity
Heel, lateral foot
Scapula
Popliteal fossa

Supine

Occiput
Scapula
Spinous processes
(especially dorsal–thoracic)
Elbow
Greater trochanter
Sacrum
Ischial tuberosity
Lower leg
Lateral malleolus
Heel
Scrotum

Prone

Ear/Cheek
Breast
Genitalia (men)
Iliac crest
Thigh
Knee (patella)
Acromial process
Metatarsals

Lateral

Head (lateral aspect)
Ear
Acromial process
Ribs
Ischium
Greater trochanter
Knee (medial/lateral condyles)
Malleolus (medial/lateral)
Foot (lateral)

clinicians who have been trained in proper photographic techniques. Photographs also provide a means of communication among care providers, patient/significant other(s), as well as insurance payers. Thorough reassessment of the wound and surrounding tissue should be made weekly and staff should be instructed to evaluate and report any deterioration during routine

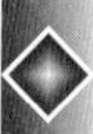

DISPLAY 14-5. *Strategies to Reduce or Relieve Pressure, Shear, Friction, and Maceration*

Timely cleansing following incontinence and routine cleansing for the patient who is ADL dependent.

Implement bowel and bladder management techniques.

Minimize exposure of skin to moisture secondary to incontinence, ostomy, diaphoresis, and wound drainage. Consider consulting the wound, ostomy, continence specialist to provide interventions to control urinary and fecal incontinence and excessive wound drainage, as well as ostomy concerns.

Minimize factors leading to dry skin. **See Protocol on Pruritus and Chapter on Special Hygiene Needs.**

Avoid massage over bony prominences.

Avoid patient positioning on the pressure ulcer.

Use the 30° lateral tilt position to minimize the number of pressure points.

Use positioning and seating devices appropriate to the patient's needs.

Avoid air-filled, donut-type devices.

Individualize the patient's turning schedule.

Maintain the head of the bed at the lowest level unless contraindicated by the patient's medical condition. Enterally fed patients and patients at risk of aspiration often present a challenge.

Use lifting devices, slide boards with movable parts, or properly instruct the patient to lift and sit while transferring, with a standard slide board, to prevent friction and shear.

Use drawsheets or other bed mobility devices (such as trapeze or transfer board with moveable parts) to prevent friction and shear when repositioning in bed.

Consider sheep skin booties and elbow protectors to decrease friction and commercial heel elevators while patient is bedridden to prevent pressure.

Elevate the heels off the bed with pillows placed horizontally between the knee and the ankle when commercial heel elevators are unavailable or are too costly.

Use support surfaces (beds/mattresses/cushions) appropriate to patient's needs.

Correct nutritional deficits by correcting the source of the problem when possible (financial concerns, immobility, dementia, lack of transportation, dentition, appetite, food preferences, vitamin/mineral supplementation, food supplementation, or consideration of enteral feeding).

Involve the patient and caregiver in the development of a rehabilitation plan appropriate to the patient's needs.

Educate the chairbound patient to shift weight every 15 min.

Eliminate sources of pressure (see Display 14-3).

Control muscle spasms.

Prevent contractures.

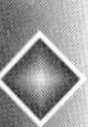

DISPLAY 14-6. *Pressure Ulcer History and Laboratory Considerations Affecting Treatment Outcomes*

Onset? Duration? How did it start? Changes over time? Interventions trialed? Pain or discomfort associated with the wound?
Comorbidities?
Medications: OTC/prescribed? Polypharmacy? Sedating/agitating agents?
Vitamins?
Nutritional status? Include: appetite, weight gain/loss, dentition, transportation means of obtaining groceries, financial concerns, functional status.
Tobacco use?
EtOH/drug abuse?
Stressors? Anxiety? Depression?
Mental status evaluation.
Incontinence?
Social support? Health and functional status of significant other(s), their availability and involvement?
Life-style? Review of a "typical day."
Sexuality?
Education?
Laboratory determinations:
- Albumin/prealbumin
- Blood urea nitrogen (BUN), creatinine, blood glucose, sodium, potassium
- Complete blood count
- Thyroid-stimulating hormone (TSH)/T4

Consider:
- Erythrocyte sedimentation rate (if osteomyelitis is suspected).
- Wound/blood cultures.
- X-ray of underlying bony structures to rule out suspicion of osteomyelitis. Bone biopsy is the only definitive diagnostic procedure to rule out osteomyelitis.

local wound care. When documenting the progressive healing of the wound, it is important to remember that ulcers do not heal by reverse staging from Stage IV to Stage I.

Pain associated with wound assessment, debridement, and treatment has received little attention. The pain has been classified as:

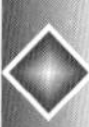

DISPLAY 14-7. *Assessment and Documentation of Pressure Ulcers and the Surrounding Tissue*

A thorough assessment includes the following descriptions:

WOUND

Etiology
Anatomical location
Shape (e.g., linear, round, irregular)
Size: length, width, and depth, measured in centimeters
Tunneling, sinus tracts, undermining
Stage/thickness
Exudate/drainage: amount, color, consistency, odor
Wound odor: assess only after thoroughly cleansing the wound with saline.
Color of wound bed
Necrotic tissue: slough, soft/dry, or hard eschar. Describe the percentage of wound bed coverage.
Granulation/epithelialization
Border/margins: edges that have thickened and rolled under prevent healing. Application of silver nitrate reinitiates the healing process.

SURROUNDING TISSUE

Erythema	Swelling/edema
Warmth	Tenderness
Induration	Pallor/dark red or purple discoloration

Accompanying photographs or tracings are helpful to further document findings and follow the outcomes of wound management.

1. Nonrecurrent acute pain that occurs with instrumentation such as sharp debridement.
2. Recurrent acute pain that occurs with daily manipulation during wound assessment, dressing changes, and repositioning.
3. Chronic wound pain occurs with or without wound manipulation.

The management of pressure ulcer pain follows the principles of pain management in general. **See Chapter on Pain Management.** For less severe pain, nonopioids such as salicylates, NSAIDs, and acetaminophen are provided on a scheduled rather than a prn basis. If ineffective, opioids should be used. Muscle relaxants, imipramine, nortriptyline, and doxepin are often used as adjunct therapy. Amitriptyline is generally avoided in the elderly due to stronger anticholinergic side effects. Transcutaneous electrical nerve stim-

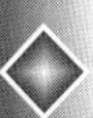

DISPLAY 14-8. *NPUAP/AHCPR Staging Guidelines*

Stage I: Nonblanchable erythema of intact skin.

The heralding lesion of skin ulceration. In individuals with darker skin, discoloration of the skin, warmth, edema, induration, or hardness may be indicators.

Stage II: Partial thickness skin loss involving epidermis, dermis, or both.

The ulcer is superficial and presents as an abrasion, blister, or shallow crater.

Stage III: Full thickness skin loss involving damage to or necrosis of subcutaneous tissue that may extend down to, but not through, underlying fascia.

The ulcer presents as a deep crater with or without undermining of adjacent tissue.

Stage IV: Full thickness skin loss with extensive destruction, tissue necrosis, or damage to muscle, bone, or supporting structures (e.g., tendon, joint capsule).

Undermining and sinus tracts may also be present.

Pressure ulcers do not necessarily progress from Stage I to Stage IV in an orderly manner, nor do they heal from Stage IV to Stage I.

ulation (TENS) has also been used effectively. Opioids are often given for predictable pressure ulcer pain. It is imperative to administer pain medication in a timely manner prior to wound manipulation and repositioning if indicated.

MANAGEMENT

Management is multifaceted and requires the expertise of an interdisciplinary team. As previously noted, treatment of the wound in isolation of the patient as a whole is of little value. Likewise, treatment of the ulcer should not be based on "stage" alone. The strategies used in prevention of pressure ulcers are also used in their management (see Display 14-5).

Management issues include: local wound care (see Display 14-9 and Table 14-1); nutritional supplementation (see Display 14-10); comorbidities; cognitive status; management of pressure, friction, and shear; multiple psychosocial issues (see Display 14-6); pain management; prevention/treatment of

(text continues on page 420)

DISPLAY 14-9. *Essentials of Local Wound Care*

DEBRIDEMENT

Necrotic tissue (slough/eschar) delays wound healing. Heel ulcers with dry eschar do not need debridement unless there is surrounding erythema, edema, or induration or there is wound fluctuance or drainage.

The types of debridement are listed below:

Sharp

Involves use of a scalpel and/or scissors. It is the quickest technique of removing necrotic tissue.
Indicated in presence of sepsis or progressing cellulitis.
May be done conservatively at bedside.
Timely pain management must be considered prior to procedure.

Mechanical

Commonly involves use of saline wet-to-dry dressings or whirlpool.
Removes necrotic tissue but may also damage epithelialized tissue.
Wet-to-dry dressing should not be moistened prior to removal when used for debridement.
Wet-to-dry dressings are usually dry in 6 to 8 hr; if found to be moist, extend the interval of dressing change.
Whirlpool should be discontinued once necrotic tissue is debrided, to prevent damage to newly developing tissue.
Timely pain management must be considered prior to dressing change or whirlpool procedure.

Enzymatic

Involves use of topical enzymatic products.
Will not penetrate hard, dry eschar. Consider cross-hatching eschar or softening eschar using a hydrogel or semipermeable transparent dressing.
Some products damage vitalized as well as necrotic tissue. Newer products are selective for necrotic tissue.
Not advisable in presence of infection.

Autolytic

Commonly involves the use of hydrocolloidal, transparent film dressings, and hydrogels.
Necrotic tissue is liquefied by the normal enzymatic activity of the wound.
Contraindicated in presence of infection.

(continued)

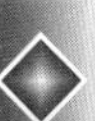

DISPLAY 14-9. *Continued*

CLEANSING

The healing process cannot be optimized in the presence of debris.

Cleansing should be done at the time of assessment and prior to acquisition of cultures.

Benefits of routine cleansing, in the absence of residual topical agents, debris, or wound exudate, must be weighed against potential trauma.

The process involves a wound cleansing solution and a solution delivery system.

A 0.9% sodium chloride solution is the safest cleansing solution.

Avoid cleansing with iodophor, hydrogen peroxide, povidone iodine, sodium hypochlorite (Dakin's), and acetic acid. These agents are cytotoxic and are potentially systemically toxic.

Safe irrigating pressures range from 4 to 15 psi. The desired pressure of 8 psi is achieved by using a 35-cc syringe and a 19-gauge IV catheter.

Margins are gently patted dry following cleansing.

DRESSINGS

The goal of the dressing is to provide:

- a moist environment;
- protection from trauma, bacteria;
- thermal insulation.

Removal should be atraumatic to wound and surrounding tissue.

Common generic categories include: gauzes, nonadherent, semi-permeable transparent films, hydrogels, hydrocolloids, foams, and exudate absorptive. See Table 14-1.

Treat cutaneous fungal infections prior to using transparent films or hydrocolloidals. Fungus thrives in warm/moist environment.

Expense and nursing time must be considered. Some dressings are individually more expensive but extended dressing change interval leads to cost-effectiveness.

Wound dead space must be packed; avoid packing too firmly, as increased ischemia can occur.

Extend transparent films and hydrocolloidals at least 2 cm beyond wound edges.

Metronidazole gel can be used for malodorous ulcers. **Caution:** Hydrocolloids, especially, interact with wounds to produce a characteristic odor. Thoroughly cleanse wound prior to determining malodorous state.

(continued)

DISPLAY 14-9. *Continued*

Dressings (continued)

Skin protectant/skin barrier applied to surrounding tissue prevents maceration.
To prevent trauma at dressing removal:
Apply skin protectant/skin barrier beneath tape and all adherent dressings.
Stretch transparent films laterally and let go until all edges are free.
Gently remove skin from hydrocolloidals; avoid pulling hydrocolloidal to remove.
For heavily draining wounds, consider use of ostomy wound drainage bags or urinary/fecal incontinence bags.

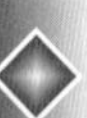

DISPLAY 14-10. *Nutritional Supplementation in Treatment of Pressure Ulcers*

In addition to correcting anemias, folic acid deficiency, and Vitamin B_{12} deficiency, consider the following if not contraindicated by the patient's medical status:

Multivitamin with minerals: 1 tablet PO daily.
Ascorbic acid (Vitamin C): 500 mg PO bid.
Vitamin A: 25,000 Units PO daily × 7 days.
Zinc: 220 mg PO tid × 6–8 weeks.

secondary complications (Display 14-11); surgical repair; patient rehabilitation; and patient/caregiver(s) education.

The number of marketed products for the treatment of pressure ulcers is in excess of 2,000. Availability of products varies within localities, institutions, and among insurance payers. The wound, ostomy, continence specialist is knowledgeable about products used directly on/in the wound, pressure relief/reduction products, and appropriate support surfaces, their costs, and availability in a variety of settings. The physical and occupational therapists are invaluable in determining proper positioning, seating, lifting, transferring, and adaptive devices. The pharmacy reviews the effects of prescribed medications and the consequences of polypharmacy on the healing process. The nutritionist develops a plan for correcting protein-calorie malnutrition and vitamin deficiencies. The social worker is often involved in the assessment of psychosocial factors that affect the outcome of management (see Dis-

TABLE 14-1. General Guidelines for Dressing Selection According to Wound Characteristics

	Moisture					Depth			
Dressing category	**Dry**	**Mini-mal**	**Mod-erate**	**Heavy**	**+ Infec-tion**	**Shal-low**	**Cavity**	**De-brides**	**Dressing change**
Gauzes	X	X	X	X	X	X	X	X (12 ply)	2–6 times daily
Nonadherent	X	X			X	X			Daily
Transparent films	X	X			Avoid	X		X	3–5 days
Hydrogel	X	X	X		Avoid	X	X	X	2 times daily to every 3 days
Hydrocolloid	X	X	X		Avoid	X		X	3–5 days
Foams		X	X	X	Avoid	X	X	X	3–5 days
Exudate absorptive: e.g., calcium alginates, Multidex		X	X	X	X	X	X	X	2 times daily to daily

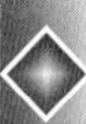

DISPLAY 14-11. *Issues in Management of Wound Colonization and Infection*

All wounds are colonized.
Not all wounds are infected.
Effective wound cleansing/debridement minimizes colonization.
Signs of infection: malodorous or purulent drainage, surrounding tissue erythema, heat, edema, induration, or tenderness. Fever may be absent in the elderly. Elevated leukocytes, neutrophils.
Necrotic tissue supports bacterial growth.
Avoid routine swab cultures.
Culture best obtained through needle aspirate or tissue biopsy.
Commonly prescribed wound antiseptics are discouraged. When used limit to 48-hr intervals due to destruction of macrophages:

- **Acetic acid** 0.25%: used for wound pseudomonas.
- **Dakin's:** used for wound staph or strep, liquefies slough.

Suspect infection/osteomyelitis of underlying bone in nonhealing ulcer.
Consider 2-week trial of topical antibiotic in nonhealing ulcer:

- **Polysporin:** covers gram-negative organisms.
- **Silvadene** (silver sulfadiazine): covers gram-negative and gram-positive organisms.
- **Bactroban** (mupirocin): covers staphylococci and streptococci.
- **Baciguent** (bacitracin): covers gram-positive organisms.
- **Polysporin (polymyxin B, bacitracin):** covers gram-negative and gram-positive organisms. May sensitize leading to allergic reaction.

Elevation of WBC and erythrocyte sedimentation rate along with a plain x-ray suggestive of osteomyelitis have >50% predictive value for osteomyelitis.
Strict adherence to institution's infection control policies.
Obtain blood culture for suspected infection.
Systemic antibiotics for progressive cellulitis, osteomyelitis, and positive wound cultures. Consult infectious disease specialist to determine treatment course (IV/PO).

play 14-6). As an interdisciplinary team, collaborative efforts define an individualized treatment plan.

Once a treatment plan is in place there should be evidence of a progressive healing process. If after 2 weeks there is no improvement or deterioration is noted, compliance to the plan must be determined. If there has been adherence to the treatment plan, the patient's medical, functional, and cognitive status, medication profile, and local and systemic interventions should be reassessed and an alternative plan implemented.

If healing continues to be prolonged, circulatory deficits, infection, and underlying osteomyelitis must be considered (see Display 14-11). Surgery consult for aggressive debridement or potential revascularization and plastic surgery consult for direct closure, skin flaps, and skin grafts should also be considered. Bone biopsies are often done during one of the above surgical procedures to rule out osteomyelitis.

Once healed, the tensile strength of the skin reaches only about 80% of its original state. The principles of assessment and prevention continue to apply since the patient remains at risk of redeveloping a pressure ulcer.

Chapter 15

Special Hygiene Needs

The preservation of health is important across the life-span. The elderly have special needs related to skin, nail, and foot care; dental and mouth care; and sleep. These needs can be particularly challenging in the elder who experiences cognitive and/or functional decline.

SKIN, NAIL, AND FOOT HYGIENE

As the skin ages, it becomes drier. This condition is not pathological unless there is xerosis and pruritus (**see Protocol on Pruritus**). Management includes adequate fluid intake; limit generalized bathing to 2–3 times a week, with daily bathing of perineal and axillary areas; bathing with a nonfragranced superfatted soap that contains no dye; and daily moisturizing. Emollients are best for moisturizing and are most effective when applied to damp skin, just after bathing. Lanolin- and aloe-containing products are widely used and very effective; however, both have been shown to be sensitizing agents and must be considered in the presence of a new rash.

The bladder and/or bowel incontinent patient requires monitoring at least every 2 hr. Consider prompted voiding and bowel management. A protective skin barrier should be considered to prevent maceration and breakdown.

The cognitively impaired patient may become aggressive or resistive at bath time. Many such patients are fearful. Often the patient requires verbal cueing or gesturing to complete the bathing process. A calm approach, calling the patient by name, providing eye contact, and informing him or her what is going to be done before doing it often assists with the process. A hand-held shower is often less agitating than a regular shower because the water can be directed away from the face. **See Chapter on Management of the Alzheimer's Patient and Protocols on Depression, Delirium, and Anxiety.**

Toe nails become dry, brittle, hard, and thick. The soles and heels may become excessively dry and keratotic, and corns, calluses, pressure areas, and bunions may develop as a result of poorly fitted shoes. Vascular compromise may occur; therefore, a thorough assessment of the pulses should be done routinely by the health care provider. Functional and visual decline often lead to an inability of the elder to carry out foot and nail hygiene. Because foot disorders can lead to further functional decline, infections, and possibly falls, a thorough examination of the feet should be incorporated into the comprehensive geriatric assessment. Foot clinics can be used in ambulatory care, residential and senior care centers, as well as extended care facilities.

Education of the patient and caregiver regarding foot care should include:

- ✦ Daily inspection—especially important in the patient with diabetes. Patient can be taught to visualize the soles using a mirror.
- ✦ Wash feet daily, avoid soaking longer than 10 min to prevent maceration. Use tepid to warm water with bath oil to help moisturize (use with caution, could lead to falls due to slick surface).
- ✦ Dry well between the toes.
- ✦ Apply moisturizer after soaking.
- ✦ Clip toenails straight across. Proper equipment is necessary for cutting excessively thick nails.
- ✦ Inspect shoes for areas of excessive wear. Inspect the inside of the shoe for worn seams and foreign objects.
- ✦ Avoid walking in bare feet and avoid walking in shoes without socks. This is especially important in the presence of edema.
- ✦ Avoid use of OTC agents for corns and calluses.
- ✦ Avoid use of heating pads and hot water bottles.

Referral to a podiatrist is encouraged for the diabetic foot, and removal of corns, calluses, and ingrown nails.

DENTAL/ORAL HYGIENE

Poor dental hygiene, not age itself, leads to dental caries. Malnutrition is often a consequence of caries, temperature-sensitive teeth, absence of teeth, or ill-fitting dentures or partial plates. Halitosis of oral etiology is common in the elderly secondary to decreased salivary production at night along with the potential for oral breathing and drying of the mucus membranes secondary to many medications. The saliva normally has a detergent action that controls the bacterial growth of gram-negative and anaerobic bacteria that are responsible for the production of odorous gases. Maintaining oral hygiene becomes especially important in the patient receiving tube feeding and the otherwise dysphagic patient because the bacteria, when aspirated, is a source of nosocomial infections. Aggressive oral hygiene (4 times a day and as needed) should be routine in this patient population.

Patients receiving radiation therapy and chemotherapy are another group of patients who experience halitosis secondary to the development of mucositis and candidiasis. Other systemic causes of halitosis include parotid disease, gastroesophageal reflux, cancer, rhinitis, sinusitis, pneumonia, diabetes, uremia, liver disease, dehydration, and autoimmune disorders. Foreign bodies in the nares (more commonly seen in the patient with dementia) is another cause of halitosis that needs to be considered.

Treatment should be aimed at correcting the underlying cause. Medications known to promote xerostomia should be discontinued if possible. Oral hygiene includes brushing the teeth with a fluoride-containing toothpaste and a soft-bristled brush; the tongue and hard palate can also be brushed at least 2 times a day. Flossing should follow. When manual dexterity is impaired, occupational therapy (OT) referral is indicated to assist in selection of toothbrush and flossing aides. Elders should undergo professional teeth cleaning twice a year. Commercial products to clean partials and dentures are readily available but may be costly over time. A dilute vinegar solution (1 teaspoon of vinegar in 8 ounces of water) or a 1:10 dilution of bleach can be substituted for these commercial products. Partial plates and dentures should be removed at night to prevent atrophy of the maxillary and mandibular ridges, which hold the dentures in place. To prevent loss of dentures in an acute or extended care facility, it is helpful for them to be engraved with the patient's social security number.

Mouthwashes should be used with caution because many contain alcohol, which further dries the oral mucosa. Peridex (chlorhexidine) is an effective antimicrobial oral rinse. One-half ounce of this agent is used 2 times a day for best results and is particularly helpful in the control of aerobic and anaerobic bacteria in patients who are at risk of aspiration. Staining of the teeth can occur but can be removed during routine professional cleaning. Saliva substitutes are often helpful and are most effective when used before meals. Each application lasts for approximately 30 min. Salagen (pilocarpine HCl) increases salivary flow, not without possible side effects, and is often used in conjunction with radiation therapy of the head and neck areas. Chewing gum and stimulation of saliva with tart sugar-free candies are also helpful in some cases.

Dental referrals are appropriate in extended care for dental pain, periodontal disease, caries, ill-fitting dentures and partials, and loose teeth. Routine dental care should be maintained but is often difficult to access.

SLEEP HYGIENE

Although reports vary, it is estimated that as many as 50% of community-dwelling elders and 70% of those in extended care facilities have insomnia. Many receive sedatives or hypnotics. Unfortunately, the use of these agents is associated with residual daytime somnolence, functional and cognitive decline affecting activities of daily living, an increased incidence of accidents, falls, hip fractures, and ultimately, a reduction in quality of life.

There are several changes that occur normally in the sleep pattern of the elderly. There are two types of sleep: rapid eye movement (REM) and non-REM, which has four stages. REM sleep is associated with dreaming and

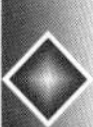

DISPLAY 15-1. ***Internal and External Factors Affecting Sleep***

Fear related to altered perception of night-time environment secondary to sensory loss (vision/hearing)
Fear of nightmares or fear of dying during sleep
Anxiety related to anticipated insomnia
Worry/concern(s) that may surround multiple losses (role, function, finances, home, significant other, friend[s], health, pet, independence, etc.)
Pain
Orthopnea
Pruritus
Nocturia
Actual or feared urinary and/or fecal incontinence
Constipation
Nausea
Tinnitus
Noise
Excess or too little environmental lighting
Caregiving responsibilities
Tending the needs of a pet
Relocation
Staff awakenings for completion of tasks—in extended care/hospital setting

decreases slightly with aging, whereas non-REM stages 1 and 2 increase and stages 3 and 4 decrease with aging. These changes result in a sleep that is easily disturbed by internal and external factors (see Display 15-1). Although the quality of sleep declines, the need for sleep does not change from younger years. The elder may get a total of 6–7 hr of sleep but these may not be continuous, nor occur only at night.

Sleep disturbances are typically described by the elder as:

- inability to fall asleep;
- inability to stay asleep;
- early awakening; or
- excess daytime somnolence, fatigue, and napping.

Changes in the circadian rhythm result in an advanced sleep phase syndrome in which sleepiness may occur earlier in the evening. If the elder chooses to go to sleep at this time, awakening is expected earlier in the morning hours.

A sleep history is aided by developing a sleep log for the patient, and requesting it be used for at least 1 week. Included is information on time of going to

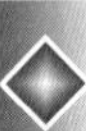

DISPLAY 15-2. *Common Causes of Insomnia*

ILLNESSES

Depression	Dementia
Delirium	Anxiety
Congestive heart failure	Chronic obstructive pulmonary disease
Peripheral neuropathy	Gastroesophageal reflux disease
Restless leg syndrome	Periodic leg movement disorder
Sleep apnea	Coronary artery disease/angina
Hyperthyroidism	Any pain-producing illness
Infection	Substance abuse

Psychiatric illness other than those listed

DRUGS

Caffeine	Albuterol	Epinephrine
Theophylline	EtOH	Phenytoin
Thyroid	Diuretics	Nicotine
Steroids		

bed; the time it took to go to sleep; the time and reason for each awakening; the time it took to return to sleep; the time of getting up for the day; and descriptions of the perceived quality of sleep and perceived state of restfulness upon awakening. Also included should be any interventions the patient used to promote sleep at any time during the night, daytime fatigue, somnolence, or napping. A review of this information is invaluable. Not only are internal and external factors revealed, but also information on the impact of medical conditions, pharmaceutical use, and poor sleep habits/hygiene may be helpful for the patient and the health care provider (see Display 15-2). A similar process can be achieved by staff recordings in an extended care facility.

If sleep apnea or periodic limb movement disorder is suspected, referral to a sleep specialist for further work-up is indicated. When these conditions are not reported or observed to be present, sleep hygiene techniques should be reviewed and a plan developed with the patient (see Display 15-3).

Chronic use of anxiolytics, sedatives, or hypnotics should be avoided in the elderly. Short-term use of these agents may be indicated during a period of acute anxiety or other psychiatric condition or during a period of grieving. When these agents are used, selection of the drug should be based on the drug's profile of onset and half-life and the patient's sleep disturbance history. The patient, significant other, and/or caregiver should be informed that tolerance develops quickly. The agent should be used once every 2–3 nights and then for only 2–3 weeks at a time. These agents are contraindicated in any patient found to have sleep apnea.

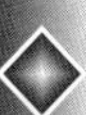

DISPLAY 15-3. *Techniques of Good Sleep Hygiene*

Engage in an exercise program.
Spend time out of doors in the sunlight each day.
Avoid exercise within 3–4 hr of bed time.
Engage in relaxing activities near bed time.
Increase light exposure during evening hours (especially during fall and winter months).
Avoid EtOH (may cause initial drowsiness but promotes early awakenings).
Drink any caffeinated beverages before mid-afternoon (stimulant effects may last 4–5 hr).
Limit fluid intake after the dinner hour if nocturia is a problem. (Caution: avoid decreasing the total fluid volume in 24 hr; consume most of the total earlier in the day).
Avoid tobacco at bed time.
Limit daytime naps to 30 min or less.
Avoid using the bed for watching TV, writing bills, and reading.
Get out of bed if awake longer than 30 min (the longer awake in bed, the more fragmented sleep becomes).
Try reading, listening to music, or watching TV (out of bed) if unable to sleep.
A warm bath, back/foot massage often promote sleep.
Try drinking a cup of warm milk at bed time if not otherwise contraindicated.
Establish an environment that is quiet, not too cool or too warm, with lighting only to orient to environment during night-time awakening.
Try white noise if quiet is not effective (such as electric fan or radio static at a very low volume).
Anticipate recurrent night-time pain and establish a plan of control.
Try using relaxation and visual imagery techniques (may take several weeks to develop the techniques and establish a habit).
Develop a routine time to go to bed and awaken each day.
Avoid the temptation of going to bed earlier in the evening.

Melatonin is a product recently introduced to the public as a natural sleep enhancer. Patients should be informed that although it is an OTC product, its safety continues to be investigated. Emphasis should be made on sleep hygiene techniques as they enhance natural sleep.

Chapter 16

Pain Management

Pain is common in the elderly but is often under-reported and commonly under-assessed. It is estimated that the prevalence of pain among the community-dwelling elderly is between 25% and 50%, and in the extended care population, between 45% and 80%. Pain may be considered a normal part of the aging process by the elder and may be minimized by the professional care provider due to atypical presentations and the unsupported belief that pain decreases or is better tolerated as one ages. Pain increases health care utilization as well as health care costs.

Optimal pain management is especially important in the elderly because pain can negatively impact quality of life, function, and ultimately, independence. Secondary complications such as deconditioning, falls, cognitive impairment, delirium, depression, anxiety, anorexia, insomnia, delayed wound healing, increased coagulability, water retention, and decreased gastrointestinal motility have all been associated with unresolved pain. Recognition and treatment of pain by health care providers is imperative and supported by published protocols on the treatment of acute pain as well as cancer pain by the Agency for Health Care Policy and Research (AHCPR). Principles of managing acute pain and chronic cancer pain have also been published by the American Pain Society (APS).

ASSESSMENT

Pain is a subjective, complex, multifaceted experience composed of physiological, psychological, behavioral, social, cultural, and religious components. There are multiple barriers to effective assessment in the elderly (see Display 16-1). The clinical history defines pain by: location, onset, relationship to activity or position, duration, quality, intensity, precipitating and alleviating factors, concomitants, and, most importantly, the effect the pain has on activities of daily living, appetite, sleep, and socialization. It is often helpful to interview the significant other, caregiver, and/or acute or extended care staff. If the pain is described as changing in character, deterioration or pain of a different etiology must be considered. The elder's ability to cope with pain may change if there are additional personal losses such as death of a significant other or pet, loss of finances, loss of transportation or the ability to drive, multiple chronic illnesses, or an unplanned or unwanted relocation.

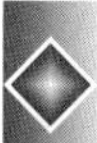

DISPLAY 16-1. *Barriers to Effective Pain Assessment and Management in the Elderly*

Myth that pain is a normal process of aging.
Underestimation of pain by the health care provider.
Overestimation of addiction rate and depressed respiration by the health care provider.
Lack of education regarding both assessment and management by the health care provider.
Underused pharmaceutical agents by the patient due to fear of addiction, concerns about what others may think, or adverse side effects.
Hearing/visual deficits.
Cognitive impairment.
Depression.
Conditions decreasing the ability to communicate.
Financial constraints.
Accessibility of resources.

Pain is classified as malignant or nonmalignant, acute or chronic. Acute pain has a distinct onset and is the consequence of injury or pathology (e.g., infection, cancer, fracture, trauma, pressure ulcers or dressing changes associated with skin breakdown, burns, surgical intervention, or herpes zoster), and generally has a duration of less than 3 months. Physiological (autonomic) changes usually accompany this type of pain, making it easier to assess. These changes include changes in blood pressure, an elevated pulse rate, and possibly, diaphoresis. Treatment is focused on the underlying condition. Chronic pain is characterized by a gradual onset and may be a continuation of acute pain that has never resolved. It can be constant or intermittent, lasts longer than 3 months, and is usually not associated with autonomic responses. Common chronic, nonmalignant conditions in the elderly include musculoskeletal conditions (such as osteoarthritis, compression fractures, rib fractures, spinal stenosis, gout, and pseudogout), vascular conditions (such as claudication and angina), and neuropathic conditions (such as peripheral and diabetic neuropathies, phantom pain associated with amputation, trigeminal neuralgia, and postherpetic pain). **See protocols on specific conditions.** Chronic pain can be an exhausting experience (physically, functionally, and psychologically) for both the patient and the significant other/caregiver. The pain becomes the focus of treatment because the underlying condition remains chronic and is rarely resolved.

The physical examination is directed at observation and palpation of the painful area(s) and dermatome(s) and examining for trigger points and tenderness. Range of motion is carried out, noting restrictions and movements/positions that enhance the pain. Functional assessment is especially important. Screening for depression, especially in the presence of chronic pain, is also often helpful in developing treatment options. Because financial strain is, at times, identified as the rationale for not seeking treatment, financial resources should be considered carefully prior to requesting diagnostic studies to confirm or rule out disease processes. These same issues should also be considered when providing treatment options.

Use of a standardized pain assessment instrument further documents the subjective report of the patient regarding present severity or intensity of pain as well as the patient's desired outcome. These instruments are classified as numerical; verbal descriptor; visual analog, both vertical and horizontal; or pictorial facial expressions of varying degrees of comfort and discomfort. The choice of the instruments must take into consideration the patient's ability to see, hear, understand, and communicate. Enlarging the scale and printing it on yellow paper may aid those with visual impairment. There is some evidence that the elderly seem to understand a vertical scale better than a horizontal format. Fatigue, anxiety, and the pain itself may create an inability for the patient to concentrate on one scale or another. Several of these scales should be offered to best meet the patient's specific needs. Ideally, the same scale should be used consistently to adequately treat and determine effectiveness of treatment interventions for that patient.

Special considerations must be made for patients who are mentally challenged, have delirium, are psychotic, or who have dementia and are unable to communicate their needs. There are estimates of 1.8 million+ persons with advanced dementia. Instruments have recently been developed that hold promise in the assessment of this subset of patients. Pain in patients with dementia is often identified through nonverbal communication. Regressive behaviors of early childhood and infancy may be the only indicators of discomfort or pain. These behaviors may include: a change in the tenseness or pitch of the voice, being easily startled, crying, rocking, holding a particular area of the body, screaming, clinging, withdrawal, resistance to care and/or combativeness, and flailing. Other indicators may be a noticeable decline in function or socialization, change in posture or gait, change in appetite or sleep pattern, weight loss, or new onset incontinence. This group of patients is particularly vulnerable to discomfort associated with falls, aspiration, degenerative joint disease, urinary tract infection, constipation, and skin breakdown. If there is uncertainty about the presence of pain, an analgesic agent should be initiated with close monitoring of behavioral outcomes.

MANAGEMENT

The goals of pain management include: prevention of acute pain, control of chronic pain, optimizing function, and improving the quality of life as the patient, not the health care provider, defines it. As pain is a complex, multifaceted experience, assessment and treatment are best approached and carried out by an interdisciplinary team. Pain center referrals are indicated when standard protocols are ineffective or when an interdisciplinary team is unavailable.

Effective management requires the health care provider to be aware of personal biases surrounding pain and its management in the older population. In addition, effective management involves pharmacological and nonpharmacological interventions; assessment of the patient's pain using a standardized tool before and after intervention; and education of patient, significant other, and health care providers (see Display 16-2).

Nonpharmacological interventions should be considered prior to initiating pharmacological interventions. When these interventions are not solely effective, a pharmaceutical agent should be added. Pharmacological management is frequently enhanced by nonpharmacological adjunct therapy. Refer to Display 16-3 for suggested nonpharmacological interventions.

The World Health Organization has developed a stepwise approach using pharmaceutical agents. The initial step is the use of a nonopioid such as aspirin, acetaminophen, or a nonsteroidal antiinflammatory drug (NSAID). When pain continues, the next step is to try another nonopioid agent in the same class; if this agent is also unsuccessful, an opioid is added for mild to moderate pain. If pain continues or increases, the opioid dose is increased or the patient is switched to a stronger agent. Cancer and chronic pain as well as pain in the patient with dementia or delirium are best managed by routine scheduling rather than prn dosing. The goal is to anticipate and prevent pain rather than unsuccessfully "catching" and attempting to control the pain.

The elderly require close monitoring of side effects from the nonopioid agents. Aspirin, even in small doses, can produce gastrointestinal bleeding, acetaminophen can produce liver dysfunction, and NSAIDs can result in gastric ulceration and renal insufficiency/failure. When NSAIDs are indicated in a high-risk patient, Cytotec (misoprostol) may be considered to decrease gastric irritation. Alternatives such as Trilisate (choline magnesium trisalicylate) could also be considered in the high-risk patient. Adjuvant agents are often helpful in enhancing the analgesic effect of nonopioids as well as opioids. The agents most commonly used in the elderly are anticonvulsants for neuropathic pain; antidepressants; and anxiolytic agents such as hydroxyzine. Other adverse side effects to both nonopioid and opioid agents are nausea, vomiting, orthostasis, constipation, urinary retention, sedation, and cognitive changes. **See Protocols on Nausea and Vomiting; Dizziness; Constipation; Delirium; and Depression.**

Normal physiological and pharmacokinetic changes occur with aging and require alteration in dosing of many agents. Renal and hepatic function should be determined and dosing altered appropriately. The risk of polypharmacy and drug–drug interactions are increased in the elderly because there is often more than one chronic illness being treated at any given time. **See**

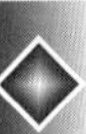

DISPLAY 16-2. *Pain Management Strategies for the Elderly*

1. The health care provider must be aware of personal biases regarding pain and the management of pain in the elderly.
2. Inquire about pain/discomfort using direct and open-ended questioning.
3. Accept the patient's pain experience and share this acceptance with the patient.
4. Encourage an interdisciplinary team approach.
5. Use standardized pain assessment tools to determine present severity or intensity and the level of pain acceptable to the patient.
6. Determine baseline functional, cognitive, and emotional status.
7. Involve the significant other(s) as well as other caregivers in determining their interpretation of the patient's pain.
8. Ask the patient to participate in the interpretation of the pain and determine the expectations of further diagnostic work-up and management.
9. Ask the patient to define his or her role and responsibility in the treatment plan.
10. Educate the patient and significant other(s) to a rehabilitative rather than a curative model of care.
11. Prevent "excess disability" by promoting proper dietary intake, mobility, socialization, and exercise.
12. Ask the patient to assist in the selection of nonpharmacologic interventions.
13. Educate the patient on the proper use of pharmaceutical agents and their potential side effects.
14. When ordering pharmaceutical agents: "start low and go slow."
15. Add one pharmaceutical agent at a time, provide for stabilization prior to increasing the dose or adding another agent.
16. Be alert to nonverbal indicators of pain in the patient who cannot communicate or who has dementia.
17. The chemically dependent or recovering chemically dependent patient has the right to receive pain management using an interdisciplinary approach.
18. Routinely re-evaluate treatment outcomes. Alter appropriately to optimize function and quality of life as defined by the patient.
19. Anticipate and initiate timely interventions for nausea, vomiting, and constipation. These side effects are particularly noted in patients receiving opioids.

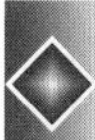

DISPLAY 16-3. ***Nonpharmacologic Interventions***

Physical or occupational therapy	Counterirritation
Transcutaneous electrical nerve stimulation (TENS)	Hydrotherapy
Biofeedback	Psychotherapy
Visual imagery	Prayer
Relaxation exercises	Meditation
Yoga	Music
Heat/cold applications	Recreational activities
Massage	Magnetic therapy
	Nerve blocks

Chapter on Medication Issues. Demerol (meperidine HCl) and Talwin (pentazocine lactate) are generally avoided in the elderly due to their potential to produce CNS toxicity and acute delirium. Use of an equianalgesic dosing table is encouraged when switching or titrating opioids. The standard

TABLE 16-1. Commonly Used Analgesics and Suggested Dosing in the Elderly: Nonopioids

	Geriatric dosing	Dosing interval	Maximum daily dose
For mild to moderate pain			
Capsaicin is a topically applied analgesic agent shown to deplete free nerve endings of substance P by blocking its reuptake. It is particularly helpful in the treatment of postherpetic pain, diabetic neuropathy, and musculoskeletal discomfort. Application is suggested at least 3 times a day and preferably, 4. There are no drug–drug interactions; a local burning sensation may be intolerable.			
Acetaminophen	325–650 mg PO	q4–6h	4,000 mg
Aspirin	325–650 mg PO	q4–6h	4,000 mg
Salsalate	500 mg PO	q12h	2,000 mg
Trilisate (choline magnesium)	500–750 mg PO	q12h	2,000 mg
Advil, Motrin, Nuprin (ibuprofen)	200–400 mg PO	q4–12h	2,400 mg
Naprosyn (naproxen)	250 mg PO 750 mg SRPO	q12h q24h	500 mg 750 mg
For moderate pain			
Tolectin (tolmetin sodium)	200 mg PO	q6–8h	1,200 mg
Clinoril (sulindac)	100 mg PO	q12h	300 mg
Lodine (etodolac)	200 mg PO	q8–12h	800 mg

TABLE 16-2. Commonly Prescribed Equianalgesic Dosing and Suggested Dosing in the Elderly: Opioids and Mixed Nonopioids/Opioids

	Approximate equianalgesic dose	Initial dosing	Dosing interval
OPIOIDS			
For moderate pain			
Oxycodone	30 mg PO	5 mg PO	q6h
Codeine	180–200 mg PO	15–30 mg PO	q4h
MIXED NONOPIOIDS/OPIOIDS			
For moderate pain			
Codeine with aspirin or acetaminophen	180–200 mg PO	15–30 mg PO	q4h
Lorcet, Lortab, Vicodin (hydrocodone bitartrate with acetaminophen)	30 mg PO	5–10 mg PO	q4h
Percocet, Percodan, Tylox (oxycodone with aspirin or acetaminophen)	30 mg PO	5–10 mg PO	q4h
For moderate to severe pain			
Dilaudid (hydromorphone HCl)	7.5 mg PO 1.5 mg IV	4–6 mg PO 1 mg IV	q4h
Morphine sulfate IR (immediate release)	30 mg PO 10 mg IV	10 mg PO 2 mg IV	q4–6h
Morphine sulfate SR (sustained release MS)	30 mg PO	15–30 mg PO	q12h
OxyContin (oxycodone SR)	30 mg PO	10–20 mg PO	q12h
For severe pain			
Fentanyl transdermal (Duragesic patch)	*	25 μg	q72h

*Fentanyl does not have a dose equianalgesic to a single morphine dosage. Fentanyl is approximately three times more potent than morphine. To convert from morphine to fentanyl: calculate the 24-hr total morphine dose and divide by 3. Select the fentanyl patch nearest this final result.

rule of "start low and go slow" holds true for a safe and effective stepwise approach to pain management in the elderly. Refer to Tables 16-1 and 16-2 and Display 16-4 for suggested dosing of commonly prescribed nonopioids and opioid equianalgesic dosing information.

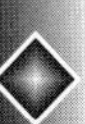

DISPLAY 16-4. *Special Considerations in Administration of Pain Medications*

Patients on a scheduled dose of opioids should have a rescue dose available that is equal to 10% of the 24-hr total dose.

Stable pain is defined as 4 or fewer rescue doses during any 24-hr period.

When titrating for mild to moderate pain levels, increase the total 24-hr dose by 25%.

When titrating for severe pain, increase the total 24-hr dose by 50%.

Titration can also be done by adding rescue doses, adding to the scheduled 24-hr dose and dividing by 2. A new rescue dose should then be figured based on the new scheduled dose.

When converting from PO to IV morphine or dilaudid, calculate the 24-hr dose, then divide by 6 (for the opioid-naive patient) **or** by 3 (for the patient receiving and tolerating an opioid). This result should further be divided by 24 to obtain the hourly IV rate.

There is no ceiling for most opioids. Combination nonopioid/opioid drugs have ceilings associated with the nonopioid component.

Sustained-release agents should not be broken, dissolved, or crushed.

Chapter 17

Management of the Postmenopausal Woman

The period surrounding menopause is an opportune time to counsel the older woman regarding health care concerns that will affect the remaining years of life. **See Chapter on Prevention and Health Maintenance.** Issues of increased concern for the postmenopausal woman include the following:

- **Risk for osteoporosis (see Protocol on Osteoporosis).**
- **Risk for cardiovascular disease.**
- **Cancer (breast, cervix, endometrial, and colon)**—7% of women >60 years will develop breast cancer; endometrial cancer occurs most frequently in women >50 years.
- **Risk for depression (see Protocol on Depression).**
- **Domestic violence (see Chapter on Special Issues/Elder Abuse).**
- **Caregiver burden.**
- **Medication use**—Women >45 years have recently been targeted by the Federal Drug Administration for an educational initiative because this group makes most medication-related decisions for American families (**see Chapter on Medication Issues**).

Women in America can expect to live one-third of their lives after completion of menopause because the average age for the female climacteric is 51 years while the average life expectancy for females is 81 years. The number of women older than 50 years in the United States is expected to rise to more than 40 million by the end of the 1990s. Some older women perceive the passage through menopause as a time of lost capabilities and function. Education and therapy can support maintenance of good health, functional status, and personal fulfillment for the postmenopausal woman.

TRANSITION THROUGH MENOPAUSE

Menopause is defined as the end of ovarian function that results in permanent cessation of menses. In the vast majority of women, the change occurs over a period of several years. The perimenopausal stage usually begins during the mid-to-late 40s. Decline in ovarian function causes a decrease in production of estrogen and androgen. Troublesome clinical symptoms begin that often lead the perimenopausal woman to seek treatment (see Display 17-1). Irregular menstrual cycles may occur with heavy, prolonged cycles as well as bleeding between periods. Hot flushes present as an acute feeling of heat sensed in the head, neck, and upper chest that may spread over the total body. Reddening of the skin is characteristic. The flush ends with perspiration that is sometimes intense. Frequency varies from very few per day to several per hour. Episodes may be as brief as a few seconds to as long as 60 min. Flushes frequently happen at night and disrupt sleep. Waning of estrogen results in thinning of the vaginal lining and loss of vaginal elasticity that may cause atrophic vaginitis, stress incontinence, urge incontinence, and dyspareunia.

It is generally accepted that menopause has been reached when no menstrual period occurs for 6 consecutive months. Follicle-stimulating hormone levels are elevated. Clinical symptoms of menopause often subside 1–2 years following cessation of periods.

During the first 5 years after menopause, silent changes caused by lack of estrogen begin to take place. Bone mineral density begins to decrease, and estrogen's cardioprotective effects are no longer present. Women who do not receive hormone replacement may experience accelerated osteoporosis, atherosclerosis, angina, and increased incidence of myocardial infarction during the late postmenopausal period.

LONG-TERM IMPLICATIONS OF ESTROGEN LOSS

Osteoporosis

Bone mass declines quickly with the loss of estrogen, placing postmenopausal women at increased risk for osteoporosis and fractures. Fifty percent of postmenopausal women have osteoporosis. It is estimated that by the year 2015 osteoporosis-related health care costs will be more than $38 million per day. Replacement of estrogen has been shown to decrease the risk for both hip and wrist fractures in elderly women. Estrogen supplementation is indicated in postmenopausal women at risk for osteoporosis unless otherwise contraindicated. **See Hormone Replacement Therapy (HRT) and Protocol on Osteoporosis.**

Cardiovascular Disease

Coronary artery disease is the leading cause of mortality in American women. Following menopause, more women die from cardiovascular disease than from all malignancies combined. The risk for cardiovascular disease increases in women after menopause because of the loss of estrogen's protective effect. Estrogen decreases total cholesterol, decreases vascular tone, decreases low-

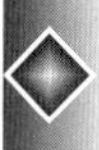

DISPLAY 17-1. *Clinical Symptoms of the Hormonal Changes of Menopause*

VASOMOTOR SYMPTOMS

Hot flushes
Night sweats

LOCAL SYMPTOMS OF UROGENITAL ATROPHY

Vaginal dryness	Dyspareunia
Pruritis	Urinary urgency/incontinence
Vaginal burning	Dysuria

density lipoprotein (LDL) levels, and increases high-density lipoprotein (HDL) levels. There is evidence that estrogen protects the arterial wall, perhaps by acting as an antioxidant and by decreasing LDL uptake.

Screening for cardiovascular disease/risks should be provided to all postmenopausal women (**see Protocol on Hypertension**). Even though smoking incidence rates have declined in men in recent years, rates are increasing in women. Estrogen replacement was found to be associated with decreased incidence of acute myocardial infarction and 50% reduction in mortality from cardiovascular disease in the Nurses' Health Study. HRT is indicated for women with cardiac disease risk unless otherwise contraindicated. **See Hormone Replacement Therapy.**

Effects on Central Nervous System

Estrogen maintains vitality of neurons, and estrogen replacement has been shown to slow memory loss after oophorectomy. Estrogen replacement may have preventive benefit or slow the progression of Alzheimer's disease.

HORMONE REPLACEMENT THERAPY

Counseling regarding the long-term effects of estrogen loss should be provided to women at mid-life, ideally before the onset of menopause. Benefits versus risks of HRT must be considered along with individual risk factors to enable educated decision-making by each woman regarding HRT.

Many women fear estrogen replacement because of associated increased risk of breast and endometrial cancer. The risk for postmenopausal women of having an osteoporosis-related hip fracture is greater than the combined risk of breast, ovarian, and endometrial cancer. Decisions regarding initiation of HRT must be made on an individual basis with consideration of all risk factors.

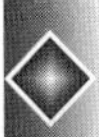

DISPLAY 17-2. *Contraindications to Estrogen Replacement**

ABSOLUTE CONTRAINDICATIONS

Abnormal, undiagnosed genital bleeding
Presence/history of estrogen-dependent neoplasia of breast, uterus, or kidney
Malignant melanoma
Active deep vein thrombosis/embolism

RELATIVE CONTRAINDICATIONS

Estrogen therapy-associated hypertension
Presence/history of gallstones
Active pancreatitis/liver disease
Hypertriglyceridemia
Presence/history of migraines
History of thrombosis
Congestive heart failure
Endometriosis

*Adapted from Greendale and Judd.

Risks (see Display 17-2)

An increase in risk of developing breast cancer of 1–2% per year of estrogen replacement has been estimated based on several population studies. The risk may be higher in women with a family history of breast cancer. More studies are needed to clarify the relationships between breast cancer risk and length of estrogen therapy and the effect on risk of concomitant progestin or androgen use. Long-term estrogen use unopposed by progestin increases the risk for cancer of the endometrium. Addition of progestin stimulates shedding of the uterine lining and removes the increased risk of endometrial cancer. Progestin opposes the favorable effects of estrogen on circulating lipoproteins but is dose- and potency-dependent. Most studies have shown that addition of progestin does not negate the protection against cardiovascular disease provided by estrogen alone.

Risk for resumption of uterine bleeding causes many women to decline HRT. When cyclic regimens are used, bleeding is usually predictable and of short duration, but many women decline HRT due to fear of uterine bleeding. Change in formulation may be needed to avoid side effects (see Display 17-3).

Selective estrogen receptor modulators (SERMs) are pharmacological agents that produce estrogen-like effects in some tissues while blocking estrogen in other tissues. SERMs do not stimulate breast or uterine tissue but prevent osteoporosis and possibly cardiac disease.

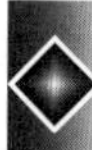

DISPLAY 17-3. ***Potential Side Effects of Hormone Replacement Therapy***

ESTROGEN

Fluid retention	Skin irritation—dermal delivery systems
Breast tenderness, pain, or swelling	Libido changes
Irregular bleeding or spotting	Changes in skin color
Weight gain or loss	Anorexia
Nausea/vomiting	Gingival bleeding/tenderness
Headaches	

PROGESTERONE

Irregular bleeding or spotting	Nausea
Fluid retention	Depression
Weight gain or loss	Insomnia

ANDROGEN

Irregular bleeding or spotting	Acne
Fluid retention	Hirsutism
Elevation of cholesterol	Nausea
Voice change/deepening	

Oral estrogen preparations may increase triglyceride levels. This rise is usually clinically insignificant, but non-oral preparations should be used in women with hypertriglyceridemia. A twofold to fourfold increase in gallstones is associated with oral estrogen use. Fluid retention is a potential side effect of estrogen therapy that must be carefully monitored in patients with cardiac dysfunction, renal dysfunction, and migraine headaches.

Benefits

HRT is often begun during the perimenopausal stage to alleviate clinical symptoms and continued after menopause to prevent the long-term implications of estrogen loss.

THERAPY FOR MENOPAUSE

For Vaginal Atrophy/Dryness

- ✦ Replens vaginal moisturing cream, OR

✦ KY Jelly, OR

✦ Premarin (conjugated estrogen) vaginal cream; 0.5–2 g/day; 3 weeks on/1 week off, OR

✦ Ortho Dienestrol (dienestrol) 0.01% vaginal cream; begin with 1–2 applicatorsful qd for 1–2 weeks; reduce dose by one-half × 2 weeks; then maintenance with 1 applicatorful 1–3 times per week; for short-term use only, OR

✦ Estring (estradiol vaginal ring) insert 1 ring high into vagina every 90 days; provides estradiol dose of only 7.5 μg/24 hr after initial 24 hr; additional progestin treatment is not required.

For Symptom Relief and Prevention of Osteoporosis and Cardiovascular Disease

✦ **Women with intact uterus:** A regimen of estrogen on the 1st through 25th days of each month plus progesterone on days 13 through 25 may be used for women with an intact uterus. Alternatively, a combined use of estrogen and progesterone, continuously or cyclically, is also appropriate. Addition of progesterone prevents endometrial hyperplasia and elevation of triglycerides. Women with an intact uterus who begin estrogen replacement without progesterone should undergo pretreatment endometrial biopsy with annual biopsies throughout duration of estrogen therapy. Referral to a gynecologist for endometrial biopsy is recommended if breakthrough bleeding occurs. When a 12-day regimen of progesterone is used, irregular bleeding and spotting of short duration usually occur, and biopsy may be reserved for heavy or prolonged bleeding.

✦ **Women status-post (S/P) hysterectomy:** Progesterone is not recommended for use in women who have undergone hysterectomy except in specific cases of endometrial cancer. Addition of androgen to estrogen replacement may increase libido and prevent elevated triglycerides.

✦ **Women with history of breast cancer:**

✧ **For vasomotor symptoms:**

✧ Recommend exercise, avoidance of alcohol (EtOH), avoidance of caffeine.

✧ Clonidine or low-dose Megace (megestrol acetate) may be used, but significant weight gain is often side effect of megestrol therapy.

✧ **To prevent osteoporosis and fractures: See Protocols on Osteoporosis and Falls.**

✧ **To prevent cardiovascular disease:** Recommend exercise, avoidance of excessive EtOH or caffeine use, smoking cessation, cholesterol-lowering agents if indicated.

✦ **Women with hypercoagulability:** Risk for thromboembolic event is not as great with HRT preparations as with oral contraceptives. The amount of estrogen present in oral contraceptives is six times greater than that in HRT formulations. Hypercoagulability may result from a primary state (deficiency of proteins C or S, or inherited mutation of factor V), malignancy, liver disease, nephrotic syndrome, hyperlipidemia, or diabetes mellitus. Risk for thromboembolism may be higher in these patients, indicating potential risks for use of HRT. Transdermal estrogen may be considered for women with hypercoagulable states, as there appears to be less hepatic effect with transdermal delivery. After consideration of the severity of a previous thromboembolic event and the passage of time since it occurred, lower-risk patients may elect to use HRT after education regarding benefits versus risks.

For Prevention of Osteoporosis in Oldest Old Women (Frail Elderly)

Many elderly women have never taken HRT. Others may have taken HRT that was discontinued because of concern about increased cancer risk with more than 5 years' duration of therapy. Osteoporosis may be established in these patients, but HRT is recommended to slow progression of bone degeneration. A Pap smear should be obtained before initiation of HRT in these patients when the uterus remains intact. A baseline pap smear is not required in patients who are S/P hysterectomy. Follow-up is required for breakthrough bleeding. Consider beginning therapy with the lowest possible dose of estrogen, e.g., Premarin 0.3 mg qod.

Estrogen Preparations

- **Vaginal ring:** Estring (estradiol vaginal ring) insert 1 ring every 90 days.
- **Tablets:**
  - Premarin (conjugated estrogen) 0.3–2.5 mg; for cyclic regimen 3 weeks on/1 week off.
  - Estinyl (ethinyl estradiol) 0.02 mg–0.05 mg qd to qod cyclically; 3 weeks on/1 week off.
  - Estrace (estradiol) for menopausal symptoms: 1–2 mg qd cyclically (3 weeks on/1 week off); for osteoporosis prevention: 0.5 mg qd for 3 weeks, then 1 week off.
  - Tace (chlorotrianisene) 12 mg and 25 mg tablets available; given cyclically (3 weeks on/1 week off); discontinue or taper dose q 3–6 months during menopause.
- **Transdermal delivery system:**
  - Estraderm (estradiol transdermal) 0.05 mg/day or 0.1 mg/day patch; beginning dose—one 0.05 mg/day patch applied to the trunk twice per week; cyclic regimen for maintenance 3 weeks on/1 week off; advise patient to rotate sites and to avoid breasts and waistline for application.

✧ Vivelle (estradiol transdermal system) 0.0375 mg/day–0.1 mg/day patch; beginning dose—0.05 mg/day patch applied two times per week to trunk area; use lowest effective dose; given cyclically (3 weeks on/1 week off) with intact uterus; without uterus, may use continuously.

✧ Climara (estradiol transdermal system) 0.05 mg/day–0.1 mg/day patch; beginning dose—one 0.05 mg/day patch applied to trunk area; advise patient to rotate sites; administer cyclically.

Progestin/Progesterone Preparations

✦ Provera (medroxyprogesterone acetate): 2.5–10 mg tablets available.

✦ Cycrin (medroxyprogesterone acetate): 2.5–10 mg tablets available.

✦ Aygestin (norethindrone acetate): 5 mg tablets available.

Combination Preparations

✦ **May be more economical than two separate prescriptions. If patient has health care plan, consider advantage of one co-pay versus two co-pays.**

✦ **Estrogen and progestin:**

✧ CombiPatch (estradiol/norethindrone acetate) provides continuous dose of estrogen plus a progestin; good choice for relief of moderate to severe vasomotor symptoms in women with intact uterus.

✧ Premphase (conjugated estrogen 0.625 mg/medroxyprogesterone acetate 5 mg) tablet; for cyclic regimen; provides immediate relief for hot flushes and night sweats and eventual relief for vaginal dryness; patient may experience predictable bleeding at the end of month's supply of pills.

✧ Prempro (conjugated estrogen 0.625 mg/medroxyprogesterone acetate 2.5 mg) tablet; for continuous regimen; provides immediate relief for night sweats and hot flushes and eventual relief of vaginal dryness; advise patient that irregular bleeding and spotting will occur.

✦ **Estrogen and androgen:** Estratest (esterified estrogen 1.25 mg/methyltestosterone 2.5 mg) tablet; cyclic regimen: ½–1 tablet daily × 3 weeks, then 1 week off.

Chapter 18

Palliative Care

Palliative care is defined by the World Health Organization as "the active total care of patients whose disease is not responsive to curative treatment." The goal is quality of life for both patients and families with the focus on physical, psychological, social, and spiritual care. Palliative care enhances quality of life when therapy focused on cure is inappropriate or futile.

The hospice organization implements palliative care through an interdisciplinary team, which develops a treatment plan and supports a peaceful and comfortable death. Hospice accepts patients whose prognosis is 6 months or less if the disease runs its natural course. Many but not all hospice patients have a diagnosis of cancer. The average age of a patient in their care is in the 70s. Many elderly patients with end-stage disease other than cancer may benefit from hospice care; however, it is often difficult to determine their life expectancy. Too frequently, patients are referred very late in their disease, and do not receive the full benefit of hospice care.

The first step in deciding on palliative care is communication with the patient and family. Sharing a terminal diagnosis is difficult. In many cases, with elderly patients, the discussion is ongoing as they progress through the last years or months of their life. At some point, the patient, family, or health care provider may raise the issue of futility with continued treatment. Acceptance of this by the patient and family is a process often requiring many discussions. It is helpful, when available, to bring other team members into these discussions to support and counsel the patient and family.

If a decision is made to shift from curative to palliative care, a referral to hospice may be appropriate. A representative from hospice is often willing to meet with the patient and family and further explain the philosophy of care, what services hospice provides, and any limitations in services. Hospice care can be provided in the home, assisted living settings, extended care, or acute care settings.

Symptom management is a primary goal of palliative care. Most symptoms have not only physical components but psychological, social, and spiritual components as well. Treating the whole person is imperative; however, it is difficult to deal with spiritual or psychological issues the person may be experiencing when he or she is in severe pain or is extremely short of breath. Managing distressing physical symptoms, therefore, becomes a primary goal.

SYMPTOM MANAGEMENT

Symptoms associated with a terminal illness are often multifactorial in etiology. A carefully focused history and physical examination should help identify the cause(s) and focus the treatment plan. Harmful side effects of treatment must be weighed with the possible benefit to symptom control. Treatment goals and modalities must be negotiated with the patient and family. For example, a patient may want to avoid pharmacological control of pain to the point of sedation even though that means he or she will continue to experience some degree of pain or discomfort. Common symptoms seen in terminally ill patients are discussed in this chapter.

PAIN MANAGEMENT

Pain is an individual and subjective phenomenon that has psychological, social, spiritual, and cultural components. Use of appropriate team members to help address these issues is recommended.

✦ Reassess positioning of patient and order appropriate bed and chair surface for maximum comfort, i.e., static air chair cushion, alternating pressure mattress, low air loss mattress, water bed, sheepskin overlay.

✦ Consider application of heat or ice to specific areas of pain.

✦ Consider use of massage therapy or biofeedback.

✦ Teach relaxation techniques, i.e., visual imagery, self-hypnosis, meditation.

✦ Consider use of music, pets, humor.

✦ Consider use of a transcutaneous electrical nerve stimulation (TENS) unit.

✦ Manage other symptoms that may exacerbate pain, i.e., anxiety, depression, nausea/vomiting, constipation.

✦ **See Chapter on Pain Management.**

✦ Consult with physician on alternative measures, i.e., palliative radiation, patient-controlled analgesia (PCA), epidural infusions.

NAUSEA AND VOMITING

Common causes of nausea and vomiting in a terminal illness include but are not limited to: (1) constipation, (2) CNS effects, (3) renal failure, (4) fluid and electrolyte abnormalities, (5) vestibular causes, (6) medications, (7) radiation therapy, and (8) anxiety.

✦ Address underlying cause(s) as appropriate.

✦ Adjust diet, i.e., serve food at room temperature, offer clear liquids, avoid sweet, salty, spicy, or fatty foods.

✦ Control odors, sights, and sounds that bring on nausea.

✦ Provide fresh air or use a fan in the room.

✦ Provide distractions, i.e., music, reading, conversation.

✦ Teach and encourage the use of relaxation techniques, i.e., rhythmic breathing, meditation, or visual imagery.

✦ Use antiemetics as needed. **See Protocol on Nausea and Vomiting.** Antiemetic agents may be administered in a variety of routes: oral (PO), sublingual (SL), rectal (PR), transdermal (TD), subcutaneous (SQ), intramuscular (IM), intravenous (IV), or continuous subcutaneous infusion (CSI). Doses must be clinically titrated to produce desired results.

✦ **Antihistamines:**

✧ Benadryl (diphenhydramine HCl) 25–50 mg PO, IM, or IV q 6 hr;

✧ Marezine (cyclizine HCl) 50 mg PO or IM q 6–8 hr, 50–100 mg CSI q 24 hr;

✧ Vistaril (hydroxyzine pamoate) 10–50 mg PO or IM q 4 hr;

✧ Robinul (glycopyrrolate) 1–2 mg PO q 8 hr;

✧ Periactin (cyproheptadine HCl) 2–8 mg PO q 4 hr.

✦ **Anticholinergics:**

✧ Hyoscine (scopolamine hydrobromide) 250–800 μg PO prior to nausea-invoking activity; 0.8–20 mg CSI q 24 hr; TD behind ear q 72 hr;

✧ Donnatal (atropine, scopolamine, hyoscyamine, phenobarbital) 0.125–0.25 mg SL q 4 hr; 0.25–0.50 mg SQ q 6 hr; 1–2 mg CSI q 24 hr.

✦ **Corticosteroids:**

✧ Decadron, Hexadrol (dexamethasone) 1–4 mg PO q 6–8 hr; 2–8 mg IV q 6 hr; 2–12 mg CSI q 24 hr;

✧ Deltasone, Meticorten (prednisone) 5–20 mg PO q 6 hr.

✦ **Benzodiazepines:**

✧ Ativan (lorazepam) 1–2 mg PO, SL, or IV q 6–8 hr;

✧ Valium (diazepam) 2–10 mg PO, SL, or IV q 6–8 hr.

✦ **Dopamine antagonists:**

✧ Compazine (prochlorperazine) 5–10 mg PO or IM q 4–6 hr; 25 mg PR q 4–8 hr;

✧ Levoprome (methotrimeprazine HCl) 10–20 mg IM q 4–6 hr; 50–300 mg CSI q 24 hr;

✧ Haldol (haloperidol) 0.5–2 mg PO or IM q 4–6 hr; 5–15 mg CSI q 24 hr;

✧ Reglan (metoclopramide) 10–20 mg PO or IV q 6 hr; 20–80 mg CSI q 24 hr.

✦ **Serotonin antagonists:**

✧ Zofran (ondansetron HCl) 8 mg PO or IV q 8 hr; 24 mg CSI q 24 hr.

DYSPNEA

Dyspnea is a commonly seen symptom especially as death approaches, often described as air hunger. Common causes include: (1) underlying disease, i.e., chronic obstructive pulmonary disease (COPD) or congestive heart failure (CHF); (2) acute episodic illness, i.e., pneumonia, pulmonary embolus; (3) cancer-related complications, i.e., superior vena cava syndrome; (4) radiation therapy; (5) concomitant disease, i.e., anemia, uremia, ascites; and (6) anxiety or depression.

✦ Address underlying cause(s) as appropriate.

✦ Consider checking hemoglobin and transfusing if anemic and with patient/family consent.

✦ Assess oxygen saturation by pulse oximetry. Consider oxygen therapy; may have placebo benefit even if dyspnea is not actually caused by hypoxia.

✦ Consider use of a bedside fan.

✦ If signs of CHF, consider Lasix (furosemide) 20–40 mg PO or IV; may give one time only or routinely as appropriate. Also, consider Nitrostat (nitroglycerine SL) or Nitro-Dur (nitroglycerine TD).

✦ **Opioids:**

✧ Morphine 5–10 mg PO or PR q 1–4 hr, may be given SQ, or IV if oral route is not tolerated. Use a 3:1 oral-to-parenteral ratio. Titrate dose and frequency as needed. If morphine is being used for pain management, may need to adjust dose for control of dyspnea.

✧ Nebulized morphine 5 mg in 2 ml normal saline q 4 hr via a hand-held nebulizer.

✦ **Corticosteroids:**

✧ Decadron or Hexadrol (dexamethasone) 4–8 mg PO or IV daily;

✧ Deltasone or Meticorten (prednisone) 20–60 mg PO daily;

✧ Medrol (methylprednisolone) 48–128 mg PO or IV daily.

✦ **Benzodiazepines:**

✧ Ativan (lorazepam) 1–2 mg PO, SL, or IV q 1–4 hr;

✧ Valium (diazepam) 2.5–25 mg PO, IM, or IV daily in divided doses,

✧ Versed (midazolam HCl) 5–10 mg bolus SQ followed by 10–30 mg CSI q 24 hr.

✦ **Phenothiazine:**

✧ Thorazine (chlorpromazine HCl) 12.5 mg IV q 4–6 hr.

✦ **Inhalation therapy:**

✧ Vanceril (beclomethasone dipropionate) metered dose inhaler (MDI) 1–2 inhalations tid or qid;

✧ Ventolin (albuterol) MDI 1–2 inhalations or 2.5 mg in 3 cc normal saline by nebulizer tid or qid;

✧ Atrovent (ipratropium bromide) MDI 1–2 inhalations or 0.5 mg (500 mcg) in 3 cc normal saline by nebulizer tid or qid.

COUGH

Coughing is a defense mechanism to maintain airway patency; however, it can exacerbate dyspnea and nausea, cause musculoskeletal pain, and fracture ribs. Common causes include: (1) underlying cardiopulmonary diseases, i.e., COPD, CHF; (2) GI conditions, i.e., gastroesophageal reflux disease; (3) medications; and (4) aspiration events.

✦ Address underlying cause(s) as appropriate.

✦ **Opioids:**

✧ Codeine 15–30 mg PO q 4 hr as needed,

✧ Morphine 2.5–5 mg PO, PR, SQ, IM, or IV q 1–4 hr as needed.

✦ **Corticosteroids:**

✧ Decadron or Hexadrol (dexamethasone) 4–8 mg PO daily or Deltasone or Meticorten (prednisone) 20–60 mg PO daily if cough is related to tumor growth; titrate as needed.

✦ Consider palliative radiation. Consult with physician; refer to radiation oncologist.

✦ Nebulized anesthetics: Marcaine (bupivacaine) 0.25% 5 ml q 4–6 hr. Refrain from eating 30 min after administration due to persistent oral numbness and risk for aspiration. Avoid use of lidocaine; reported to cause bronchospasm.

CONSTIPATION

Most palliative care patients will require laxatives to maintain bowel function. Constipation can contribute to increased pain, nausea and vomiting, urinary retention, and mental status changes, further decreasing quality of life. Be alert to the possibility of bowel obstruction.

✦ Prescribe bowel regimen with decrease of mobility and/or initiation of opioids.

✦ **See Protocol on Constipation.**

DIARRHEA

Less common than constipation in palliative care patients, diarrhea is often due to aggressive laxative use. Diarrhea may, however, be associated with the underlying disease itself, i.e., often occurs with mesenteric ischemia associated with end-stage cardiovascular disease.

- Treat underlying cause(s) as appropriate.
- Adjust laxative dose.
- **See Protocol on Diarrhea.**

XEROSTOMIA

Common causes of xerostomia in terminal patients include: (1) medications, i.e., morphine; (2) infections; (3) dehydration; (4) chemotherapy; and (5) radiation therapy.

- Encourage oral fluid intake.
- Encourage frequent oral hygiene.
- **See Protocol on Mouth Lesions.**

PRURITUS

Common causes of pruritus include (1) underlying diseases, i.e., liver or renal failure; (2) dehydration; and (3) anxiety.

- **See Protocol on Pruritus and Chapter on Special Hygiene Needs.**
- **See Chapter on Pressure Ulcers.**

ANOREXIA

Eating is highly connected to social and cultural beliefs. Loss of appetite commonly occurs with terminal illness but may be difficult for the patient and family to accept. Negotiation of withholding or withdrawing food and fluids can be an emotionally charged discussion.

- Manage distressing symptoms that can impact appetite, i.e., pain, nausea/vomiting, dyspnea, oral lesions.
- Consider antidepressant. **See Protocol on Depression.**
- Consider Megace (megestrol acetate) 80–160 mg PO qid; available as a 40 mg/cc concentrate.
- Support family in decisions related to withholding or withdrawing food and fluids. **See Chapter on Legal and Ethical Issues.**
- Consider referral to nutritionist for further recommendations.
- Provide small portions of calorie-dense foods/supplements as tolerated.
- Encourage favorite foods/liquids for pleasure.
- Consider short-term IV fluids if patient/family insistent on hydration.

TERMINAL ANXIETY

Patient may exhibit signs of extreme restlessness and anxiety with onset of "active dying." These signs may be very distressing to family and caregivers. Symptoms may be alleviated with use of transdermal opioids (Fentanyl transdermal patch 25 μg as initial dose), neuroleptics (chlorpromazine and haloperidol are available in rectal form), or benzodiazepines.

OTHER ISSUES

In addition to appropriate management of the physical symptoms associated with a terminal illness, the health care provider should be alert to the psychological, social, spiritual, and financial issues the patient and family are facing. Providing mechanisms for meeting these patient needs is very important.

- Utilize other team members when available, i.e., social worker, medical ethicist, chaplain, psychologist.
- Enlist ethics committee for complex cases as appropriate.
- Provide adequate time as needed for family support.

Chapter 19

Management of the Alzheimer's Patient

Dementing illnesses affect 5–10% of individuals age 65 and older in the United States. The incidence is increased with increasing age. The most common cause of dementia is Alzheimer's disease which is discussed in this chapter as the prototype for dementia management.

Frequency of follow-up visits will depend on the patient's comorbid conditions, the progression of symptoms, the incidence of troublesome behaviors, or other issues requiring monitoring or adjustment of treatment modalities. Adequate time must be allotted for discussion with the caregiver(s) as education and counseling are important treatment modalities in dementia management. Involvement of an interdisciplinary team is recommended if possible, especially with patients who are difficult to manage.

For initial dementia assessment, **see Protocol on Dementia.** For each follow-up visit, consider the following key components of history, physical examination, and diagnostic testing.

HISTORY

✦ Changes in patient's physical, functional, or cognitive status since last examination?

✦ Recent acute illness or infection?

✦ Mood? Signs of depression? Vegetative symptoms?

✦ Status of comorbid conditions?

✦ Troublesome behaviors: repetitive behaviors or speech, delusions, hallucinations (visual or auditory), paranoia, wandering, sleep disturbances, agitation, combativeness, lack of inhibitions, incontinence, inappropriate toileting, sexual aggressiveness, or yelling?

✦ Safety concerns? Is patient cooking, driving, home alone for periods of time?

✦ Changes in appetite? Weight loss or gain?

✦ Medications? **Note any adverse effects, i.e., oversedation, increased agitation. Assess compliance.**

✦ Caregiver status? Caregiver stress?

✦ Changes in level or location of care?

PHYSICAL EXAMINATION

✦ Weight. **Malnutrition and weight loss are common problems as dementia progresses.**

✦ Vital signs.

✦ Assess skin, especially as patient becomes less mobile. Note presence of bruising, excoriations, pressure ulcers. **See Chapters on Special Hygiene Needs and on Pressure Ulcers.**

✦ Cognitive assessment. Repeat mental status examination as necessary to document status, especially if patient is on Aricept (donepezil HCl) or Cognex (tacrine HCl).

✦ Depression screening. **Maintain a high degree of suspicion for depression; can occur concomitantly with Alzheimer's disease. Use standardized instrument such as the Beck Depression Screening or Geriatric Depression Scale. See Protocol on Depression.**

✦ Functional assessment. Note changes since last examination. Repeat Functional Activities Questionnaire as appropriate. Consider use of the Global Deterioration Scale for assessment of primary degenerative dementia.

✦ Focused examination based on other acute or chronic health problems.

DIAGNOSTIC TESTS

✦ Drug levels as appropriate, e.g., Depakote, Dilantin, digoxin, theophylline, phenobarbital.

✦ Serum albumin or prealbumin at least annually to document nutritional status.

✦ Consider electrolytes, blood urea nitrogen if dehydration suspected.

✦ **See Protocol on Delirium** for recommended diagnostic tests if acute worsening of symptoms is reported.

✦ Monitor comorbid conditions as appropriate.

STAGES OF ALZHEIMER'S DISEASE

Alzheimer's disease is generally described as a condition that progresses through a number of stages. The National Alzheimer's Association defines early, middle, and late stages. Following is a description of each stage with suggested management strategies.

Early Stage

Individuals in the early stage of Alzheimer's disease experience memory loss that affects work, daily routine, and social activities. They may exhibit poor judgment, a lack of initiative, difficulty performing ordinary tasks, and changes in mood, behavior, and personality. They often get lost in familiar places, and forget appointments, errands, or names of familiar people. They may be easily frustrated, become withdrawn, or experience depression.

✦ Focus assessment and education on patient's need for assistance with activities of daily living (ADLs) and instrumental activities of daily living (IADLs).

✦ Educate caregiver/family on dementia, common causes, means of evaluating and diagnosing, community resources, management techniques. Provide educational materials. Refer to local chapter of the Alzheimer's Association and other resources in the community.

✦ Begin discussion on advance directives, and legal and financial issues. **See Chapter on Legal and Ethical Issues.**

✦ Recommend trial of memory aids, i.e., calendar, notebook, notes in strategic places around the house, medication aids, phone calls to remind patient to take medication/eat a meal.

✦ Address issues related to driving, hobbies involving power tools, cooking, managing finances, managing medications, and living independently as appropriate.

✦ Consider referral for driving evaluation through occupational therapy if available.

✦ Listen to and support caregiver(s).

✦ Consider referral of caregiver to social worker for assessment, education, and counseling, and referral to community services, i.e., support groups, adult day care centers, respite programs.

✦ Address troublesome behaviors. **Educate on behavioral management techniques. Consistency is important. See Table 19-1.**

✦ Consider trial of an antidepressant if appropriate. **See Protocol on Depression.**

✦ Consider need for bowel regimen. **See Protocol on Constipation.**

✦ Consider trial of Aricept (donepezil HCl). Begin at 5 mg daily for 1 month; advance to 10 mg daily if patient tolerates. Have family/caregiver keep a daily diary to document effect on cognition and behavior. Advise family that it generally takes 4–6 months to determine if medication is effective.

(text continues on page 458)

TABLE 19-1. Behavioral Management Strategies

Behavior	Common causes	Management strategies
Uncooperative with ADLs	Process is too confusing Sees as invasion of privacy Fearful of process	Simplify tasks Avoid "why" questions Do one step at a time Use a calm, consistent approach Speak in low pitch Don't rush the patient Use simple clothing Lay out clothes in the order to put on Praise for success Maintain independence as long as possible Approach with a statement rather than a question, i.e., "It is time for your bath"
Feeding	Cannot remember whether they ate or not As disease advances, may forget how to eat	Use simple, one-step instructions Repeat instructions as necessary Limit choices Put one utensil and one food in front of the patient at a time Try finger foods Remind patient to chew and swallow Offer fluids frequently Observe for swallowing difficulties Use adaptive equipment when appropriate, i.e., plate guards, suction cups and plates
Toileting	Unable to recognize signals of toileting need Cannot remember where the bathroom is Cannot remember what to do once in the bathroom	Post an identifying sign on the bathroom door Set a regular schedule and remind patient Be alert to signs of restlessness, which may indicate a toileting need

(continued)

TABLE 19-1. Continued

Behavior	Common causes	Management strategies
Toileting *(continued)*		Assist with adjusting clothing but respect privacy **See Protocol on Urinary Incontinence and Chapter on Special Hygiene Needs**
Wandering	May feel lost or that they are searching for something or someone May be overstimulated, anxious, uncomfortable May be bored or need exercise May be the result of life-style pattern of coping with stress	Observe for any prompting events that precede wandering Assess for unmet needs, i.e., hunger, need to toilet, pain, thirst Redirect patient if lost Put familiar pictures, items on door or outside room to remind patient Offer frequent, gentle reassurances to the patient Consider use of wander guard devices Provide a safe environment for patient to pace if needed
Sundowning—increased agitation or other behavioral problems in the late afternoon and evening	May be tired after activities of the day, less able to cope with stress	Provide rest periods throughout the day to prevent the patient from getting overtired Limit overstimulation in the late afternoon and evening Observe for precipitating events and alter as appropriate Observe for signs, i.e., pacing, wringing hands, agitation Provide "quiet time" to avoid catastrophic reaction
Suspiciousness/paranoia	Inability to understand the environment around them	Reduce hiding places Check wastebaskets before emptying Do not argue with patient or try to rationally explain disappearances Avoid whispering

(continued)

TABLE 19-1. Continued

Behavior	Common causes	Management strategies
Suspiciousness/ paranoia *(continued)*		Use distraction Keep an extra set of glasses, keys, hearing aid batteries available
Delusions/ hallucinations	Visual and auditory stimuli may be distorted resulting in distorted perceptions	Do not argue with or try to convince the patient that the belief is untrue Use reassurance and distraction Reduce clutter; eliminate large mirrors and shadows in the room Avoid television

✦ If patient is on Cognex (tacrine HCl), monitor liver function weekly to every other week for the first 18 weeks of therapy. Initial dose is 10 mg qid increased by 40 mg daily every 6 weeks to maintenance dose of 40 mg qid.

✦ Consider hormone replacement therapy (HRT) for women, vitamin E 400 IU daily, antioxidants, and/or ibuprofen.

✦ Consider medications for symptom management (see Display 19-1).

Middle Stage

The middle stage of Alzheimer's disease is the longest stage, often lasting as long as 20 years. Individuals in the middle stage have increased difficulty in performing ADLs, problems recognizing close friends and family, and difficulty carrying on a conversation. Nutrition often becomes a major concern with either anorexia and weight loss or a huge appetite, especially for junk food. Gradually, however, they will exhibit a loss of interest in food. At some point during this stage, the patient will require full-time supervision. Troublesome behaviors, including repetitious statements and actions, sleep disturbances, hallucinations, paranoid thoughts, agitation, wandering, loss of impulse control, combativeness, and uncooperative behavior with ADLs, become more frequent.

✦ Assess for increasing need for assistance with ADLs.

✦ Address troublesome behaviors. See Table 19-1 on behavioral management.

✦ Manage incontinence to decrease number of incontinent episodes. **See Protocol on Urinary Incontinence.**

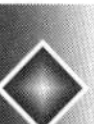

DISPLAY 19-1. *Symptom Management*

Agitation

Desyrel (trazodone HCl) 25–50 mg daily initial dose
Depakote (divalproex sodium) 250 mg bid initial dose

Psychosis

Clozaril (clozapine) 6.25–150 mg. Consult with physician on use.
Haldol (haloperidol) 0.5 mg daily initial dose (range 0.5–3 mg daily)
Risperdal (risperidone) 0.25 mg daily initial dose (range 0.25–3 mg daily)
Zyprexa (olanzapine) 2.5–20 mg daily. Consult with physician on use.

Anxiety

Ativan (lorazepam) 0.5 mg daily initial dose (range 0.5–6 mg daily)

Insomnia

Ambien (zolpidem tartrate) 5 mg at night
Noctec (chloral hydrate) 250–500 mg at night (short term only)
Restoril (temazepam) 7.5–15 mg at night
Desyrel (trazodone HCl) 25–50 mg at night initial dose

Depression

See Protocol on Depression

✦ Consider need for bowel regimen. **See Protocol on Constipation.**

✦ Consider referral to nutritionist for recommendations to meet daily nutritional needs.

✦ Educate on available care options; encourage and support caregiver(s) to visit adult day care centers, assisted living residences, and extended care facilities and develop a plan if they are no longer able to care for patient at home.

✦ Discuss available community resources. Refer to social worker as needed.

✦ Continue discussion on advance directives, and legal and financial issues. The ability of the patient to participate in making a living will or appointing a durable power of attorney will be lost as the dementia progresses.

✦ Consider antidepressant if indicated. **See Protocol on Depression.**

✦ Consider medications for symptom management (see Display 19-1).

Late Stage

As individuals enter the late stage of Alzheimer's disease, they begin to experience difficulty walking, increased incontinence of bladder and bowel, and weight loss even with a good diet. They usually lose interest in food, have increased problems with constipation and skin care due to immobility, and become dependent in all ADLs. Many become bedridden, noncommunicative, and assume the fetal position.

✦ Address skin care issues. Prevention is key. **See Chapters on Special Hygiene Needs and on Pressure Ulcers.**

✦ Maintain mobility; teach range of motion/positioning, use splinting to prevent contractures.

✦ Address risk for aspiration pneumonia, dehydration, malnutrition with family. Educate on preventive measures.

✦ Continue discussion regarding appropriate level of care with family/caregiver. Refer to social worker for education and counseling on care options.

✦ Continue discussion regarding end of life/palliative care issues, i.e., feeding, pain management, resuscitation. **See Chapters on Legal and Ethical Issues and on Palliative Care.**

Chapter 20

Alternatives to Living Alone

Older individuals generally equate health with maintaining function. As people age, however, many are faced with physical and cognitive changes that affect their ability to function independently. These changes are the result of normal aging, lifestyle choices, chronic disease, and/or acute illness or trauma (see Display 20-1).

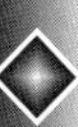

DISPLAY 20-1. *Aging Factors That Affect Functional Status*

NORMAL AGING CHANGES

Decreased vision and hearing
Decreased muscle strength and flexibility
Loss of reserve in all organ systems

LIFESTYLE CHOICES

Sedentary lifestyle
Tobacco use
EtOH use

CHRONIC DISEASES

Arthritis
Osteoporosis
Parkinson's disease
Dementia
Heart disease
Respiratory disease
Renal disease

ACUTE ILLNESS/TRAUMA

Cerebrovascular accident
Infections:
- Pneumonia
- Urinary tract infections
- Influenza

Falls
Fractures
Motor vehicle accidents

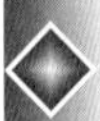

DISPLAY 20-2. *In-Home Services*

Equipment: Cane, walker, wheelchair, hospital bed, lifts, trapeze, special mattress, oxygen, nebulizer, suction machine, ramp, adaptations for bathroom/kitchen, adaptive utensils for cooking/eating. Apartments for the disabled may be available; structural adaptations to the home are not generally covered under insurance; for equipment covered under Medicare, patient must meet specified criteria and have an order from health care provider.

Safety: Emergency call system, telephone check-in, medication reminders

Intermittent nursing services: Skilled nursing care, home health aide, homemaker services, social worker, physical therapy, occupational therapy, speech therapy, respiratory services, hospice. Must meet specified criteria for reimbursement under Medicare and have an order from health care provider; requires prior authorization under Medicare HMO; services are time limited and of decreasing frequency based on continued need.

Private duty: Sitter, companion, nursing aide or technician, LPN or RN up to 24 hr a day. Services are private pay only. Some long-term care insurance policies may have provisions for these services.

As these changes occur, most elderly try to adapt to maintain their function and independence. Most prefer to do so in their own home. In fact, only 5% of the over 65 population reside in nursing homes, although it is expected that one in five will spend some time in a nursing facility during their lifetime. Most long-term nursing home residents are in the over-85 age group and 75% are women.

Four of five persons age 65 and older have at least one chronic condition and many have multiple chronic diseases. The most common chronic conditions reported are arthritis, hypertension, sensory impairments, and heart disease. The degree of functional impairment or disability varies greatly in the elderly population, with the over-85 group reporting the greatest number of limitations in activities of daily living (ADLs) and instrumental activities of daily living (IADLs).

As people "age in place" it is often possible to import services and equipment to support them in remaining in their own home. These services range from arranging a walker or setting up Meals on Wheels to 24-hr nursing support (see Display 20-2). Availability, cost, and third party reimbursement for services vary from state to state. In addition to in-home services, there are community services available to help support continued independent living. Examples of community services include congregate meals, senior's programs, adult day centers, phone checks and reminders for medication administration, outpatient rehabilitation programs, and transportation.

Alternatives to living alone in one's own home also vary in cost and availability across the country. Many options are private pay and may be prohibitively expensive for some elders. See Display 20-3 for examples of these alternatives.

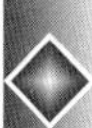

DISPLAY 20-3. *Alternatives to Living Alone*

Senior Apartments

Independent apartments for congregate living
Rent subsidy available if income guidelines met, often have long waiting lists
May be handicap adapted
May have emergency call systems
May provide limited transportation
May have additional services on premises for additional fee, i.e., beauty shop, grocery, housekeeping
Can import in-home services to help maintain independence (see Display 20-2)

Shared Housing

Independent living for small group of elderly
May provide housekeeping, meals, and prompts to take medications
Often sponsored by religious organizations

Matched Housing

Matches elderly with another person, often younger
Usually live in elder's home
Individual arrangement made regarding finances and services

Assisted Living

Vary from small, independently run homes to larger facilities
Provide an array of services including ADL and medication assistance, meals, housekeeping, social programs
Do not provide skilled nursing care
Monthly fee, wide range in cost, usually private pay
Licensing varies from state to state
May be able to import in-home services (see Display 20-2)

Intermediate Level

Licensed nursing facility
Resident requires 24-hr care but does not meet skilled criteria under Medicare*
Private pay, long-term care insurance, or Medicaid *(continued)*

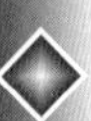

DISPLAY 20-3. *Continued*

Skilled Level

Licensed nursing facility
Must meet medically necessary skilled criteria under Medicare*
Requires 3-day hospital stay within 30 days prior to admission to the skilled facility for Medicare reimbursement
Medicare pays 100% of first 20 days, all but set fee for days 21–100 as long as resident continues to meet skilled criteria*
With Medicare HMO, requires prior authorization but no 3-day hospital stay

Subacute

Licensed nursing facility
Skilled level care
May be affiliated with a hospital or part of an extended care facility
Must meet medically necessary skilled criteria under Medicare* or have authorization under HMO for reimbursement
Often used as a "step-down" from acute hospital to complete complex treatments, i.e., IV antibiotics, wound care, prior to return home

Inpatient Rehabilitation

Intensive rehabilitation covered under Medicare Part A hospital benefits
Provides 24-hr care with physical, occupational, and/or speech therapy
Patient must need at least two rehabilitative modalities and be able to participate in a minimum of 3 hr of therapy daily
May provide cardiac and pulmonary rehabilitation

Specialized Alzheimer's Unit

Available in some extended care facilities
Provide 24-hr care at intermediate level
Staff and programs geared to Alzheimer's patients
Private pay, long-term care insurance or Medicaid

Hospice Units

Must meet criteria for hospice
Can provide respite care

*Examples of skilled criteria under Medicare include: need for physical, occupational, or speech therapy; wound care more frequently than once daily; intravenous antibiotics.

Chapter 21

Legal and Ethical Issues

The care of elderly patients often involves complex legal and ethical issues. Care providers must be knowledgeable in many arenas that relate to the health of aging individuals. Beyond understanding the physiological changes and special health concerns associated with aging, care providers must understand the benefits and limitations of Medicare, Medicaid, and Medigap insurance and help educate their patients in these issues. Care providers must be proactive in raising issues related to a patient's wishes in the event he or she faces a life-threatening situation, can no longer live independently, or loses the capacity to make decisions. Studies have shown that most patients have thought about these concerns and want to have these issues raised by their health care provider but often will not initiate the conversation themselves.

INFORMED CONSENT

Before health care providers can treat patients, they must obtain informed consent to the treatment. Informed consent is usually interpreted to mean that the practitioner has given adequate information to the patient (and when appropriate, the patient's family) so that the patient may make an "informed decision" about any treatment recommended. The Joint Commission on the Accreditation of Healthcare Organizations (JCAHO) has suggested that "adequate information" includes: data about the diagnosis and prognosis, reasonable treatment options with potential benefits and drawbacks, inherent problems related to recuperation, the likelihood of success, the possible results of nontreatment, and any significant alternatives.

Each patient encounter may bring the need and opportunity to obtain informed consent, e.g., starting a new antihypertensive medication, initiating treatment for depression, referral to a gastroenterologist to evaluate persistent epigastric pain or place a percuanteous endoscopic gastrostomy (PEG) tube, or scheduling a dual energy x-ray absorptiometry scan to screen for osteoporosis. The patient's ability to fully understand the pending medical decision and participate in making that decision must be assessed. **See Decision-Making Capacity.** Some treatments are fairly commonplace, readily explained and understood, and decisions can be made relatively easily. The consent for these treatments is often given informally, i.e., agreeing to the substitution of one medication for another. Some require written informed consent, i.e., consent for a surgical procedure. In long-term care settings, written informed consent is required for the use of any psychoactive medication or restraints. More complex decisions, particularly those related to end-of-life issues, require multiple, often lengthy discussions and are more burdensome to patients, family members, and health care providers.

THE RIGHT TO REFUSE MEDICAL TREATMENT

The right to refuse medical treatment is a necessary corollary to the legal doctrine of informed consent. Because patients must consent before treatment is provided, patients must also have—by implication—a corresponding right to refuse treatment, even life-sustaining treatment.

DECISION-MAKING CAPACITY

All competent adults have the right of self-determination, i.e., the right to consent as well as the right to refuse medical treatment. All adults are presumed to be legally competent. Only a court with proper jurisdiction can declare a person legally incompetent.

Decision-making capacity is an informal assessment usually made by a physician. An inability to make health care decisions is not necessarily an "all or none" situation. A person's decision-making ability may change over time and should be reassessed frequently. For example, an elderly person may experience postoperative delirium and be temporarily unable to understand and participate in decisions regarding his or her care. When the delirium clears, however, his or her ability to make decisions may return.

There may be circumstances in which a person has been declared legally incompetent and has a court-appointed guardian or conservator yet retains decision-making capacity related to health care decisions.

Key considerations in assessing decision-making capacity and suggestions for putting these into practice include the following:

- Can the patient receive and comprehend information about a specific situation or issue? Have the patient repeat his or her understanding of the situation in his or her own words.
- Can the patient deliberate on available alternatives? Does he or she recognize that he or she has a choice? Have the patient repeat the alternatives as he or she understands them.
- Can the patient make a choice and provide reasons for the choice? It is important to consider the decision-making process rather than the content of the decision. Refusal of treatment, failure to make what the health care provider considers the "right" decision, declaration of unusual or idiosyn-

cratic beliefs, or even refusal to communicate does not necessarily mean the patient lacks decision-making capacity.

SURROGATE DECISION MAKING

If a patient lacks decision-making capacity, either temporarily as with a post-operative delirium or permanently as with advanced Alzheimer's disease, the health care provider must inquire if the patient has a representative or surrogate to speak for him or her. It is common medical practice to rely on family members, "next-of-kin," in the absence of an identified surrogate. Many states have now recognized this with health care proxy statutes, which delineate the hierarchy of family members who are considered to be the "proxy" if no one is legally identified. In the absence of family, it may be necessary to involve the state adult protective services and initiate guardianship/conservatorship proceedings.

For competent older patients, the health care provider should discuss the patient's wishes with him or her and encourage him or her to identify a surrogate through a durable power of attorney (DPOA) for health care.

Even in situations in which there is an identified family member who is the spokesperson or "surrogate," every effort should be made to discuss issues with others to avoid family disagreements over a particular decision. A patient/family conference is a useful tool. When possible, include the physician, nurse practitioner, and social worker as well as any other team members who would help provide a clear picture of the situation to the patient and family.

PATIENTS' WISHES AND ADVANCE DIRECTIVES

Treatment decisions should be based on patient preferences. If the patient has decision-making capacity, preferences may be obtained directly from the patient. In the absence of decision-making capacity, preferences may be elicited from the patient's surrogate or from advance directives.

Advance directives are legal instruments that permit patients to make their preferences about health care treatment options known in the event they lose decision-making capacity.

A Living Will is a statutory declaration that details a patient's wishes regarding treatment options when he or she has a terminal illness. A DPOA is a statutory instrument that permits appointment of another person to make decisions for the patient in the event the patient loses the ability to make his or her own decisions. Nondurable powers of attorney (POAs) lapse when the declarant loses decision-making capacity. DPOAs may specify the patient's wishes on issues such as artificial nutrition and hydration (ANH) or may give the surrogate named broad authority to act in the patient's behalf. Generally, the surrogate should base decisions on the patient's expressed preferences ("substituted judgment" standard). If the patient's preferences are not known, then the decision should be made that is in the best interest of the patient ("best interests" standard). Some combination of these two standards is often necessary, as it is virtually impossible to anticipate all potential medical circumstances and associated decisions.

A copy of any pertinent legal document should be kept in the patient's medical record.

DO-NOT-RESUSCITATE (DNR) ORDERS

✦ Prehospital do-not-resuscitate (DNR) orders are authorized in some states to otherwise prevent emergency medical personnel from attempting resuscitation of a terminally ill person. Assisting with the completion of these documents and educating the family on the importance of keeping the original with the patient at all times is an important role of the health care provider.

✦ In-hospital DNR orders are generally completed by the physician unless the nurse practitioner has admitting privileges; however, the nurse practitioner as the primary care provider should be involved in the discussions regarding these decisions. The actual DNR order should be dated, timed, signed by the appropriate person, and contain certain essential elements.

✦ The essential elements of the DNR order and accompanying chart notes include:

✧ the diagnosis and prognosis,

✧ the patient's preferences regarding treatment options,

✧ an assessment of the patient's decision-making capacity,

✧ the name and relationship of the surrogate if the patient lacks decision-making capacity,

✧ the method of decision making by the surrogate, i.e., substituted judgment or best interests standard, and

✧ presence or absence of an advance directive.

✦ It may be useful to include the following information in the DNR order documentation as well:

✧ the names and relationships of other family members present during discussions,

✧ pertinent psychosocial information,

✧ spiritual issues, if addressed, and

✧ the discharge plan.

ARTIFICIAL NUTRITION AND HYDRATION (ANH)

ANH may be delivered by enteral feeding, i.e., feeding tube or total parenteral nutrition (TPN). Hydration alone can be given by an IV route, either peripherally or centrally. Any decision regarding the use of ANH should take into consideration the medical goals of therapy, the patient's preferences, and the patient's quality of life. As with any therapy, the benefits vs. the risks or burdens must be weighed.

- ✦ Benefits to consider include:
  - ✧ sustaining life,
  - ✧ supporting the patient through an acute illness,
  - ✧ meeting nutritional and hydration needs when the patient can no longer meet his or her needs orally,
  - ✧ providing a means to administer necessary medications,
  - ✧ preventing or correcting malnutrition and dehydration,
  - ✧ preventing complications associated with malnutrition and dehydration, i.e., pressure ulcers, confusion.
- ✦ Risks/burdens to consider include:
  - ✧ prolonging life and associated suffering,
  - ✧ possible need to restrain patient to prevent tube dislodgment, especially with nasogastric tube,
  - ✧ risks associated with tube placement, i.e., nasogastric tube inadvertently placed into lungs or bleeding/infection associated with PEG or surgically placed tube,
  - ✧ recurrent aspiration pneumonia,
  - ✧ refeeding syndrome,
  - ✧ line infection with peripherally or centrally placed intravenous lines,
  - ✧ fluid and electrolyte imbalance,
  - ✧ hyperglycemia associated with TPN,
  - ✧ premature nursing home placement due to inability of family to care for patient at home.

RISK MANAGEMENT

The nurse practitioner should be knowledgeable of the state laws governing the scope of practice and take appropriate measures to ensure compliance with those regulations. In collaborative practice situations, ongoing close communication with the physician partner is imperative. Documentation should be based on clinical, professional, and Health Care and Financing Administration (HCFA) guidelines.

The care of elderly patients occurs in many different settings. Areas of risk management concern in extended care settings include injuries related to falls, which account for two-thirds of all claims filed against nursing homes. The nurse practitioner practicing in this setting should consider close involvement in the development and implementation of the fall prevention program, ongoing review of incidents, staff education, and participation in other quality review initiatives.

Development of clinical parameters that prompt notification of the nurse practitioner and/or physician should also be considered. Examples of clinical parameters that trigger a call to the health care provider include a change in mental status, chest pain, seizures, pressure ulcers, falls, and changes in vital signs. These clinical parameters along with specific management protocols should be negotiated with the collaborative physician or medical director of the facility.

Other areas of risk management prevention include involvement in development and implementation of the restraint policy, frequent and clear communication with the resident and his or her family, and adherence to assessment and documentation standards under the Omnibus Budget Reconciliation Act (OBRA). Use of available patient ombudsman in long-term care facilities may be helpful, especially with patients without family.

Chapter 22

Medication Issues

Multiple medication use and the potential for iatrogenesis in the elderly are issues of growing concern. Age-related changes, the existence of multiple comorbidities, and psychosocial issues that accompany aging predispose the elderly to increased risk for adverse drug reactions. The geriatric population uses one-fourth of all drugs prescribed in the United States and are prescribed an average of 13–14 medications each year. The institutionalized elderly use the greatest number of medications, yet the average older American takes 4.5 prescription drugs at a time. The elderly use 40% of all over-the-counter (OTC) preparations. The incidence of adverse drug reactions is two-to-three times higher in the geriatric population than in the young. Drug therapy in the elderly requires a unique approach and management plan.

AGE-RELATED CHANGES

Organ Reserve

Organ reserve declines at a rate of 0.8–0.9% per year beyond age 30 but maintains adequacy in the healthy older adult until the end of the life-span. Reserved organ function enables the body to compensate for insults that may be invoked by medication use. When concomitant disease is present (as frequently occurs in the elderly), decline in organ reserve accelerates so that compensatory mechanisms are further reduced. Pharmacokinetics (absorption, distribution, metabolism, and excretion) and pharmacodynamics are affected by aging (see Display 22-1).

Absorption

Absorption is the parameter of pharmacodynamics least affected by normal aging. If there is decreased gastric acid production, absorption of coated tablets is decreased. Because of the elderly's propensity to multiple medication use, drug–drug interactions may occur that decrease absorption. Use of antacids and laxatives creates potential for decreased absorption of drugs

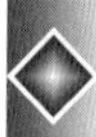

DISPLAY 22-1. *Age-Related Changes in Pharmacodynamics and Pharmacokinetics*

PHARMACOKINETICS

Absorption

Delayed gastric emptying may alter absorption (increase or decrease depending on drug and where most is absorbed).

Thinning of intestinal mucosa and diminished gastric acid production may decrease absorption of weak-acid drugs.

Increase in body fat may decrease absorption of transdermal preparations.

Distribution

Increased tissue binding of some drugs due to increase in ratio of body fat to lean tissue.

Reduction in total body water decreases distribution and increases plasma concentration of water-soluble drugs.

Decrease in serum albumin affects highly protein-bound drugs.

Decrease in Vitamin K clotting factors.

Metabolism

Prolonged half-life of some drugs due to decreased hepatic blood flow.

Reduction in liver enzymes involved in Phase I drug metabolism.

Excretion

Reduction in renal blood flow.

Decreased glomerular filtration rate.

Decline in creatinine clearance despite normal serum creatinine.

PHARMACODYNAMICS

Changes in number of receptors.

Decreased or increased receptor binding.

Changes in end-organ reserve.

such as cimetidine, tetracycline, digoxin, ciprofloxin, and iron. Consumption of alcohol (EtOH) may accelerate absorption of drugs such as chloral hydrate. Greater effects may be seen from drugs used concomitantly with anticholinergics that slow gastric emptying.

Distribution

Distribution of a drug is determined by body composition and the volume of drug available for delivery to body tissues.

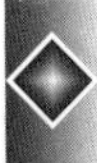

DISPLAY 22-2. ***Drugs Potentiated by Decreased Hepatic Blood Flow***

Quinidine	Morphine	Nitrates
Propanolol	Meperidine	Isoproterenol

The ratio of adipose tissue to total body weight increases with aging. Lipophilic drugs (benzodiazepines, phenytoin) that are well-distributed into adipose tissue exhibit increased tissue binding, prolonged action, and greater risk for toxicity in the elderly. Total body water decreases with age because the increase in body fat reduces the space for water. Higher serum levels of water-soluble drugs (digoxin, EtOH, lithium, phenytoin, theophylline, morphine) occur because there is smaller space for distribution. The elderly are more sensitive to anticoagulants because of a decrease in Vitamin-K clotting factors; therefore, doses of these agents should be reduced by 30–40%.

There is an age-related decrease in the binding protein albumin. Elderly who are acutely ill, chronically ill, or malnourished are at high risk for drug toxicity from reductions in albumin concentration, because hypoalbuminemia increases the circulating volume of free drug. Because a normal range for serum drug level is based on a constant proportion of free to bound drug, a normal value may not indicate toxicity in the presence of hypoalbuminemia.

Many drugs frequently prescribed in the elderly are highly protein bound. When several of these medications are taken concomitantly, one drug may displace another from its binding site. Competition for binding sites results in increased volume of unbound drug in the circulation and greater risk for toxicity. Some medications often affected include warfarin, digoxin, furosemide, phenytoin, meperidine, cimetidine, theophylline, indomethacin, and salicylates.

Metabolism

Drug metabolism by the liver is affected by the age-related decrease in hepatic blood flow. Medications that are administered orally pass directly into the portal circulation before entering the systemic circulation. Drugs that undergo extensive metabolism through this first pass through the liver will have greater availability in the systemic circulation when hepatic blood flow is decreased. Dosing must be reduced in the elderly to prevent side effects and toxicity from the potentiation of these medications (see Display 22-2).

Drugs are biotransformed by the liver by two reactions, Phase I and Phase II. The enzymes involved in Phase I metabolism are reduced in the elderly, causing prolonged half-lives and more frequent side effects of drugs metabolized primarily by Phase I reaction. In the elderly, normal hepatic metabolism cannot be implied from liver enzyme levels (alkaline phosphatase, SGOT, SGPT) within normal range. Many medications frequently prescribed for use

DISPLAY 22-3. *Drugs with Prolonged Metabolism by the Liver*

Warfarin	Captopril	Furosemide
Theophylline	Digoxin	Lithium
Diazepam	Cimetidine	Propranolol
Phenytoin	Enalapril	Tolbutamide
Atenelol	Famotidine	

in the elderly have prolonged metabolism by the liver (see Display 22-3). Phase II metabolism is not known to be significantly affected by aging so that medications metabolized primarily during Phase II do not exhibit prolonged action.

Excretion

Renal excretion declines with aging. Even though approximately one-third of the elderly retain normal kidney function, the glomerular filtration rate (GFR) in older adults may be decreased by as much as 35%. Altered clearance results in increased serum level and prolonged half-life of medications cleared by the kidney (see Display 22-4).

Normal kidney function should not be assumed from normal serum creatinine level in an elderly individual. Because creatinine production decreases with the age-related loss of muscle mass, an increase in GFR may be masked. The elderly are a heterogeneous group whose true renal function is difficult to discern, but the Cockcroft–Gault equation (provided below) adjusts for age and sex and provides a better approximation of renal function than serum creatinine level. Dosages and dosing intervals must be individualized based on estimated renal function.

$$\text{Creatinine clearance} = \frac{(140 - \text{age}) \times \text{weight (kg)}}{\text{serum creatinine (mg/dL)} \times 72}$$

(Multiply × 0.85 for women)

Pharmacodynamics

Age-related effects on pharmacodynamics are not as clearly understood as pharmacokinetic changes, but it is certain that the elderly may exhibit either decreased or increased sensitivity to certain drugs. Changes in the number of receptors, receptor binding, and end-organ reserve result in a narrowed therapeutic index of many medications requiring more exact dosing in the elderly than in the younger population. Aging may lead to a decreased sensitivity to beta-blockers and beta-agonists. The elderly exhibit increased sen-

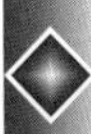

DISPLAY 22-4. ***Drugs Cleared by Renal Excretion***

Sulfa drugs	Lithium
Methotrexate	Digoxin
Cimetidine	Phenobarbital
Chlorpropamide	Aminoglycoside antibiotics

sitivity to diazepam, nitrazepam, EtOH, anticholinergics, narcotics, and coumadin that is likely due in part to pharmacodynamic changes.

SPECIAL CONSIDERATIONS FOR PRESCRIBING IN THE ELDERLY

Polypharmacy/Adverse Drug Reactions (ADRs)

Numerous factors must be considered in assessing risk for polypharmacy. It is not uncommon for an elderly individual to seek treatment and receive prescriptions from several providers who are not aware of other drugs being used. The elderly may self-medicate to avoid encounters with the health care system and use OTC preparations that they do not consider to be medications. OTC agents such as acetaminophen, eye drops, aspirin, laxatives, and sleep aids are used by as many as 75% of the elderly. The infirm elderly population often are transferred between care settings (e.g., acute care to nursing home) without adequate or appropriate information regarding changes in medications.

The likelihood and the risk of an ADR increases as the number of drugs used increases. ADRs account for as many as 30% of hospital admissions in the elderly. Ageism may cause ADRs to be attributed to older age. ADRs may be misdiagnosed because the elderly often present atypically. Elderly women may be at greater risk for ADRs because they have a greater reduction in muscle mass and generally receive more medications than elderly men. Drug substitutions required for reimbursement by health maintenance organizations may contribute to the incidence of ADRs. The exclusion of elders from pharmaceutical trials often makes it necessary to adjust doses recommended for a younger population to avoid ADRs.

Inappropriate use of medications occurs when medications are continued when they are no longer needed. Definite therapeutic goals should be established, and benefits versus risks considered before prescribing (see Display 22-5). Use of an additional drug to treat an ADR should be avoided. Sedative-hypnotics and antipsychotics are frequently inappropriately given. Antipsychotics are prescribed to more than one-fourth of all nursing home residents even though the Omnibus Budget Reconciliation Act (OBRA) established guidelines to avoid use of these agents as chemical restraints.

DISPLAY 22-5. *Risks Associated with Drugs Used Frequently in the Elderly*

Digoxin

High risk for toxicity especially in frail elderly

Loop Diuretics

Decreased total body clearance in the elderly
May cause ototoxicity especially in large doses

Thyroid hormone

Inappropriate dosing may lead to thyrotoxicosis

Antipsychotics

Use increases risk for hip fracture
High incidence of anticholinergic side effects: hypotension, dry mouth, constipation, urinary retention, blurred vision
Risk for tardive dyskinesia and dystonia (side effects that do not resolve with withdrawal of drug)

Tricyclic Antidepressants

Risk for ECG changes and orthostatic hypotension
Anticholinergic side effects greatest with use of amitriptyline

Sedative-Hypnotics

Increased risk for hip fracture

NSAIDs

May induce renal failure especially in patients with heart failure, cirrhosis, diabetes mellitus, volume depletion, or sodium depletion

Neuroleptics

Drug-induced Parkinsonianism (Compazine, Mellaril)

Anticholinergics

When used as adjuvant to anesthestics, increases risk for post-operative confusion

Diuretics

Increased risk of hypotension related to volume depletion

Antihypertensive Medications

Increased risk of hypotension due to age-related impairment in vasomotor response

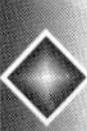

DISPLAY 22-6. *Factors Determining Medication Compliance in the Elderly*

Presence of symptoms
Belief that medication will work or prevent disease
Number of medications
Inadequate education of patient regarding medication regimen
Caregiver education/understanding/support
Fear of side effects or toxicity
Duration of therapy
Complexity of regimen
Packaging of medication (difficulty/ease of opening)
Cost
Cognitive status
Visual acuity

Underuse of needed medications (antidepressants, vaccines) is frequently seen in the geriatric population.

Use of digoxin is one of the most common causes of drug toxicity in the geriatric population. The elderly may present with atypical manifestations of toxicity such as anorexia, depression, delirium, psychosis, or confusion. Digoxin is often given concomitantly with diuretics for heart failure in the elderly. Hypokalemia resulting from diuretic use predisposes to digoxin toxicity. Addition of quinidine or a calcium-channel blocker may increase digoxin levels. Digoxin is eliminated mainly by glomerular filtration so renal function is an important consideration. Careful clinical monitoring is required because side effects or toxicity may occur with normal serum levels.

Compliance

The problem of noncompliance is more common in the elderly population but is related to the increase in number of medications used rather than age alone. Multiple factors influence whether an elder can or will comply with recommended regimens (see Display 22-6).

Psychosocial Considerations

Functional and sensory deficits may hinder medication use. Vision, motor dexterity, and cognitive status are major determinants of whether an individual is capable of taking medications. Many elderly live alone or do not have access to transportation for filling prescriptions or financial resources to pay for drugs. Literacy level and cultural background may create barriers to appropriate medication use.

GUIDELINES FOR DRUG THERAPY IN THE ELDERLY

✦ **Consider management with nonpharmacological interventions before prescribing drugs:**

✧ Dietary interventions (change in diet before antacids or laxatives);

✧ Physical therapy (before use of NSAIDs);

✧ Relaxation techniques (before anxiolytics/sleep aids);

✧ Behavior modification (diversion before use of antipsychotics).

✦ Conduct a thorough history and physical examination before prescribing.

✧ Assess for signs of:

✧ dehydration, edema, or ascites—may alter drug distribution.

✧ chronic liver disease—adjust dosing for drugs that require hepatic transformation.

✧ renal insufficiency.

✧ swallowing difficulty.

✧ Measure height and weight.

✧ **Always consider medication use as first probable cause of a change in functional or cognitive status in the elderly.**

✦ Obtain from patient/caregiver a list of allergies (prescription medications, OTCs, environmental agents) with specific description of reaction. Advise patient/caregiver to carry a wallet card or wear identification that lists allergies.

✦ Individualize dosing based on body size and known organ function (kidney and liver). Begin with smallest dose possible (usually one-fourth to one-half of recommended adult dose) and titrate to larger dose based on response. Consult physician as needed.

✦ Assess risk for drug–drug interactions. Consult physician and refer to pharmacological resources. A complete listing of possible interactions is beyond the scope of this book, but many resources are available for clinical use. Caution patients about the risk for medication interactions with EtOH and illicit drugs. Avoid use of another drug to treat an ADR. The offending agent should be removed from the patient's regimen whenever possible.

✦ Encourage patient to bring all medications, including OTC preparations, for review at every visit. Provide a written list of medications and doses and suggest that the patient keep this list on his or her person at all times. Use a screening tool to assess patient's knowledge of medications, doses, how to take, and barriers to taking medications.

✦ Advise patient/caregiver of potential side effects of medications and the importance of reporting any changes in status. Caution patients against assuming that symptoms are related to aging or disease process.

✦ Inform patient/caregiver of doses and administration of medications. Include discussion of correct use of prn medications.

✦ Establish goals for efficacy of medication before prescribing. Advise patient/caregiver of desired outcome and reassess continued use of every medication at every visit. Discontinue medications that are no longer needed. When antipsychotics or sedative-hypnotics are used chronically, reassess need every 30–60 days. Consider a drug holiday to determine need for medication and to avoid tardive dyskinesia and dystonia.

✦ Emphasize that OTCs (including herbal preparations) must be considered as medications. Provide education regarding OTCs:

  ✧ Possible side effects;

  ✧ Possible interactions with other medications.

✦ Simplify regimen to increase compliance whenever possible. Consider qd dosing rather than bid–qid.

✦ Adjust only one aspect of regimen at a time to better evaluate effects of change.

✦ Encourage the use of one pharmacy.

✦ Monitor drug levels. Remain alert to the possibility of side effects/toxicity even while levels are within normal range.

✦ Evaluate capability to take medications as prescribed. Assess dexterity, vision, memory, and judgment. Periodically observe the patient set up medications. Assess for barriers such as childproof caps. Recommend use of medicine box or other memory aids.

✦ Assess financial situation to determine ability to buy medications. Refer to formularies for reimbursement and consider least expensive therapeutic option. Refer to social work services as needed.

Chapter 23

Rehabilitation Issues

Loss of independence and premature placement in an extended care facility is a common fear among the elderly. The risk of a potentially disabling condition, and often more than one, increases with age (see Display 23-1). Bed rest associated with these surgical, acute, and chronic conditions often leads to additional complications (see Display 23-2). As deconditioning, cognitive, and functional decline occur, loss of independence often follows. The loss of independence may be prevented by the timely implementation of rehabilitation.

Rehabilitation focuses on function rather than illness or disease and adaptation rather than cure. The common goal is to optimize function; physiological, psychological, and spiritual wellness; and quality of life as specified by the patient. Although prevention and treatment of illness, disease, or injury continues, it becomes secondary to the rehabilitative focus.

Geriatric rehabilitation requires an interdisciplinary approach with knowledge of gerontology and rehabilitation. An interdisciplinary approach implies the members interact collaboratively, advocating for the patient, and coordinating care to meet specific goals. Alternatively, a multidisciplinary approach is one in which the members represent multiple disciplines, each functioning independently of other team members. Geriatric interdisciplinary teams may include a geriatrician; physiatrist; gerontological nurse practitioner; social worker; nutritionist; pharmacist; psychologist; psychiatrist; chaplain; ethicist; rehabilitation nurses; and physical, occupational, kinesio, speech, and recreational therapists. Unfortunately, some of these specialties may be accessible only by consult. Other team members often called upon as consultants may include a podiatrist, audiologist, ophthalmologist, dentist, and wound/ostomy/continence nurse.

Rehabilitation involves cognitive and functional assessment, realistic goal setting, counseling, and intensive education of the patient and significant other(s) (see Display 23-3). Standardized assessment instruments provide consistency in outcome determinations throughout the continuum of care. Interventions are focused on energy conservation, coping skills, and adaptive mechanisms (see Display 23-4). Assessment of function includes activities of daily living (ADLs), instrumental activities of daily living (IADLs) such as transportation, grocery shopping, banking, and laundering, and executive activities of living (such as financial planning, volunteer, vocational, and recre-

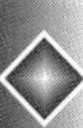

DISPLAY 23-1. *Potentially Disabling Conditions Seen in Geriatric Rehabilitation Settings*

NEUROLOGICAL

Cerebrovascular Accident
Multiple sclerosis
Head injury secondary to falls/accidents
Parkinson's
Spinal stenosis

CARDIOVASCULAR

Unstable angina
Valvular disease
Congestive heart failure
Postoperative: Valve replacement/coronary artery bypass graft

PULMONARY

Chronic obstructive pulmonary disease
Tuberculosis

ORTHOPEDIC

Joint replacement
Arthritis
Fractures

OTHER

General deconditioning commonly associated with pneumonia, urinary tract infection, or sepsis
Depression
Cancer
Pressure ulcers
Amputation
Complications of diabetes mellitus
Acquired immunodeficiency syndrome
Substance abuse
Pain
Falls
Peripheral vascular disease

ational skills), as appropriate. Adaptive needs are evaluated and equipment is issued with appropriate education of the patient and significant other(s) for safe use. Commonly, modifications are required in the patient's home environment (see Display 23-4).

(text continues on page 484)

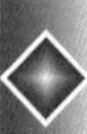

DISPLAY 23-2. *Complications of Bed Rest*

Generalized weakness	Orthostasis
Pneumonia	Pressure ulcers
Contractures	Malnutrition
Urinary tract infections	Constipation
Functional incontinence	Depression
Falls	Osteoporosis
Calcium renal calculi	Muscle wasting
Gait abnormalities	Dehydration

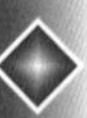

DISPLAY 23-3. *Rehabilitation Techniques*

Patient/family/interdisciplinary rehabilitation team conferences: To clarify goals, discuss expectations, provide explanations, and present progress reports.

Environment: Pleasant, supportive, safe, and stimulating settings to enhance therapeutic milieu.

Motivation: Critical to maximize outcome; encouragement, reeducation, reinforcement, and identification/treatment of depression frequently required.

Understanding/empathy: Required of treatment team members toward patient/caregiver concerning losses and redirection of life goals.

Continuity of care: Enhances the rehabilitation process with care provided by primary care provider, communication between levels of care, and preferably, consistent therapists between levels of care.

Case management: Includes case manager/interdisciplinary team collaboration; movement of patient through rehabilitative process and across levels of care; appropriate use of available resources to provide cost effective services/achieve optimal rehabilitative outcomes.

Education: Of patient/family using principles of adult learning with consideration of cultural diversity.

Advocacy: For patient/family.

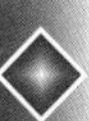

DISPLAY 23-4. *Common Adaptive Equipment and Home Modifications*

ADAPTIVE EQUIPMENT

Sensory/communication: Hearing aids, corrective lenses, low vision aids, speaking aids, specialized phone systems, and computerized programs.

Nutrition: Dentures/partials, adaptive eating utensils, plates and cups, stabilizing materials, eating surfaces.

Mobility: Crutches, straight/quad canes, walkers/hemi-walkers, wheelchairs (companion/standard/customized/electric with or without removable arms and legs with adjustable/nonadjustable leg/foot rests), motorized scooters, and adapted vans. Hospital bed (manual/electric) with or without side rails. Specialty beds. Slide boards with or without movable components. Lifts. Over-the-bed trapeze. Lift chair.

Positioning devices: Wedges, specialty seating.

Dressing/grooming aids: Reachers, button hooks, sock/stocking aids, Velcro closures, elastic shoe laces, long-handled sponges.

Orthotics: Slings, splints, braces, shrinkers, ankle/foot and ankle/knee orthotics (AFOs and AKOs), specialty shoes.

Prostheses.

Bathing: Shower/bathtub chairs, hand-held shower heads, grab bars.

Bladder: Devices designed for urinary incontinence, bladder drainage, and adapted self-intermittent catheterization (SIC). Commode chairs of various designs, high rise toilet seats, and versa frames.

Bowel: Devices designed for bowel incontinence and bowel management, including pulsed irrigation devices.

Respiratory: Suction apparatus, oxygen, nebulizers, ventilatory support devices, as well as mechanical ventilation.

COMMON HOME MODIFICATIONS

Ramps
Grab bars
Elevated commode seat
Versa frame
Transfer tub bench
Shower chair
Hand-held shower head
Removal of doors to permit walker or wheelchair entry
Transition of an inaccessible sleeping area to an accessible area

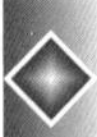

DISPLAY 23-5. *Rehabilitation Settings*

Acute hospital
Subacute/transitional units
Specialized rehabilitation facility
Outpatient rehabilitation center
Skilled extended care facility
Adult day health facility
Veteran's Administration medical and extended care facilities
Assisted living
Home with home health rehabilitation nursing, PT/OT/speech therapies

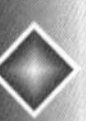

DISPLAY 23-6. *Factors Influencing the Rehabilitative Process*

Comorbidities—especially end-stage cardiac, pulmonary, or renal disease
Sensory loss—especially vision, hearing, and touch
Cognitive deficits preventing carry over (new learning)
Literacy
Level of education
Patient motivation
Nutritional status
Culture
Patient's values and beliefs regarding illness and self-care
Inaccessibility of home environment
Pressure ulcers
Substance abuse
Pain
Expectations of caregiver by patient
Unrealistic goals/expectations of significant other(s)
Health status and availability of significant other(s)
Physical reserve—especially when considering prosthesis for amputee
Predictable social support/resources
Transportation
Finances

Rehabilitative services are provided in a number of settings (see Display 23-5). Selection of the appropriate setting is based on the patient's medical stability, cognitive status, motivation, rehabilitative nursing needs, the intensity of therapy required, patient preferences, and the payer.

A number of factors influence the rehabilitation process (see Display 23-6). These factors must be considered prior to acceptance into a rehabilitation program. The availability/support of family/significant other(s) is an important consideration in the elder's rehabilitation and ultimate disposition. Normal physiological changes of aging impact the rehabilitative process; however, chronic comorbidities have the most influence. Normal physiological reserve may be further compromised by multiple comorbidities and pain, resulting in an inability of the elder to tolerate aggressive rehabilitation. Pain management (especially the timely administration of analgesics prior to therapy), bladder and bowel management, and prevention of skin breakdown are emphasized. Goal setting must be specific, measurable, realistically attainable, and time limited. The geriatric rehabilitation process requires more time and may require treatment in more than one setting over time.

Chapter 24

Special Issues

ELDERS AS CAREGIVERS

The geriatric population is a heterogeneous group who live in a variety of settings and family environments. Societal and demographic changes in recent decades have resulted in more elderly persons serving as caregivers for spouses, siblings, grandchildren, and adult children. Caring can be one of the most rewarding aspects of the human experience. At the same time, caregiving often places a burden on older individuals at a point in their lives when they, themselves, require increased assistance and care to maintain health and viability.

Much has been written in the literature to address the needs of the elderly who are serving as caregivers for spouses with chronic illnesses and Alzheimer's disease. In these settings, the aged spouse is the most frequent caregiver with middle-aged daughters often assisting in this role. In-home care is often continued beyond the point of practicality to avoid exorbitant costs of institutionalization. Healthcare professionals who provide case management to elderly caregivers should provide counseling regarding various care options that are available. Community-based assistance to elderly caregivers is presently inadequate in the United States, but legislation is pending to increase the scope of services as well as financial aid.

Grandparents as Primary Caregivers

As many as 2.4 million children are living in homes headed by grandparents, and as many as 1 million children are being raised by grandparents alone. These staggering numbers reflect a 44% increase between 1980 and 1990 in the numbers of children living with grandparents or other relatives. Causes for this increase have been attributed to teen pregnancy, AIDS, drug and alcohol (EtOH) abuse, poverty, the increase in the number of single-parent homes, the necessity for families to pursue dual incomes, and imprisonment of parents.

Children may be placed with their grandparents by state agencies when parents are deemed unfit; or parents may willingly transfer care of their children to grandparents. Often the responsibility is transferred suddenly, leaving grandparents with no time to prepare for the role. Both grandmothers and grandfathers are assuming the role of primary caregiver, and many provide simultaneously for the needs of adult children and grandchildren. Grandmothers often view themselves as more successful than grandfathers at caregiving, but little difference exists between grandmothers and grandfathers in role satisfaction. Sociocultural influence may cause children to turn to grandmothers more frequently for assistance and cause grandfathers to expect less involvement. Some grandparents are themselves unmarried or widowed and must fulfill the role without the support of a partner. There is evidence that grandparents are more likely to be rearing boys than girls, and care for disruptive rather than compliant children is more likely to have been transferred to grandparents.

The greatest concern for most elderly grandparents is that they will not live long enough to be able to take care of their grandchildren until the children reach maturity. Many elderly caregivers express fear that their grandchildren will return to neglectful or abusive parents. Legislation has been adopted in many states that guarantees grandparents' rights should unfit adult children attempt to interfere with caregiving. Another frequent worry is that the children will not be able to overcome the emotional burdens that have been placed on them at an early age by their parents' dysfunction. The elderly may experience shame associated with feelings that they failed their own children but remain devoted to providing their grandchildren with better opportunities. Grandparents often experience ambivalent feelings toward their new role, i.e., they love their grandchildren but did not expect to be responsible for their upbringing.

Older adults may find themselves in the position of providing care to multiple generations. Younger grandmothers are often taking care of their elderly parents and their grandchildren at the same time. This level of responsibility is exhausting and leaves little or no time for contacts with peers or outside interests. Many grandparents caring for grandchildren neglect their own health and have more health-related problems than their peers who are not caring for grandchildren. Some are unwilling to report their own health problems for fear that grandchildren will be taken away or placed in foster care. Role reversal poses a serious problem when adult children remain in the household while a grandparent is the principal caregiver/authority for grandchildren. The relationship between the grandparent and the adult child may undermine the grandparent's relationship with grandchildren. The adult child may actually compete with the grandchildren for the elderly caregiver's attention.

Grandparents are serving as primary caregivers for grandchildren in all ethnic groups. Variation has been found to exist between the significance assigned to the grandparenting role by African-American versus Anglo-American grandparent-caregivers. In both groups, most grandparents view themselves as having more strengths than weaknesses; however, many African Americans perceive themselves as more involved in teaching their grandchildren. African-American culture often encourages greater cross-generational involvement in families.

Grandparents are serving as primary caregivers for grandchildren in all socioeconomic groups. In one study of grandparent-caregivers, one-fourth were found to live below the poverty level. For many, the ability to make a living is compromised by child-rearing tasks. The 1995 White House Conference on Aging called for increased financial assistance for grandparent-caregivers. Laws need to be changed to qualify grandparents for aid similar to that received by individuals who provide foster care for children.

Despite many problems, not all families are impaired by the challenges of grandparents rearing grandchildren. Many grandparents find great fulfillment in maintaining family values and passing family history to succeeding generations. Grandparents can dispel myths held by their grandchildren about aging and the geriatric population. Some elderly have been motivated to improve their own health behaviors (smoking and EtOH cessation) in order to exhibit a positive influence on their grandchildren.

The interdisciplinary geriatric healthcare team can take a proactive role in assisting the elderly who serve as primary caregivers for their grandchildren. Screening tools are available to inventory strengths and needs of grandparents. Regular, thorough history and physical examination will enable monitoring of the grandparent's health status and ability to care for his or her own needs and manage chronic illnesses. Grandparents should be encouraged to voice ambivalent feelings about the burden of responsibility and assured that they are not alone in their feelings. Referrals should be encouraged for psychiatric evaluation and management of children with emotional disturbances.

Social work services can provide contacts for community assistance. More than 400 support groups for grandparents now exist in the United States. By attending these groups, not only do grandparents receive support but grandchildren may often find an opportunity to play and share with other children who live in similar situations. Many grandparents may need financial assistance and help in obtaining health insurance for grandchildren. Senior centers and churches now offer opportunities for grandparenting education. The cultural background of grandparents should be considered; the church is a strong influence in the African-American community. Anticipatory guidance regarding custodial and financial planning is available from legal services agencies.

Caregivers of Adults With Learning Disabilities/Mental Retardation

Aging adults with learning disabilities/mental retardation experience the same age-related changes as do their cohorts. Because of technological advances, the life-span of adults with disabilities has increased. It is now projected that 44% of adults with Down's syndrome will reach age 60, and 14% will reach age 68.

The trend in the past 20 years to deinstitutionalize individuals with learning disabilities/mental retardation has transferred the setting of care to community-based group homes or to private homes. Many elderly parents continue to care for adult children who have always been cared for in the home.

Both the caregiver and the impaired adult are aging, and the elderly caregiver may have reached frailty or near-disability from chronic illness. Physical limitations and financial burden may overcome the elder's ability to provide care. Some elderly caregivers have cited examples of their adult children being easier to care for as they age because they have the physical capacity and have acquired skills to assist their parents when needed. Elder caregivers may have to cope with decision-making regarding long-term care for themselves and their adult children at the same time. Like grandparents caring for grandchildren, these elderly caregivers fear death because of worry about what will happen to their adult children who are not capable of caring for themselves. At a time when they are dealing with their own aging, many elderly caregivers have unresolved grief related to the child's disabilities.

Most elderly caregivers of adults with mental disabilities have not made plans for placement at the time of the caregiver's death and wait for a crisis (impending death) to occur before plans are made. Inappropriate placements are often made under "last-minute" circumstances. Responsibility for the disabled adult child is often passed to a spouse or sibling on the death of the elder caregiver, unfortunately with no time for preparation or resolution of grief. Many elderly caregivers express concern for the disabled adult child's sibling who they anticipate will assume the role, but with whom they often never discussed long-range plans. Elderly caregivers may fear that the unpredictability of the disabled child's behavior will pose considerable hardship for the sibling. The long-term strain of caring for adult children may have depleted the elderly caregiver's financial resources. Many elderly caregivers are uninformed regarding financial planning. They are unsure whether to leave funds to the disabled child (mental handicaps may exclude that child from full benefits) or to leave funds to a relative who is charged with caring for the adult child (which carries the risk of the relative misusing funds).

The degree of handicap in older mentally retarded adults ranges from mild to profound. Diagnostic standards in previous years may have been different, and adults >60 years with mental retardation may require reassessment. Tragically, adults with profound impairment may suffer sequelae from being restrained in the past (contractures, neck drop). Elderly caregivers who remember bad experiences may not access services or may not be aware of newer services. Some have voiced a sense of little support from medical professionals who they feel are not sensitive to their needs and frustrations.

Individuals with mild impairment may reside in community-based group homes where a resident trainer assists with grooming and preparing meals. Many attend a day care facility where they are taught daily living and vocational skills. Employment may be held in the community or at the facility. These individuals may go home with elderly caregivers on a frequent, routine basis. Some progress to permanent residence with an elderly parent-caregiver. Many elderly caregivers express concern regarding the regulations that govern community-based homes. Some elderly caregivers are reluctant to transfer care of their adult children to group home facilities because they lack knowledge regarding services.

Older adults with learning disabilities/mental retardation have unique problems that must be addressed. Adults with Down's syndrome have increased incidence of Alzheimer's disease, cardiovascular disease, hearing loss with aging, cataracts, and hypothyroidism. In a recent survey, as many as two-thirds of older adults with mental retardation were found to have chronic illnesses. Obesity is a common problem in adults with mental retardation and is likely attributable to sedentary lifestyle, use of medications that increase appetite, and use of food for behavioral modification. Iatrogenic anorexia is another potential problem when medications are changed frequently to manage behavior.

The complexity of needs for adults with mental handicaps requires an interdisciplinary approach and service coordination. Communication with these patients is difficult because of cognitive and sensory impairments and requires skill innonverbal techniques. Issues important to providing adequate health care to these patients include hygiene, exercise, nutrition, screening for sensory impairment, medication review/monitoring, contraception, and safe-sex practices. Elderly caregivers may require referral for respite and transportation assistance. Education regarding employment opportunities for the adult child, group home regulations, dementia/Alzheimer's disease, and sterilization procedures for the adult child (if indicated) is often sought by the parent caregiver. Legal services may be accessed through the local legal societies and Area Agency on Aging. Contingency plans should be discussed with the elderly caregiver to address emergent institutionalization. Elderly caregivers often possess strong problem-solving ability developed over years of caring for their disabled children. Although this skill often prevents elderly caregivers from seeking outside assistance, coping ability is clearly a strength that can be used during difficult decision-making if outside placement becomes necessary.

ELDER MISTREATMENT

Every year in the United States, approximately 1 million older adults are mistreated. Elder mistreatment includes physical, sexual, and psychological abuse; neglect by others and self-neglect; and exploitation (see Display 24-1). Findings from a recent prospective cohort study showed that elders who are abused have a 3.1 times greater risk of death than those who suffer no mistreatment. In addition to the cost of emergency room visits and medical treatment, elder mistreatment perpetuates the burden of violence in society. As the young witness mistreatment of the elderly, the cycle of violence is transmitted from one generation to the next.

Profile of the Mistreated

See Display 24-2. Most studies show elderly females to be at greater risk for mistreatment than elderly males, although gender has not been proven to

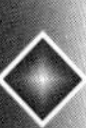

DISPLAY 24-1. *Types of Elder Mistreatment*

PHYSICAL MISTREATMENT

Infliction of pain or bodily injury
Sexual abuse
Physical or chemical restraints: Tying elders to furniture; over-medicating

NEGLECT

Intentional: Deprivation of food or care; confinement
Unintentional: Lack of care related to caregiver's knowledge deficit or inability to provide care

EXPLOITATION

Mismanagement/theft of funds: Theft of pension, savings, or Social Security checks; forcing elders to sign checks or give money to others; forcing to change will or forcing to sign power of attorney by threatening institutionalization or other measures
Misuse of medications: Medications prescribed for elder used by others; withholding medications from elders
Psychological threats, humiliation, insults
Fraudulence/scams: Recommendation of unnecessary home repairs by contractors, "get-rich-quick" schemes, solicitation of fraudulent charitable donations

determine risk for mistreatment. Increased incidence among elderly women may be due to societal influences or increased longevity in females versus males. Abuse occurs more frequently in the elderly who reside with family members who have little social support and are isolated from community resources. Intergenerational strife may provoke retaliation toward the older parent for past offenses. Because of increased mobility in American society, some elders live long distances from their children and isolation from relatives makes them easier prey for those who would exploit or mistreat.

Profile of the Abuser

Mistreatment of elders occurs in all socioeconomic and ethnic groups. A close family member or caregiver is most often the party responsible for elder abuse. Abusive behavior may be exhibited by caregivers who are strained by financial obligations or the physical burden of providing care for physically and cognitively impaired elders. The caregiver who must rely on the elderly individual for housing or other financial assistance may resent this depen-

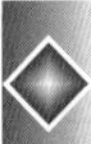

DISPLAY 24-2. *Risk Factors for Elder Mistreatment*

Advanced age
Financial dependency of caregiver on the elder
EtOH or drug abuse by the abuser
History of intergenerational conflict within family
Previous history of abuse
Impaired physical status of elder
Impaired cognitive status of abuser or elder
Social isolation

dency. Caregivers with mental illness or EtOH or drug abuse often commit abusive acts toward the elder with whom they reside.

Management of Elder Mistreatment

Elder mistreatment may present in the emergency room, primary care, extended care, or home health setting. The prospective payment system now demands early hospital discharge, but funding for adequate follow-up by home health is often unavailable. Involvement by the interdisciplinary team to assess the advisability of home care is essential. When providing care for the dependent geriatric client, the entire family/significant others also become clients of the interdisciplinary team.

HISTORY

Many individuals who become abusive toward elders are trying to fulfill the expectations of caring for a loved one. **See section above on Elders as Caregivers.** A nonjudgmental approach must be taken when interviewing patients/family members for history of violence/mistreatment, EtOH and drug abuse, and possible causes for retribution against the elder. Be aware of cultural values that may define individual/family attitudes toward treatment of elders. Appraisal of family members'/caregivers' ability to provide care while meeting their own needs can prevent elder mistreatment. Screening tools are available for assessment of the elderly individual's risk for mistreatment and the caregiver's burden. Multiple trips to the emergency room for falls, fractures, or other injuries or a pattern of frequently changing providers should raise suspicion for elder mistreatment.

When elder mistreatment is suspected, the elderly individual and suspected abuser should be interviewed both together and individually when possible. It is important to maintain a nonthreatening approach with both parties because the elder may fear retaliation from the abuser and the abuser may fear prosecution. Elders may also underreport mistreatment because of feelings of shame, guilt related to dependent status, fear of prosecution of the caregiver, or fear of institutionalization. Integrating questions as part of routine history-taking can help to alleviate anxiety. Observe the interaction between the elderly individual and the suspected abuser, noting especially the caregiver who answers all questions for the elder or when the elder looks to the caregiver before speaking. Be alert for evasive accounts of injuries and the caregiver who describes the elder as being prone to accidents.

While apart from the suspected abuser, the elderly individual should be asked direct questions regarding how much time is spent alone, accessibility to religious activities and social events, and his or her knowledge regarding available finances. During a separate interview, the suspected abuser should be questioned about stressors such as personal health, family, and financial problems, and asked if he or she ever loses control while interacting with the elderly individual.

PHYSICAL EXAMINATION

A thorough, systematic physical examination should be performed with particular attention for signs of mistreatment.

✦ **Be aware that signs of abuse may be attributed to normal age-related changes (see Appendix A. Common Changes of Aging) or disease.**

✦ **Be alert for injuries in various stages of healing and evidence of previous injuries.**

✦ Use photographs or body maps to document suspected abuse.

✦ Weight: Assess for possible sign of neglect to provide nutrition.

✦ General appearance: Assess for poor hygiene, soiled clothing.

✦ Head: Assess for absence of hair, hemorrhages below the scalp (signs of hair-pulling). Note presence of broken teeth and lacerations around mouth (sign of forced feeding or gagging). Presence of ecchymoses over the mastoid process, papilledema, or raccoon's eyes may indicate head injury. Assess integrity of tympanic membrane and note presence of fluid or blood.

✦ Neck: Assess for whiplash injury suggestive of shaking.

✦ Neurological: Mental status examination for impaired cognitive status. Note affect. Assess for agitation, depression, passiveness, withdrawal of patient from caregiver. Delirium may indicate neglect (dehydration, malnutrition).

✦ Skin: Note presence of lacerations, abrasions, bruises on breasts (females), bite marks, or ecchymoses (may reflect shape, size of striking object). Note burns: may reflect pattern of object (e.g., end of cigarette butt or shape of clothing iron); may indicate scalding of hands or feet in hot water (stocking-glove pattern); may suggest restraint with ropes or chains (friction burns). Assess for urine burns or pressure ulcers that may result from caregiver's neglect or inability to provide incontinence care.

✦ Musculoskeletal: Assess for dislocations/sprains/fractures.

✦ Genitalia: Note bleeding, ecchymoses, signs of sexually transmitted disease.

✦ Rectal: Assess sphincter tone for sign of sexual abuse.

DIAGNOSTIC TESTS

✦ Serum electrolytes for dehydration (neglect).

✦ Urinalysis for dehydration (neglect).

✦ CBC to assess for anemia of malnutrition.

✦ Serum albumin/prealbumin to assess nutritional status.

✦ Prothrombin time and partial thromboplastin time to assess for easy bleeding.

✦ Serum drug levels: Absent or below therapeutic level may indicate withholding of medication.

✦ X-rays may reveal fractures in various healing stages.

✦ Culture for chlamydia, gonococcus, VDRL for syphilis, wet mount for suspected sexual abuse.

MANAGEMENT

Elderly individuals at emergent risk for mistreatment must be removed from their potentially dangerous environment. Home health patients may be transferred for hospital admission and admitted under an alias for protection.

✦ Provide contact numbers for emergency assistance.

✦ Refer residents in extended care setting to ombudsman.

✦ Simplify medication regimen as much as possible. **See Chapter on Medication Issues.**

✦ Refer to physical therapy (PT) or occupational therapy (OT) for assistive devices to promote independence in performing activities of daily living (ADLs/IADLs).

✦ Refer to social work services for information about respite care/community resources/social supports.

✦ Refer to Area Agency on Aging or legal assistance programs for seniors.

✦ Suggest professional management of finances to avoid conflict.

✦ Recommend direct deposit of Social Security and pension checks.

✦ Educate caregivers about the needs of elderly individuals.

✦ Recommend counseling and employment training to caregivers as indicated.

✦ Assess need for alternative living situation and refer to social work services or Adult Protective Service for guidance. **See Chapter on Alternatives to Living Alone.**

✦ Encourage patients to maintain contact with others after moving to home of family member. Social contact increases the likelihood that the elderly individual will report mistreatment.

Every state in America has established Adult Protective Service (APS) programs for investigation of elder mistreatment. When APS receives a report of suspected abuse, the agency will visit the home for evaluation, but funding is often unavailable for follow-up. Healthcare providers must become familiar with specific state legislation regarding requirements for reporting of elder abuse. Some states ensure anonymity for informants and hold providers criminally responsible for failure to report. Legislation in some states protects healthcare providers from any possible liability for reporting.

Mandatory reporting poses a dilemma for the clinician who has an ethical responsibility to ensure patient confidentiality and autonomy. **See Chapter on Legal and Ethical Issues.** The decision of the competent patient to remain in a high-risk setting must be respected. If the patient lacks decision-making capacity, petition may be made for establishment of conservatorship for the elderly individual. Providers may be required to testify regarding the patient's capacity to make decisions and provide documentation of suspected abuse.

SUICIDE RISK AND PREVENTION

Most elders do not experience a decline in psychological function with aging. Depression is more common in the elderly population but often occurs as a result of age-associated losses or as recurrence of major depression first seen earlier in life. For some elders, the death of a spouse or termination of a valued, life-long career occurs simultaneously with a decreased ability to cope with such losses. Individuals >65 years are at increased risk for suicide compared with younger populations. In the United States, white males >75 years are at highest risk for suicide. There is opportunity in the primary care setting for assessment of suicide risk and prevention of suicide in the elderly population.

Suicide Risk

Presence of factors that have been identified as increasing suicidal risk in all age groups (psychological diagnoses, family history of suicide, history of prior attempts, death of a loved one) contribute to risk for the elderly. History of depression or anxiety disorder, recent relationship loss (separation, divorce, death), EtOH or substance abuse, and a recent previous attempt have been shown to increase an elder's risk for suicide. Chronic illnesses and life-threatening diagnoses such as cancer, renal failure, and cardiac/respiratory disorders may cause at-risk elders to "give up" the will to live. The decline in social roles that results with aging may further compound the hopelessness experienced by elders who ultimately complete the act of suicide.

Assessment

All elderly should be assessed for potential suicide risk. Screening tools are useful for obtaining baseline evaluation, but results must be combined with

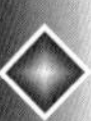

DISPLAY 24-3. *History for Assessment of Suicide Risk*

Existing plan to harm self
Existing plan to harm others
Existing means to carry out plan (guns or other weapons available)
Identification of individual who can help to prevent enactment of the plan
Identification of what is necessary to prevent plan (increased social support, improved pain management)
Family history of suicide attempt
History of previous attempts/denial of previous attempts
Past medical history
- Depression (Recent improvement may precipitate an attempt because energy level is elevated)
- Anxiety disorder
- Chronic, disabling illness (e.g., dialysis)
- Intractable pain
- Life-threatening diagnosis (cancer, AIDS, cardiac disease)
- EtOH or substance abuse

Medication history (prescribed and OTC)
- Note those medications with potential side effect of depression
- Note medications often used for suicide (antidepressants, barbiturates, sedatives)

Decline in functional status, inability for self-care

thorough history-taking from the patient and family/caregiver (see Display 24-3). All suicide threats and warning signs must be investigated and taken seriously, and appropriate action is legally required of healthcare providers when an elder voices suicidal ideation. Be aware that the elder at risk for suicide may send a mixed message (e.g., "I said I would kill myself but now I feel better"). See Display 24-4.

Intervention/Prevention

Patients who express suicidal or homicidal ideation should be referred immediately for hospitalization where constant supervision can be provided. Consultation with the physician/referral for psychological evaluation is critical to correctly assign the degree of risk and ensure hospital admission if indicated.

After it is established that a patient is not in immediate danger of harming himself/herself or others, an interdisciplinary team approach should be used to reduce risk and prevent suicide:

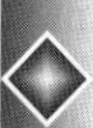

DISPLAY 24-4. *Warning Signs of Suicide Potential in the Elderly*

Overt threats
"I've thought of killing myself."
Expressions of hopelessness or uselessness
"I might as well give up."
"There's no reason to go on."
Fear of aging
"I'd rather die than grow old by myself."
Fear of painful death
Refusal of necessary medications or food (subtle sign that should be carefully monitored in extended care residents)
Farewells to family, friends, or healthcare provider
Plans in preparation for dying (making special wishes known)
Distributing possessions to family, friends

✦ Underlying conditions that alter mental status/mood should be excluded (e.g., metabolic disturbances). Consider thyroid function tests, serum electrolytes, CBC, and drug/EtOH toxicity screen.

✦ Refer for psychiatric evaluation and management.

✦ Enlist assistance from family member, friend, or other individual to prevent enactment of suicide plan by:

✧ Removing weapons from patient's environment. Potential weapons may include an item otherwise considered benign (e.g., a garden tool).

✧ Monitoring number of medications/tablets taken by patient.

✦ Provide counseling:

✧ Support use of problem-solving.

✧ Review efficacy of previous coping skills and develop new coping strategies if needed.

✦ Manage pain. **See Chapter on Pain Management.**

✦ Refer for counseling for EtOH/substance abuse if indicated. **See Protocol on Substance Abuse.**

✦ Refer to social work services for increased access to resources.

✦ Refer to PT/OT to increase functional status, thereby building self-worth.

Appendix A

Common Changes of Aging

VISUAL

Aging Changes

Yellowing, opacity, rigidity of the lens
Decreased pupil size
Decreased accommodation
Less efficient absorption of intraocular fluid
Narrowing of visual field
Decreased lacrimal secretions
Decreased number of cones in retina

Consequences

Presbyopia
Distorted depth perception
Decreased adaptation to darkness
Decreased color discrimination
Need for stronger light
Increased sensitivity to glare
Drier cornea

Adaptations

Provide adequate lighting
Decrease the glare in the environment
Avoid monochromatic color schemes
Provide large-print books, magazines, educational materials
Use black print on off-white or yellow background
Use colors that are easier to discern, i.e., red-orange rather than blue-green
Proper use of adaptive equipment
Address safety concerns in the environment

HEARING

Aging Changes

Decreased number of nerve cells in 8th cranial nerve
Increased production of cerumen
Increased amount of keratin in cerumen
Atrophy and rigidity of ossicles
Decreased elasticity of tympanic membrane

Consequences

Presbycusis
High frequency loss occurs first
Tone discrimination loss
Difficulty following conversations
Cerumen impaction
Social isolation

Adaptations

Regular hearing tests
Correct use of hearing aids or other assistive devices
Environmental modifications
Lower the pitch of your voice when speaking to older individuals
Face the older individual and get at eye level
If you are not being understood, reword
Check for and remove cerumen impaction

INTEGUMENTARY

Aging Changes

Thinning and atrophy of epidermis
Decreased strength and elasticity of epidermis
Decreased blood flow
Increased vascular fragility
Loss of subcutaneous fat
Decreased size and function of sweat glands
Decreased sebaceous secretions
"Clustering" of melanocytes
Decreased number of nerve cells
Thinning and graying of scalp, pubic, and axilla hair

Thickening of nasal and ear hair
Increased facial hair in women
Decreased blood supply to nailbed
Increased longitudinal striations in nails
Accumulation of "debris" under nails

Consequences

Increased susceptibility to infection, trauma, malignant lesions, pressure ulcers
Skin is dry, scaly, wrinkled
Decreased skin turgor
Decreased ability to maintain body temperature and homeostasis; baseline temperature may be lower than normal
Slower rate of healing
Slower absorption of drugs by subcutaneous route
"Liver spots"
Nails thicken, grow slowly, become brittle and yellowed
Increased risk of splitting, infections of the nails

Adaptations

Avoid daily baths; use tepid water rather than hot; avoid harsh soaps
Inspect skin carefully and at regular intervals
To assess hydration, check over the sternum or forehead; condition of the tongue is also a good indicator
Provide extra warmth during bathing
Apply emollients when the skin is moist
Assess nails and provide nail care when indicated

CARDIOVASCULAR

Aging Changes

Increased amount of collagen and fat in cardiac muscle
Thickening and rigidity of valves
Reduced oxygen utilization
Myocardial hypertrophy, but over-all heart size is not affected by age
Coronary artery blood flow decreased
Increased peripheral resistance
Increased myocardial irritability
Decreased blood flow to all organs
Increased amount of lipofuscin

Consequences

Decreased stroke volume, cardiac output
Decreased ability to increase heart rate in response to stress
Increased aortic volume and systolic blood pressure
No change in resting heart rate
Increased risk of extra systoles
Electrocardiogram changes

Adaptations

Be aware that anything that greatly increases the need for blood (fever, vasodilation, exercise, stress) can produce angina or syncope
Frequent small meals provide less cardiac stress
Avoid extremes and sudden changes in temperature
Provide frequent rest periods
Advise to change position gradually

RESPIRATORY

Aging Changes

Decreased elasticity of lungs
Decreased number of alveoli
Increased size of alveoli
Increased diameter of alveolar ducts and bronchioles
Decreased ciliary action
Increased anteroposterior chest diameter
Weakening of respiratory muscles
Decreased coughing reflex
Calcification of costal cartilages

Consequences

50% increase in residual capacity
Decreased vital capacity
Decreased mobility of bony thorax
Decreased blood oxygen
Decreased oxygen uptake during exercise
Increased risk of infection
Increased amount of dead air space
Decreased exercise tolerance
Decreased gas exchange

Adaptations

Patient with a superimposed infection will have a decreased reserve and often appear "sicker" than a younger patient
Allow rest periods between strenuous activities
It may take less activity to produce shortness of breath
Encourage continued mobility at a comfortable level

GASTROINTESTINAL

Aging Changes

Poor dentition
Decreased number of taste buds
Decreased muscle strength for chewing
Decreased saliva production
Decreased ptyalin in saliva
Weakened gag reflex
Decreased gastric acid secretion
Decreased emptying of esophagus and stomach
Decreased intrinsic factor
Thickened bile
Thinned gastric mucosa
Decreased ability of small intestine to absorb sugars and lipids
Decreased hepatic enzymes and storage capacity

Consequences

Decreased taste sensation
Decreased appetite
Decreased chewing ability
Decreased digestion of starch
Possible swallowing difficulty
Indigestion, flatus
Risk of pernicious anemia
Increased problems with elimination
Reduced tolerance for fats
Possible change in drug metabolism
Difficulty in gaining weight

Adaptations

Smaller, more frequent meals may be better
Advise upright position during and after meals

Bowel regimen is important
Avoid chronic use of laxatives and enemas
Careful diet instruction; try nutritional supplements

GENITOURINARY

Aging Changes

Decreased number of nephrons
Decreased glomerular filtration rate and tubular reabsorption
Change in renal threshold
Decreased blood flow to kidneys
Decrease in bladder capacity from 500 ml to 250 ml
Decreased elasticity of bladder
Decreased bladder tone
Decreased muscle tone of urethra
Benign prostatic hyperplasia common in males

Consequences

Decreased creatinine clearance
Decreased ability to concentrate urine
Increased risk of urinary retention
Increased incidence of incontinence
Increased urinary frequency; nocturia
Effects on drug clearance via kidneys

Adaptations

Medications excreted by the kidneys remain in the system longer; monitor medications closely and check creatinine clearance
Recognize incontinence as a symptom that needs investigating, not as a disease
Keep incontinence records and initiate incontinence strategies
Under stress, an elderly person is more susceptible to fluid and electrolyte imbalances; monitor closely; be aware of atypical presentations of illness
Initiate skin care protocols as needed
Advise patient to avoid atropine-like drugs
Encourage adequate fluid intake (2000 ml/day) unless directed otherwise

MUSCULOSKELETAL

Aging Changes

Muscle cells atrophy
Generalized symmetrical muscle wasting
Demineralization of bones
Deterioration of cartilage surface of joints
Thinning of intervertebral discs
Loss of cartilage in vertebral column
Loss of elastic fibers in muscle tissue
Kyphosis

Consequences

Decreased muscle strength after age 70
Two-inch loss of height between ages 20 and 70
Increased incidence of osteoporosis
Decreased joint range of motion
Decreased flexibility
Decreased mobility
Increased risk for falls
Gait changes
Changes in body image

Adaptations

Promote activity; weight-bearing activity decreases demineralization of bones
Be alert to safety issues arising from decreased strength and gait changes
Proper fitting and use of assistive devices
Proper fitting of shoes; proper nail care
Modify the environment, i.e., provide adequate lighting, handrails, bathroom aids

NEUROLOGICAL

Aging Changes

Decreased number of neurons
Decreased weight of brain
Histological changes in brain: increased intracellular pigment, decreased protein synthesis, senile plaques
Decreased rate of conduction in peripheral nerves

Change in sleep patterns
Depletion of dopamine and some of the enzymes in the brain
Increased accumulation of lipofuscin

Consequences

Decreased adaptability
Slower response to stimuli
Decreased sensation
Impaired proprioception
Gait changes
Decreased deep tendon reflexes
Slower voluntary movement
Sleep pattern disturbances
Increased susceptibility to environmental temperature changes
Decreased short-term memory

Adaptations

Be alert to safety factors
Do not rely on complaints of pain or change in temperature to indicate problems
Use memory aids
Adjust care to avoid exacerbating sleep disturbances
Patient teaching may require shorter sessions over a longer span of time

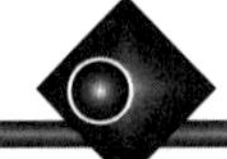

Bibliography

Chapter 1: Prevention and Health Maintenance

American Association of Retired Persons. (1990). *Health risks and preventive care among older blacks.* [Brochure].

Canadian Task Force on the Periodic Health Examination. (1979). The periodic health examination. *Canadian Medical Association Journal, 121,* 1193–1254.

Duryea, W. R. (1990). Adult health maintenance: A guide for primary care PAs. *Journal of the American Academy of Physician Assistants, 3*(8), 607–613.

Helfand, M., & Redfern, C. C. (1998). Screening for thyroid disease: An update. *Annals of Internal Medicine, 129,* 144–158.

Khaw, K. -T. (1997). Healthy aging. *British Medical Journal, 315,* 1090–1096.

Reuben, D. B. (1993). Assessment of older drivers. *Clinics in Geriatric Medicine, 9*(2), 449–458.

U.S. Preventive Services Task Force. (1989). *Guide to clinical preventive services: An assessment of the effectiveness of 169 interventions.* Baltimore: Williams & Wilkins.

Woolf, S. H., Kamerow, D. B., Lawrence, R. S., Medalie, J. H., & Estes, E. H. (1990). The periodic health examination of older adults: The recommendations of the U.S. Preventive Services Task Force: Part II, screening tests. *Journal of the American Geriatrics Society, 38,* 933–942.

Chapter 2: Head, Ears, Eyes, Nose, and Throat

Tinnitus

Alleva, M., Loch, E., & Paparella, M. (1990). Tinnitus. *Primary Care, 17*(2), 289–297.

Ciocon, J. O., Amede, F., Lechtenberg, C., & Astor, F. (1995). Tinnitus: A stepwise workup to quiet the noise within. *Geriatrics, 50*(2), 19–25.

Gulya, A. J. (1995). Evaluation of tinnitus. In A. H. Goroll, L. A. May, & A. G. Mulley (Eds.), *Primary care medicine* (3rd ed., pp. 1001–1002). Philadelphia: J. B. Lippincott.

Rubinstein, B. (1993). Tinnitus and craniomandibular disorders—Is there a link? *Swedish Dental Journal, 95*(Suppl.), 1–46.

Schleuning, A. (1991). Management of the patient with tinnitus. *Medical Clinics of North America, 75*(6), 1225–1237.

Sismanis, A., & Smoker, W. (1994). Pulsatile tinnitus: Recent advances in diagnosis. *Laryngoscope, 104*(6), 681–687.

Cerumen Impaction

Chen, D. A., & Caparasa, R. J. (1991). A nonprescription ceruminolytic. *American Journal of Otology, 12*(6), 475–476.

Fisch, L., & Brooks, D. N. (1992). Disorders of hearing. In J. C. Brocklehurst, R. C. Tallis, & H. M. Fillit (Eds.), *Textbook of geriatric medicine and gerontology* (4th ed., pp. 480–493). London: Churchill-Livingston.

Freeman, R. B. (1995). Impacted cerumen: How to safely remove earwax in an office visit. *Geriatrics, 50*(6), 52–53.

Kelly, K. (1996). The external auditory canal. Otolaryngologic *Clinics of North America, 29*(5), 725–739.

Lewis-Cullinan, C., & Janken, J. K. (1990). Effect of cerumen removal on the hearing ability of geriatric patients. *Journal of Advanced Nursing 15*(5), 594–600.

Mahoney, D. F. (1993). Cerumen impaction. Prevalence and detection in nursing homes. *Journal of Gerontological Nursing, 19*(4), 23–30.

Meador, J. A. (1995). Cerumen impaction in the elderly. *Journal of Gerontological Nursing, 21*(12), 43–45.

Meyers, A. D. (1997). Managing cerumen impaction. *Postgraduate Medicine, 62*(1), 207–209.

Spiro, S. R. (1997). A cost-effectiveness analysis of earwax softeners. *The Nurse Practitioner, 22*(28), 30–31, 166.

Zivic, R. C., & King, S. (1993). Cerumen-impaction management for clients of all ages. *The Nurse Practitioner, 18*(3), 29, 33–36, 39.

Orofacial Pain

Epstein, J. B., & Marcoe, J. H. (1994). Topical application of capsaicin for treatment of oral neuropathic pain and trigeminal neuralgia. *Oral Surgery, Oral Medicine, Oral Pathology, 77*(2), 135–139.

Gouda, J. J., & Brown, J. A. (1997). Atypical facial pain and other pain syndromes. *Neurosurgery Clinics of North America, 8*(1), 87–100.

Gremillion, H. A., & Reams, M. T. (1997). Comprehensive orofacial pain analysis: A structured approach to patient history. *General Dentistry, 45*(3), 237–241.

Kaplan, A. S. (1997). History and examination of the orofacial pain patient. *Dental Clinics of North America, 41*(2), 155–166.

Okeson, J. P. (1995). *Bell's orofacial pain* (5th ed.). Chicago: Quintessence Publishing Co, Inc.

Turp, J. C., & Gobetti, J. P. (1996). Trigeminal neuralgia versus atypical facial pain. *Oral Surgery, Oral Medicine, Oral Pathology, 1*(4), 424–431.

Nasal Congestion

Amedee, R. G., Baraniuk, J. N., Bardana, E. J., Bunton, S., Juniper, E. F., Kaiser, H. B., Meltzer, E. O., Pearlman, D. S., Schoenwetter, W. F., Smith, S. P., & Spector, S. L. (1996). Part II: Practical guidelines for recognition, treatment, and prevention. *The Chronic Airway Disease Connection Redefining Rhinitis. Consensus Conference Proceedings, UCLA School of Medicine.*

Barbey, J. T., Meltzer, E.O., & Weinreb, L. (1996). *Antihistamine update: April 1996.* CME University of Massachusetts, 1–5.

Dolen, W. K., Juniper, E. F., Nelson, H. S., Weinreb, L. F., & Busse, W.W. (1997). Seasonal versus perennial rhinitis: Achieving symptom relief. *Dialogues In Redefining Allergy, UCLA School of Medicine 1*(4), 1–16.

Douville, L., & Fitzgerald, M. (1995). Pharmacologic highlights: Management of acute sinusitis. *Journal of the American Academy of Nurse Practitioners, 7*(8), 407–411.

Fireman, P., Fischer, T. J., Gellman, E. F, Pransky, S. M., Busse, W. W., & Brunton, S. (1997). Allergic rhinitis, associated disorders, and nasal congestion: Combination therapy. *Dialogues in Redefining Allergy, UCLA School of Medicine, 2*(1), 1–16.

Griffith, C. J. (1994). Allergic rhinitis: Practical guide to diagnosis and management. *Physician Assistant, 18*(7), 19–36.

Rachelefsky, G. S., Naclerio, R. M., Schocket, A. L., Slavin, R. G., & Williams, J. W., Jr. (1996). Investigating the allergy–sinusitis connection. *Dialogues in Redefining Rhinitis, UCLA School of Medicine, 1*(4), 1–14.

Rudy, S. F. (1997). Preventing and treating rhinitis medicamentosa. *The Nurse Practitioner, 22*(13), 115–116.

Schwartz, R. (1994). The diagnosis and management of sinusitis. *The Nurse Practitioner, 19*(12), 58–63.

Smith, L. J. (1995). Diagnosis and treatment of allergic rhinitis. *The Nurse Practitioner, 20*(10), 58–66.

Spector, S. L., Barbey, J. T., Bardana, E. J., Schoenwetter, W. F., & Uy, S. (1996). Management and safety issues in special populations with allergic rhinitis. *Dialogues in Redefining Rhinitis, UCLA School of Medicine, 1*(3), 1–16.

Spector, S. L., Moulton, B. W., Nolen, T. M., Slavin, R. G., & Busse, W. W. (1996). Sedation and safety issues. *Dialogues in Redefining Allergy, UCLA School of Medicine, 1*(2), 1016.

Stool, S. E. (1985). Diagnosis and treatment of sinusitis. *American Family Practitioner, 32*(6), 101–107.

Wilder, B. (1996). Pearls of practice: Management of sinusitis. *Journal of the American Academy of Nurse Practitioners, 8*(11), 525–529.

Willett, L. R., Carson, J. L., & Williams, J. W. (1994). Current diagnosis and management of sinusitis. *Journal of General Internal Medicine, 9*(1), 38–45.

Headache

Bruckenthal, P. (1997). A guide to the diagnosis and management of migraine headaches for the nurse practitioner. *American Journal for Nurse Practitioners, 1*(3), 12–18.

Gur, H., Rapman, E., Ehrenfeld, M., & Sidi, Y. (1996). Clinical manifestations of temporal arteritis: A report from Israel. *Journal of Rheumatology, 23*(11), 1927–1931.

Lamonte, M., Silberstein, S. D., & Marcelis, J. F. (1995). Headache associated with aseptic meningitis. *Headache, 35*(9), 520–526.

Lipton, R. B., Pfeffer, D., Newman, L. C., & Solomon, S. (1993). Headaches in the elderly. *Journal of Pain and Symptom Management, 8*(2), 87–95.

Oates, L. N., Scholz, M. J., & Hoffert, M. J. (1993). Polypharmacy in a headache centre population. *Headache, 33*(8), 436–438.

Pascual, J., & Berciano, J. (1994). Experience in the diagnosis of headaches that start in elderly people. *Journal of Neurology, Neurosurgery, & Psychiatry, 57*(10), 1255–1257.

Raskin, N. (1998). Options for preventing migraine in women who take HRT. *Consultant, 38*, 16.

Silberstein, S. D., & Merriam, G. R. (1991). Estrogens, progestins, and headache. *Neurology, 41*, 786.

Solomon, G. D. (1993). Treatment considerations in headache and associated medical disorders. *Journal of Pain and Symptom Management, 8*(2), 73–80.

Trachtenbarg, D. E. (1994). Tension headaches: Relieving pain without creating dependence. *Postgraduate Medicine, 95*(6), 44–46, 49–52, 55–56.

Glaucoma

Alward, W. L. M. (1998). Medical management of glaucoma. *New England Journal of Medicine, 339*(18), 1298–1307.

Epstein, D. L., Allingham. R. R., & Schuman, J. S. (Eds.), (1997). *Chandler and Grants' glaucoma* (4th ed.). Baltimore: Williams and Wilkins.

Pavan-Langston, D. (Ed.), *Manual of ocular diagnosis and therapy* (4th ed.). Boston: Little, Brown and Co.

Shoemaker, J. A. (1997). Adult vision screening by nonphysicians. *Journal of Ophthalmic Nursing & Technology, 16*(5), 244–250.

Weisbecker, C. A., Fraunfelder, F. T., & Naidoff, M., et al. (Eds.), (1999). *Physicians desk reference for ophthalmology* (27th ed.). Montvale, NJ: Medical Economics Co., Inc.

Whitaker, R. Jr., Whitaker, V. B., & Dill, C. (1998). Glaucoma: What the nurse practitioner should know. *Nurse Practitioner Forum, 9*(1), 7–12.

Cataract

Butler, R. N., Guazzo, E., & Kupfer, C. (1997). Keeping an eye on vision: Primary care of age-related ocular disease. *Geriatrics, 52*(8), 30–36.

Castor, T. D., & Carter, T. L. (1995). Low vision: Physician screening helps to improve patient function. *Geriatrics, 50,* 51–57.

Christen, W. G., Glynn, R. J., & Hennekens, C. H. (1996). Antioxidants and age-related eye disease: Current and future perspectives. *Annals of Epidemiology, 6*(1), 60–66.

Felson, D. T., Anderson, J. J., Hannan, M. T., Milton, R. C., Wilson, P. W., & Keil, D. P. (1989). Impaired vision and hip fracture: The Framington study. *Journal of the American Geriatrics Society, 37,* 494–500.

Javitt, J. C., Wang, F., & West, S. K. (1996). Blindness due to cataract: Epidemiology and prevention. *Annual Review of Public Health, 17,* 159–177.

Klein, B., Klein, R., & Ritter, L. (1994). Is there evidence of an estrogen affect on age-related lens opacities? *Archives of Ophthalmology 112,* 85–91.

Kollarits, C. R. (1992). The aging eye. In E. Calkins, A. B. Ford, & P. R. Katz, (Eds.), *Practice of geriatrics* (2nd ed., pp. 236–246). Philadelphia: W. B. Saunders Company.

Litwack-Saleh, K. (1993). Practical points in the care of the patient undergoing cataract surgery. *Journal of Post Anesthesia Nursing, 8*(2), 113–115.

U.S. Department of Health and Human Services. (1993). Management of cataracts in adults. *Quick Reference Guide for Clinicians: Number 4.* [Brochure].

Wood, S. L., Thiese, S. M., & Haines, J. H. (1990). Cataract detection and management: An update. *Physician Assistant, 14*(10), 69–70, 79–81, 85–86.

Age-Related Macular Degeneration

Butler, R. N., Faye, E. E., Guazzo, E., & Kupfer, C. (1997). Keeping an eye on vision: Primary care of age-related ocular disease. *Geriatrics, 52*(8), 30–41.

Faye, E. E. (1998). Living with low vision. *Postgraduate Medicine, 103*(5), 167–178.

Hampton, G. R., & Nelson, P. T. (1992). Office evaluation. In G. R. Hampton & P. T. Nelson (Eds.), *Age related macular degeneration.* New York: Raven Press.

Newsome, D. A. (1992). Medical treatment of age related macular degeneration. In G. F. Hampton & P. T. Nelson (Eds.), *Age related macular degeneration.* New York: Raven Press.

Starr, C. E., Guyer, D. R., & Yannuzzi, L. A. (1998). Age related macular degeneration: Can we stem this worldwide public health crisis? *Postgraduate Medicine, 103*(5), 153–163.

Trudo, E. W., & Stark, W. J. (1998). Lifting the clouds on an age-old problem. *Postgraduate Medicine, 103*(5), 114–126.

Red Eye

American Academy of Ophthalmology. (1996). *Eye facts about: Blepharitis* [Brochure]. San Francisco, CA: Author.

Hara, J. H. (1996). The red eye: Diagnosis and treatment. *American Family Physician, 54*(8), 2423–2430.

Johns, K. J. (1998). Evaluation of the red eye. Presentation, Department of Ophthalmology, Vanderbilt University Medical Center.

Michelson, P. E. (1997). Red eye unresponsive to treatment. *The Western Journal of Medicine, 166*(2), 145–147.

Morrow, G. L., & Abbott, R. L. (1998). Conjunctivitis. *American Family Physician, 57*(4), 735–746.

Mortemousque, B., Williamson, W., Poirier, L., Brousse, D., & Verin, P. (1995). Floppy eyelid syndrome. *Journal Français d'Ophtalmologie, 18*(8–9), 542–547.

Rosenbloom, A. A., Jr., & Morgan, M. W. (1993). *Vision and aging* (2nd ed.). Boston: Butterworth-Heinemann.

Soparkar, C. N., Wilhelmus, K. R., Koch, D. D., Wallace, G. W., & Jones, D. B. (1997). Acute and chronic conjunctivitis due to over-the-counter ophthalmic decongestants. *Archives of Ophthalmology, 115*(1), 34–38.

Trudo, E. W., & Stark, W. J. (1998). Cataracts: Lifting the clouds on an age-old problem. *Postgraduate Medicine, 103*(5), 114–126.

Mouth Lesions

Fantasia, J. E. (1997). Diagnosis and treatment of common oral lesions found in the elderly. *Dental Clinics of North America, 41*(4), 877–890.

Marder, M. Z. (1998). The standard of care for oral diagnosis as it relates to oral cancer. *Compendium of Continuing Education in Dentistry, 19*(6), 569–572, 574, 576 passim.

Mobley, C., & Saunders, M. J. (1997). Oral health screening guidelines for nondental health care providers. *Journal of the American Dietetic Association, 97*(10, Suppl. 2), S123–S126.

Reynolds, M. W. (1997). Education for geriatric oral health promotion. *Special Care in Dentistry, 17*(1), 33–36.

Shugars, D. C., & Patton, L. L. (1997). Detecting, diagnosing, and preventing oral cancer. *The Nurse Practitioner, 22*(6), 105, 109–110, 113–115 passim.

Chapter 3: Skin

Pruritus

Burdette-Taylor, S. R. (1995). Eczema, ichthyosis, psoriasis. Conditions of cornification. *Ostomy/Wound Management, 41*(7), 36–42.

Burdette-Taylor, S. R. (1995). Vignette: Eczema, ichthyosis, and psoriasis. *Ostomy/Wound Management, 41*(8), 64–65.

Chotzen, V., Crowell, J. E., & Metzler, C. (1998). Aging skin: Best approaches to common problems. *Patient Care Nurse Practitioner, 1*(5), 28–39.

Cox, P. (1994). Dermadilemma. *Physician Assistant, 18*(5), 79.

Eaglstein, W. H., McKay, M., & Pariser, D. M. (1994). The problems that plague aging skin. *Patient Care, 28*(7), 89–119.

Federal Practitioner. (1997). New drugs, drug news. *14*(12), 44–45.

Fenske, N. A., Grayson, L. D., & Newcomer, V. D. (1992). Tips for treating aging skin. *Patient Care, 26*(6), 61–72.

Kleinsmith, D. M., & Perricone, N. V. (1989). Common skin problems in the elderly. *Clinics in Geriatric Medicine, 5*(1), 189–211.

Krenek, G., & Rosen, T. (1996). Eczema: The nuts and bolts of management. *Consultant, 36*(3), 486–506.

Levine, N. (1996). Winter itch: What's causing the rash? *Geriatrics, 51*(1), 20.

Phillips, T. J. (1994). O/WM commentary: A clinician's guide to common dermatology problems. *Ostomy/Wound Management, 40*(9), 70–72, 74, 76–79.

Reifsnider, E. (1997). Common adult infectious skin conditions. *The Nurse Practitioner, 22*(11), 17–33.

Yeap, S. S., Deighton, C. M., Powell, R. J., Read, R. C., & Finch, R. G. (1995). Diagnostic and management problems in complex case of connective tissue disease. *Postgraduate Medicine, 71*(842), 751–752.

Seborrheic Dermatitis

Beacham, B. E. (1993). Common dermatoses in the elderly. *American Family Physician, 47*(6), 1445–1456.

Dalziel, K. L., & Bickers, D. R. (1992). Skin aging. In J. C. Brocklehurst, R. C. Tallis, & H. M. Fillit (Eds.), *Textbook of geriatric medicine and gerontology* (4th ed., pp. 898–919). London: Churchill Livingston.

Fitzpatrick, T. B., Johnson, R. A., Polano, M. K., Suurmond, D., & Wolff, K. (1992). Common scaling eruptions of unknown etiology. In *Color atlas and synopsis of clinical dermatology* (2nd ed.). New York: McGraw-Hill Inc.

Ghadially, R. (1996). Skin. In E. T. Lonergan (Ed.), *Geriatrics, a Lange clinical manual* (pp. 354–355). Stamford, CT: Appleton & Lange.

Newcomer, V. D., & King, D. F. (1982). Geriatric dermatology: Constitutional changes invite cutaneous disorders. *Consultant, 22*(12), 210–219.

Neoplasms

Chotzen, V., Crowell, J. E., & Metzler, C. (1998). Aging skin: Best approaches to common problems. *Patient Care Nurse Practitioner, 1*(5), 28–39.

Dalziel, K. L., & Bickers, D. R. (1992). Skin aging. In J.C. Brocklehurst, R. C. Tallis, & H. M. Fillit (Eds.), *Textbook of geriatric medicine and gerontology* (4th ed., pp. 898–921). London: Churchill Livingston.

Gordon, M. L., & Hecker, M. S. (1997). Care of the skin at midlife: Diagnosis of pigmented lesions. *Geriatrics, 52*(8), 56–69.

Kauffman, A. L. (1998, March). Springbreak sun-seekers: There's no such thing as a healthy tan. *Margaret Cuninggim Women's Center Newsletter*, Vanderbilt University.

MacKie, R. M. (1990). Cutaneous cancer in old age. In F. I. Caird & T. B. Brewin (Eds.), *Cancer in the elderly* (pp. 186–202). London: Wright.

Marghoob, A. A. (1997). Basal and squamous cell carcinomas: What every primary care physician should know. *Postgraduate Medicine, 102*(2), 139–159.

Muglia, J. J., & McDonald, C. J. (1994). Skin cancer screening. *Physician Assistant, 18*(1), 21–32.

Rumsfield, J. (1990). Sunscreens: What you and your patients should know. *Dermatology Nursing, 2*(3), 139–147.

Contact Dermatitis

Beltrani, V. S., & Beltrani, V. P. (1997). Contact dermatitis. *Annals of Allergy, Asthma, & Immunology, 78*, 160–171.

Dermal Candidiasis

Shellow, W. V. Management of intertrigo and intertriginous dermatoses. In A. H. Goroll, L. A. May, & A. G. Mulley, *Primary care medicine: Office evaluation and management of the adult patient* (2nd ed., pp. 802–803). Philadelphia: J. B. Lippincott.

Lower Extremity Ulcers

Barr D. M. The Unna's boot as a treatment for venous ulcers. *Nurse Practitioner, 21*(7), 55–56, 61–62, 64, 71–72, 74–75.

Black, J. (1995). Management of venous stasis ulcers. *Plastic Surgical Nursing, 15*(2), 104, 103.

Black, S. B. (1995). Venous stasis ulcers: A review. *Ostomy/Wound Management, 41*(8), 20–22, 24–30, 32.

Bowman, P. H., & Hogan, D. J. (1999). Leg ulcers: A common problem with sometimes uncommon etiologies. *Geriatrics, 54*(3), 43, 47–48, 50, 53–54.

Brewster, D. C. (1987). Management of venous disease. In A. H. Goroll, L. A. May, & A. G. Mulley (Eds.), *Primary care medicine: Office evaluation and management of the adult patient* (2nd ed., pp. 157–161). Philadelphia: J. B. Lippincott.

Elder, D. M., & Greer, K. E. (1995). Venous disease: How to heal and prevent chronic leg ulcers. *Geriatrics, 50*(8), 30–35.

Friedman, S. J. (1995). Management of skin ulceration. In A. H. Goroll, L. A. May, & A. G. Mulley (Eds.), *Primary care medicine: Office evaluation and management of the adult patient* (3rd ed., pp. 946–948). Philadelphia: J. B. Lippincott.

Janisse, D. J. (1994). The role of the pedorthist in the prevention and management of diabetic foot ulcer. *Ostomy/Wound Management 40*(8), 54–56, 60–64.

Korstanje, M. J. (1995). Venous stasis ulcers: Diagnostic and surgical considerations. *Dermatologic Surgery, 21*, 635–640.

Lipsky, B. A. (1997). Osteomyelitis of the foot in diabetic patients. *Clinical Infectious Diseases, 25*, 1318–1326.

Lipsky, B. A., Robbins, J. M., Dahn, M. S., & Neal, D. F. (1998). New treatment approaches to management of diabetic foot ulcers. Teleconference conducted by Department of Veterans Affairs.

May, L. A. (1987). Management of stasis dermatitis, stasis ulcers, and decubitus ulcers. In A. H. Goroll, L. A. May, & A. G. Mulley (Eds.), *Primary care medicine: Office evaluation and management of the adult patient* (2nd ed., pp. 805–807). Philadelphia: J. B. Lippincott.

Rosseau, P. (1991). Managing venous leg ulcers. *Geriatric Consultant, 9*(6), 23–24.

Sieggreen, M. Y., & Maklebust, J. (1996). Managing leg ulcers: Different types of ulcers call for different treatments. *Nursing96, 26*(12), 41–46.

Cellulitis

Goldstein, E. J. (1987). Management of cellulitis. In A. H. Goroll, L. A. May, & A. G. Mulley (Eds.), *Primary care medicine: Office evaluation and management of the adult patient* (2nd ed., pp. 807–809). Philadelphia: J. B. Lippincott.

Lindbeck, G., & Powers, R. (1993). Outpatient parenteral antibiotic therapy: Management of serious infections. Part II: Amenable infections and models for delivery, cellulitis. *Hospital Practice, 28*(Suppl. 2), 10–14.

Senile Purpura

Ghadially, R. (1996). Skin. In E. T. Lonergan (Ed.), *Geriatrics, a Lange clinical manual* (p. 356). Stamford, CT: Appleton & Lange.

Newcomer, V. D., & King, D. F. (1982). Geriatric dermatology: Constitutional changes invite cutaneous disorders. *Consultant, 22*(12), 210–219.

Small, E. J., & Damon, L.E. (1996). Blood. In E. T. Lonergan (Ed.), *Geriatrics, a Lange clinical manual* (p. 283). Stamford, CT: Appleton & Lange.

Herpes Zoster

Kost, R., & Straus, S. E. (1996). Post-herpetic neuralgia—Pathogenesis, treatment, and prevention. *New England Journal of Medicine, 335*(1), 32–42.

Schmader, K. (1997). Herpes Zoster. In C. K. Cassel, H. J. Cohen, E. B. Larson, et al. (Eds.), *Geriatric medicine* (3rd ed., pp. 841–854). New York: Springer.

Tyring, S., Barbarash, R., Nahlik, J., et al. (1995). Famciclovir for the treatment of acute zoster: Effects on acute disease and post-herpetic neuralgia. *Annals of Internal Medicine, 123*(2), 89–96.

Whitley, R., Weiss, H., Grann, J., et al. (1996). Acyclovir with and without prednisone for the treatment of herpes zoster. *Annals of Internal Medicine, 25*(5), 376–83.

Chapter 4: Cardiovascular System

Chest Pain

Donat, W. E. (1987). Chest pain: Cardiac and noncardiac causes. *Clinical Chest Medicine, 8*(1), 241–252.

Fruth, R. M. (1991). Differential diagnosis of chest pain. *Critical Care Nursing Clinics of North America, 3*(1), 59–67.

Hill, G., & Geraci, S. A. (1998). A diagnostic approach to chest pain based on history and ancillary evaluation. *The Nurse Practitioner, 23*(4), 20–47.

Mukerji, B., Alpert, M. A., & Mukerji, V. (1994). Musculoskeletal causes of chest pain. *Hospital Medicine, 30*(11), 26–28, 32–33, 36–39.

Richter, J. E. (1991). Gastroesophageal reflux disease as a cause of chest pain. *Medical Clinics of North America, 75*(5), 1065–1080.

Hypertension

Black, H. R. (1998). New concepts in hypertension: Focus on the elderly. *American Heart Journal, 135*(2 Pt 2), S2–S7.

Forman, D. E., Chander, R. B., Lapane, K. L., et al. (1998). Evaluating the use of angiotensin-converting enzyme inhibitors for older nursing home residents with chronic heart failure. *Journal of the American Geriatrics Society, 46*(12), 1550–1554.

Frost, P. H., Davis, B. R., Burlando, A. J., et al. (1996). Serum lipids and incidence of coronary heart disease. Findings from the systolic hypertension in the elderly program (SHEP). *Circulation, 94*(10), 2381–2388.

Gambassi, G., Lapane, K., Sgadari, A., et al. (1998). Prevalence, clinical correlates, and treatment of hypertension in elderly nursing home residents. *Archives of Internal Medicine, 158*(21), 2377–2385.

Kostis, J. B., Davis, B. R., Cutler, J., et al. (1997). Prevention of heart failure by antihypertensive drug treatment in older persons with isolated systolic hypertension. *Journal of the American Medical Association, 278*(3), 212–216.

Krakoff, L. R. (Ed.), (1995). *Management of the hypertensive patient.* New York: Churchill Livingstone.

Olutade, B., & Hall, W. D. (1997). Systolic hypertension in the elderly. *Current Problems in Cardiology, 22*(8), 405–443.

Heart Failure

Agency for Health Care Policy and Research. (1994). *Heart failure: Management of patients with left-ventricular systolic dysfunction. Quick Reference Guide for Clinicians, Number 11.* AHCPR Publication No. 94-0613. Rockville, MD: U.S. Department of Health and Human Services.

Cusack, B. J., & Olson, R. D. (1994). Heart failure. In R. N. Winickoff (Ed.), *Strategies in Geriatrics, 2*(1), 1–6. Department of Veterans Affairs.

Gottlieb, S. H. (1995). Heart failure. In L. Barker, J. Burton, & P. Zieve (Eds.), *Principles of ambulatory medicine* (4th ed., pp. 782–803). Baltimore: Williams & Wilkins.

Guerra-Garcia, H., Taffet, G. E., & Luchi, R. J. (1994). Congestive heart failure: Special considerations for diagnosis in the elderly. *Consultant, 34,* 523–527.

Guerra-Garcia, H., Taffet, G. E., & Luchi, R. J. (1994). Congestive heart failure: Treatment modifications in the elderly. *Consultant, 34,* 528–536.

Massie, B. M., & Amidon, T. M. (1998). Cardiac failure. In L. M. Tierney, S. J. McPhee, & M. A. Papadakis (Eds.), *Current medical diagnosis and treatment 1998* (pp. 403–412). Stamford, CT: Appleton & Lange.

Miller, M. M. (1994). Current trends in the primary care management of chronic congestive heart failure. *Nurse Practitioner, 19*(5), 64–70.

Moriarty, W. (1996). Emergency care. In E. Lonergan (Ed.), *Geriatrics* (pp. 16–37). Stamford, Connecticut: Appleton & Lange.

Nagelhout, J. J. (1991). Pharmacological treatment of heart failure. *Nursing Clinics of North America, 26*(2), 401–415.

Rich, M. W., Beckham, V., Wittenberg, C., Leven, C. L., Freedland, K. E., & Carney, R. M. (1995). A multidisciplinary intervention to prevent the readmission of elderly patients with congestive heart failure. *New England Journal of Medicine, 333*(18), 1190–1195.

Atrial Fibrillation

Akhtar, W., Reeves, W. C., & Movahed, A. (1998). Indications for anticoagulation in atrial fibrillation. *American Family Physician, 58*(1), 130–136.

Cerebral Embolism Task Force (2nd report). (1989). Cardiogenic brain embolism. *Archives of Neurology, 46,* 727–743.

Dumas, M. A. (1997). Atrial fibrillation in primary care. *American Journal for Nurse Practitioners, 1*(2), 7–10, 36.

Flegel, K. M., Shipley, M. J., & Rose, G. (1987). Risk of stroke in nonrheumatic atrial fibrillation. *Lancet, 526*–529.

Onundarsun, P. T., Thorgeirsson, T., Jonmundsson, E., et al. (1987). Chronic atrial fibrillation-epidemiologic features and 14 year follow-up: A case control study. *European Heart Journal, 8,* 521–527.

Selig, P. M. (1996). Management of anticoagulation therapy with the International Normalized Ratio. *Journal of the American Academy of Nurse Practitioners, 8*(2), 77–80.

Wolf, P. A., Abbott, R. D., & Kannel, W. D. Atrial fibrillation: A major contributor to stroke in the elderly: The Framingham study. *Archives of Internal Medicine, 147*, 1561–1564.

Abnormal Heart Sounds

Cannon, L. A., & Marshall, J. M. (1993). Cardiac disease in the elderly population. *Clinics in Geriatric Medicine, 9*(3), 499–525.

Erickson, B. (1997). *Heart sounds and murmurs: A practical guide* (3rd ed.). St. Louis: Mosby-Year Book.

Jeremiah, J. (1997). Valvular heart disease. In F. F. Ferri, M. D. Fretwell, & T. J. Wachtel (Eds.), *Practical guide to the care of the geriatric patient* (2nd ed., pp. 253–256). St. Louis: Mosby-Year Book.

St. Claire, D., & Hollenberg, M. (1996). Valvular heart disease. In E. T. Lonergan (Ed.), *Geriatrics* (1st ed., pp. 59–78). Stamford, CT: Appleton & Lange.

Wilson, J. S., Hearne, S. E., Harrison, J. K., et al. (1994). How to recognize and manage aortic stenosis in the elderly. *Journal of Critical Illness, 9*(5), 429–432, 435–436.

Peripheral Vascular Disease

Cahall, E., & Spence, R. K. (1995). Practical nursing measures for vascular compromise in the lower leg. *Ostomy/Wound Management, 41*(9), 16–18, 20, 22, 24–26, 28–32.

Foley, K. T., & Palmer, R. M. (1998). In T. T. Yoshikawa, E. L. Cobbs, & K. Brummel-Smith (Eds.), *Practical ambulatory geriatrics* (2nd ed., pp. 474–481). St. Louis: Mosby.

Sieggreen, M. K., & Maklebust, J. (1996). Managing leg ulcers. *Nursing96, 26*(12), 41–46.

Wachtel, T. J. (1997). Peripheral vascular disease. In F. F. Ferri, M. D. Fretwell, & T. J. Wachtel (Eds.), *The care of the geriatric patient* (2nd ed., pp. 256–258).

Weingarten, M. S. (1993). The history and diagnosis of venous ulceration. *Ostomy/Wound Management, 39*(5), 40–42.

Wilt, T. J. (1992). Current strategies in the diagnosis and management of lower extremity peripheral vascular disease. *Journal of General Internal Medicine, 7*(1), 87–101.

Chapter 5: Pulmonary System

Chronic Obstructive Pulmonary Disease (COPD)

Addison, T. E. (1996). Pulmonary disease. In E. Lonergan (Ed.), *Geriatrics* (pp. 139–147). Stamford, Connecticut: Appleton & Lange.

Anderson, K. L. (1995). The effect of chronic obstructive pulmonary disease on quality of life. *Research in Nursing & Health, 18*(6), 547–556.

Bloom, J. W., & Barreuther, A. D. (1993). Drug therapy of airways obstructive diseases. In R. Bressler & M. D. Katz (Eds)., *Geriatric Pharmacology* (pp. 507–533). New York: McGraw-Hill.

Kradjan, W. A., Driesner, N. K., Abuan, T. H., Emmick, G., & Schoene, R. B. (1992). Effect of age on bronchodilator response. *Chest, 101*, 1545–1551.

Hahn, K. (1989). Sexuality and COPD. *Rehabilitation Nursing, 14*(4), 191–195.

Sassi-Dambron, D. E., Eakin, E. G., Ries, A. L., & Kaplan, R. M. (1995). Treatment of dyspnea in COPD: A controlled clinical trial of dyspnea management strategies. *Chest, 107*(3), 724–729.

Tiep, B. (1995). Portable oxygen therapy with oxygen conserving devices and methodologies. *Monaldi Archives for Chest Disease, 50*(1), 51–57.

Tsoukleris, M. G., & Michocki, R. J. (1995). Geriatrics for the clinician: Inhalation therapy and the elderly: What every physician should consider. *Maryland Medical Journal, 44*(12), 1049–1052.

Pneumonia

Ahkee, S., Srinath, L., & Ramirez, J. (1997). Community-acquired pneumonia in the elderly: Association of mortality with lack of fever and leukocytosis. *Southern Medical Journal, 90*(3), 296–298.

American Thoracic Society. (1993). Guidelines for the initial management of adults with community-acquired pneumonia: Diagnosis, assessment of severity, and initial antimicrobial therapy. *American Review of Respiratory Disease, 148*(5), 1418–1426.

Cunha, B. A. (1996). Community-acquired pneumonia: Cost effective antimicrobial therapy. *Postgraduate Medicine, 99*(1), 109–110, 113–114, 117–119, 122.

Davis, A. L., Kane, G. C., & Plouffe, J.F. (1998). The changing care of community-acquired pneumonia. *Patient Care Nurse Practitioner, 1*(6), 9–20.

Fein, A. M. (1994). Pneumonia in the elderly: Special diagnostic and therapeutic considerations. *Medical Clinics of North America, 78*(5), 1015–1034.

Fein, A. M., Niederman, M.S. (1994). Severe pneumonia in the elderly. *Clinics in Geriatric Medicine, 10*(1), 121–143.

File, T. M., Tan, J. S., & Plouffe, J. F. (1996). Community-acquired pneumonia: What's needed for accurate diagnosis? *Postgraduate Medicine, 99*(1), 95–106.

Hecht, A., Siple, J., Deitz, S., & Williams, P. (1995). Diagnosis and treatment of pneumonia in the nursing home. *The Nurse Practitioner, 20*(5), 24–39.

McCue, J. D. (1993). Pneumonia in the elderly: Special considerations in a special population. *Postgraduate Medicine, 94*(5), 39–47.

Mick, D. J. (1997). Pneumonia in elders: Recognition of symptoms, prompt diagnosis, and administration of appropriate antibiotics can reduce complications of pneumonia. *Geriatric Nursing, 18*(3), 99–102.

Moroney, C., & Fitzgerald, M. A. (1996). Pharmacologic update: Management of pneumonia in elderly people. *Journal of the American Academy of Nurse Practitioners, 8*(5), 237–241.

Nichol, K. L., Margolis, K. L., Wouremna, J., & von Sternberg T. (1996). Effectiveness of influenza vaccine in the elderly. *Gerontology, 42*(5), 272–279.

Warner, L. (1996). Infectious diseases. In E. T. Lonergan (Ed.), *Geriatrics, a Lange clinical manual* (pp. 123–138). Stamford, CT: Appleton & Lange.

Yoshikawa, T. (1989). Pneumonia, UTI, and decubiti in the nursing home: Optional management. *Geriatrics, 44*(10), 32–43.

Yoshikawa, T. (1991). Treatment of nursing home-acquired pneumonia. *Journal of the American Geriatrics Society, 39*(10), 1040–1041.

Tuberculosis

Bass, J. B., Farer, L. S., Hopewell, P. C., et al. (1994). Treatment of tuberculosis and tuberculosis infection in adults and children. American Thoracic Society and the Centers for Disease Control and Prevention. *American Journal of Respiratory and Critical Care Medicine, 149*(5), 1359–1374.

Centers for Disease Control and Prevention. CDC issues recommendations for screening for tuberculosis in high-risk populations. (1996). *American Family Physician, 53*(4), 1433–1434, 1436.

Davis, P. D. (1996). Tuberculosis in the elderly. Epidemiology and optimal management. *Drugs and Aging, 8*(6), 436–444.

Davis, Y. M., McCray, E., & Simone, P. M. (1997). Hospital infection control practices for tuberculosis. *Clinics in Chest Medicine, 18*(1), 19–33.

Hocking, T. L., & Choi, C. (1997). Tuberculosis: A strategy to detect and treat new and reactivated infections. *Geriatrics, 52*(3), 52–63.

Hopkins, M. L., & Schoener, L. (1996). Tuberculosis and the elderly living in long term care facilities. *Geriatric Nursing, 17*(1), 27–32.

Pettit, J. (1996). Tuberculosis in the elderly. *Journal of the American Academy of Nurse Practitioners, 8*(3), 131–134.

Chapter 6: Gastrointestinal System

Management of the Enterally Fed Patient

Bockus, S. (1991). Troubleshooting your tube-feedings. *American Journal of Nursing, 91*(5), 24–28.

Bruckstein, D. C. (1988). Percutaneous endoscopic gastrostomy. *Geriatric Nursing, 9*(2), 92–93.

Faller, N. A, Lawrence, K. G, & Ferraro, C. B. (1993). Gastrostomy, replacement, feeding tubes: The long and short of it. *Ostomy/Wound Management, 39*(1), 26, 28–29, 32–33.

Karchenfels, M. M. Home tube feedings: Gastrointestinal complications. *Home Healthcare Nurse, 5*(1), 41–42.

Sanowski, R. A. (1990). Percutaneous gastrostomy in the debilitated elderly. *Geriatric Consultant, 8*(4), 20–22.

Gastroesophageal Reflux Disease (GERD)

Bozymski, E. (1993). Pathophysiology and diagnosis of gastroesophageal reflux disease. *American Journal of Hospital Pharmacy, 50*(Suppl. 4), S4–S6.

Devalt, K. R., & Castell, D. O. (1995). Guidelines for the diagnosis and treatment of gastroesophageal reflux disease. *Archives of Internal Medicine, 155*(20), 2165–2173.

Horn, J. R. (1996). Use of prokinetic agents in special populations. *American Journal of Health-Systems Pharmacy, 53*(Suppl. 3), 27–29.

Kahrilas, P. J. (1996). Gastroesophageal reflux disease. *Journal of American Medical Association, 276*(12), 983–988.

Middlemiss, C. (1997). Gastroesophageal reflux disease: A common condition in the elderly. *The Nurse Practitioner, 22*(11), 51–59.

Morton, L. S., & Fromkes, J. J. (1993). Gastroesophageal reflux disease: Diagnosis and medical therapy. *Geriatrics, 48*(3), 60–66.

Reynolds, J. C. (1996). Influence of pathophysiology, severity, and cost on the medical management of gastroesophageal reflux disease. *American Journal of Health-Systems Pharmacy, 53*(Suppl. 22), S5–S12.

Schiller, L. R. (1996). Upper gastrointestinal motility disorders and respiratory symptoms. *American Journal of Health-Systems Pharmacy, 53*(Suppl. 3), 13–16.

Sullivan, C. A., & Samuelson, W. M. (1996). Gastroesophageal reflux: A common exacerbating factor in adult asthma. *The Nurse Practitioner, 21*(11), 82–86.

Weiss, R. A. Esophageal disease. (1996). In A. M. Gelb (Ed.), *Clinical gastroenterology in the elderly* (pp. 13–35). New York: Marcel Dekker.

Gastrointestinal (GI) Bleeding

Billingham, R. P. (1997). The conundrum of lower gastrointestinal bleeding. *Surgical Clinics of North America, 77*(1), 241–252.

Isaacs, K. L. (1994). Severe gastrointestinal bleeding. *Clinics in Geriatric Medicine, 10*(1), 1–17.

Lieberman, D. (1993). Gastrointestinal bleeding: Initial management. *Gastroenterology Clinics of North America, 22*(4), 723–736.

Papp, J. P. (1991). Management of upper gastrointestinal bleeding. *Clinics in Geriatric Medicine, 7*(2), 255–263.

Reinus, J. F., & Brandt, L. J. (1991). Lower intestinal bleeding in the elderly. *Clinics in Geriatric Medicine, 7*(2), 301–317.
Wright, I. O. (1998). Esophageal varices: Treatment and implications. *Gastroenterology Nursing, 21*(1), 2–5.

Nausea and Vomiting

Amann, S. T., DiMagno, E., & Rubin, W. (1997). Pancreatitis: Diagnostic and therapeutic interventions. *Patient Care, 21*(11), 200–202, 205–212, 215–216.
Champion, G., & Richter, J. E. (1997). Esophageal dysphagia: Differentiating benign from life-threatening causes. *Consultant, 37*(10), 2626–2628, 2633, 2636–2640.
Galen, B. A. (1997). Protocols. Acute gastroenteritis. *Lippincott's Primary Care Practice, 1*(3), 328–335.
Hayko, D. M. (1997). Clinical practice. Assessing for bowel obstruction. *Home Health Focus, 4*(2), 9, 11.
Koch, K. L. (1995). Approach to the patient with nausea and vomiting. In T. Yamada, D. H. Alpers, C. Owyang, et al. (Eds.), *Textbook of gastroenterology* (2nd ed., Vol. 1, pp. 731–749). Philadelphia: J. B. Lippincott Co.
Marcon, N. E. (1998). Management of esophageal stenosis. *Gastrointestinal Endoscopy Clinics of North America, 8*(2), xiii–xvi, 273–519.
Middlemiss, C. (1997). Gastroesophageal reflux disease: A common condition in the elderly. *The Nurse Practitioner, 22*(11), 51–52, 55, 61.
Rao, S. P. (1993). Bowel obstruction: An overview. *Applied Radiology*, (Suppl.), 18–21.

Abdominal Pain

Altman, D. F. (1996). Gastrointestinal disease. In E. T. Lonergan (Ed.), *Geriatrics* (pp. 183–206). Stamford, Conneticut: Appleton & Lange.
Brunton, S. A. (1998). Diagnosing diabetic gastropathy: A primary care challenge. *Patient Care Nurse Practitioner, Clinical Focus Supplement*, 11–16.
Koch, K. L. (1998). Diabetic gastropathy: A clinical overview. *Patient Care Nurse Practitioner, Clinical Focus Supplement*, 1–10.
Krasman, M. L, Gracie, W. A., & Strasius, S. R. (1991). Biliary tract disease in the aged. *Clinics in Geriatric Medicine, 7*(2), 347–370.
Moscati, R. M. (1996). Cholelithiasis, cholecystitis, and pancreatitis. *Emergency Medicine Clinics of North America, 14*(4), 719–737.
Sanson, T. G., & O'Keefe, K. P. (1996). Evaluation of abdominal pain in the elderly. *Emergency Medicine Clinics of North America, 14*(3), 615–627.
Siegel, J. H., & Kasmin, F. E. (1997). Biliary tract diseases in the elderly: Management and outcomes. *Gut, 41*, 433–435.
Tokunaga, Y., Nakayama, N., Ishikawa, Y., Nishitai, R., Irie, A., Kaganoi, J., Ohsumi, K., & Higo, T. (1997). Surgical risks of acute cholecystitis in elderly. *Hepatogastroenterology, 44*(15), 671–676.

Valentine, V. (1998). Diabetic gastropathy in the elderly. *Patient Care Nurse Practitioner, Clinical Focus Supplement*, 17–21.

Constipation

Abyad, A., & Mourad, F. (1996). Constipation: Common sense care of the older patient. *Geriatrics, 51*(12), 28–32, 34, 36.

Allison, O. C., Porter, M. E., & Briggs, G. C. (1994). Chronic constipation: Assessment and management in the elderly. *Journal of the American Academy of Nurse Practitioners, 6*(7), 311–317.

Fay, D. E. (1998). Constipation. *Lippincott's Primary Care Practice, 2*(4), 417–420.

Ferlotti, T. (1997). Bowel elimination. In M. M. Burke (Ed.), *Gerontologic Nursing: Wholistic Care of the Older Adult* (pp. 369–388). St. Louis: Mosby-Year Book.

Harari, D., Gurwitz, J. H., Avorn, J., et al. (1994). Constipation: Assessment and management in an institutionalized elderly population. *Journal of the American Geriatrics Society, 42*(9), 947–952.

Orr, W. C., Johnson, P., & Yates, C. (1997). Chronic constipation: A clinical conundrum. *Journal of the American Geriatrics Society, 45*(5), 652–653.

Petticrew, M., Watt, I., & Sheldon, T. (1997). Systematic review of the effectiveness of laxatives in the elderly. *Health Technology Assessment, 1*(13), i–iv, 1–52.

Schaefer, D. C., & Cheskin, L. F. (1998). Constipation in the elderly. *American Family Physician, 58*(4), 907–914.

Towers, A. L., Burgio, K. L., Locker, J. L., et al. (1994). Constipation in the elderly: Influence of dietary, psychological, and physiological factors. *Journal of the American Geriatrics Society, 42*(7), 701–706.

Diarrhea

Arduino, R. C., & DuPont, H. L. (1998). Diarrhea in the critically ill: When and how to use the lab to tailor therapy. A guide to key laboratory tests, prescriptions for cure. *Journal of Critical Illness, 13*(6), 364–369.

Bennett, R. G. (1993). Diarrhea among residents of long-term care facilities. *Infection Control & Hospital Epidemiology, 14*(7), 397–404.

Fruto, L. V. (1994). Current concepts: Management of diarrhea in acute care. *Journal of Wound, Ostomy Care Nursing, 21*(5), 199–205.

Losonsky, G. (1992). Diarrhea and gastroenteritis. *Current Opinion in Infectious Diseases, 5*(4), 576–581, 614–616.

Melillo, K. D. (1998). Clostridium difficile and older adults: What primary care providers should know. *The Nurse Practitioner, 23*(7), 25–26, 29–30, 39–40 passim.

Nordeman, L., & Hamilton, R. (1996). Dehydration and gastroenteritis. *Topics in Emergency Medicine, 18*(3), 11–20.

Ryan, M. C. (1997). Clinical puzzler: Persistent diarrhea. *Clinical Excellence for Nurse Practitioners, 1*(2), 124–126.

Peptic Ulcer Disease (PUD)

Altman, D. F. (1996). Gastrointestinal disease. In E. T. Lonergan (Ed.), *Geriatrics* (pp. 183–206). Stamford, Connecticut: Appleton & Lange.

Chiba, N., Rao, B. V., Radenmaker, J. W., & Hunt, R. H. (1992). Meta-analysis of the efficacy of antibiotic therapy in eradicating *Helicobacter pylori. American Journal of Gastroenterology, 87*, 1716–1727.

Connor, B. A. (1996). Gastrointestinal disorders of the stomach and duodenum in the elderly. In Gerb, A. M. (Ed.), *Clinical Gastroenterology in the Elderly* (pp. 37–72). New York: Marcel Dekker, Inc.

Damianos, A. J., & McGarrity, T. J. (1997). Treatment strategies for *Helicobacter pylori* infection. *American Family Physician, 55*(8), 2765–2774.

Graham, D. Y., & Smith, J. L. (1988). Gastroduodenal complications of chronic NSAID therapy. *American Journal of Gastroenterology, 83*, 1081–1084.

Kauvar, D., & Brandt, L. J. (1992). Treatment of common GI disorders in the elderly. *Physician Assistant, 16*, 105–108, 111–112.

Marshall, B. J. (1994). Epidemiology of *H. pylori* in Western countries. In R. H. Hunt & G. N. J. Tytgat, (Eds.), *Helicobacter pylori: Basic mechanisms to clinical cure* (pp. 75–84). Boston: Kluwer Academic.

McCarthy, D. M. (1991). Acid peptic disease in the elderly. *Clinics in Geriatric Medicine, 7*(2), 231–251.

Chapter 7: Genitourinary System

Urinary Tract Infection

Clague, J. E., & Horan, M. A. (1996). The diagnosis of urinary "infection" in old people. *Reviews in Clinical Gerontology, 6*(3), 225–230.

Haus, E. (1998). Urinary tract infections in the homebound elderly. *Home Healthcare Nurse, 16*(5), 323–327.

Hooton, T. M., & Stamm, W. E. (1997). Diagnosis and treatment of uncomplicated urinary tract infection. *Infectious Disease Clinics of North America, 11*(3), 551–581.

McCue, J. D. (1997). Urinary tract infection: Treatment guidelines for older women. *Consultant, 37*(8), 2135–2138, 2141–2142.

Melillo, K. D. (1995). Asymptomatic bactiuria in older adults: When is it necessary to screen and treat? *Nurse Practitioner, 20*(8), 50–66.

Ronald, A. R., & Harding, G. K. M. (1997). Complicated urinary tract infections. *Infectious Disease Clinics of North America, 11*(3), 583–592.

Ryals, J. K., Vetrosky, D., & White, G. L. (1997). Urinary tract infections. *Lippincott's Primary Care Practice, 1*(4), 442–445.

Stapleton, A., & Stamm, W. E. (1997). Prevention of urinary tract infection. *Infectious Disease Clinics of North America. 11*(3), 719–733.

Warren, J. W. (1997). Catheter-associated urinary tract infections. *Infectious Disease Clinics of North America, 11*(3), 609–622.

Wood, C. A., & Abrutyn, E. (1998), Urinary tract infection in older adults. *Clinics in Geriatric Medicine, 14*(2), 267–283.

Urinary Incontinence

Agency for Health Care Policy and Research. (1992). *Urinary incontinence in adults: Quick reference guide for clinicians* (AHCPR Publication No. 92-0041). Rockville, MD: U.S. Department of Health and Human Services.

Agency for Health Care Policy and Research. (1996). *Helping people with incontinence: Caregiver guide* (AHCPR Publication No. 96-0683). Rockville, MD: U.S. Department of Health and Human Services.

Agency for Health Care Policy and Research. (1996). *Urinary incontinence in adults: Clinical practice guidelines* (AHCPR Publication No. 96-0682). Rockville, MD: U.S. Department of Health and Human Services.

Houston, K. A. (1993). Incontinence and the older woman. *Clinics in Geriatric Medicine, 9*(1), 157–171.

Maloney, C. (1998). Urinary incontinence: A guide to the diagnosis of chronic and reversible causes in a primary care setting. *American Journal for Nurse Practitioners, 2*, 8–10, 13–15, 48.

Prostatism

Albertson, P. C. (1997). Urologic "nuisances": How to work up and relieve men's symptoms. *Geriatrics, 52*(2), 46–55.

Bauer, J. J., & Moul, J. W. (1997). Prostatitis: Diagnostic and treatment challenges. *Federal Practitioner, 14*(9), 10–15.

Krieger, J. N., Morganstern, M. D., & Nickel, J. C. (1998). Prostatitis. *Patient Care*, (Suppl. Summer), 1–20.

Mosier, W. A., Schymanski, T. J., & Walgren, K. D. (1998). Benign prostatic hyperplasia: Focusing on primary care. *Clinician Reviews, 8*(7), 55–75.

U.S. Department of Health and Human Services. (1994). *Benign prostatic hyperplasia: Diagnosis and treatment* (AHCPR Publication No. 94-0583). Rockville, MD: Author.

Van Rooyen, M. (1997). Benign prostatic hyperplasia: Diagnosis and watchful waiting as management. *Physician Assistant, 21*(1), 40–61.

Renal Disease

Kee, C. (1998). Renal disorders. In A. S. Luggen et al. (Eds.), *NGNA Core Curriculum for Gerontological Advanced Practice Nurses* (pp. 626–631). Thousand Oaks, CA: Sage.

Palmer, B. F., & Levi, M. (1996). Kidney disease in the elderly. In D. W. Jahnigen & R. W. Schrier (Eds.), *Geriatric medicine* (2nd ed., pp. 688–706). Cambridge: Blackwell Science, Inc.

Pastan, S., & Bailey, J. (1998). Dialysis therapy. *New England Journal of Medicine, 338*(20), 1428–1437.

Porush, J. G., & Faubert, P. F. (1997). Renal disease in elderly patients. *Reviews in Clinical Gerontology, 7*(4), 299–307.

Saklaayen, M. G. (1997). Renal disease. *Medical Clinics of North America, 81*(3), xi–xii, 585–822.

Thadhani, R., Pascual, M., & Bonventure, J. V. (1996). Acute renal failure. *New England Journal of Medicine, 334*, 1448–1460.

Chapter 8: Musculoskeletal System

Musculoskeletal Pain

Bridwell, K. H. (1994). Lumbar spinal stenosis: Diagnosis, management, and treatment. *Clinics in Geriatric Medicine, 10*(4), 677–701.

Emmerson, B. T. (1996). The management of gout. *The New England Journal of Medicine, 334*(7), 445–451.

Fam, A. G. (1997). Problem gout: Clinical challenges, effective solutions. *The Journal of Musculoskeletal Medicine, 14*(10), 63–77.

Healey, P. M., & Jacobson, E. J. (1994). Musculoskeletal disorders. In *Common medical diagnoses: An algorithmic approach* (2nd ed., pp. 212–219). Philadelphia: W. B. Saunders.

Jones, A. K. (1997). Primary care management of acute low back pain. *The Nurse Practitioner, 22*(7), 50–73.

Levy, H. I. (1998). Primary care management of low back pain. *The Journal of Musculoskeletal Medicine, 15*(10), 45–54.

Lipsky, P. E., & Simmons, H. C. (1997). Algorithms for the diagnosis and management of musculoskeletal complaints. *The American Journal of Medicine, 103*(Suppl. 6A), 3–81.

Pfenninger, J. L. (1991). Injections of joints and soft tissue: Part I General guidelines. *American Family Practice, 44*(4), 1196–1202.

Sack, K. E. (1996). Musculoskeletal diseases. In E. T. Lonergan (Ed.), *Geriatrics, a Lange clinical manual* (pp. 207–235). Stamford, CT: Appleton & Lange.

Watchel, T. J. (1997). Bursitis, tendinitis, and selected soft tissue syndromes. In F. F. Ferri, M. D. Fretwell, & T. J. Wachtel (Eds.), *Practical guide to the care of the geriatric patient* (2nd ed., pp. 224–227). St. Louis: Mosby.

Wiese, W., & Wortmann, R. L. (1998). Gout: Effective strategies for acute and long-term control. *The Journal of Musculoskeletal Medicine, 15*(10), 45–53.

Degenerative Joint Disease (DJD)

Creamer, P., & Hochberg, M. C. (1997). Seminar. Osteoarthritis. *Lancet, 350*(9076), 503–509.

Flemming, D. J., & Murphey, M. D. (1997). Osteoarthritis: A guide to roentgenographic findings. *Journal of Musculoskeletal Medicine, 14*(9), 15–17, 20, 22 passim.

Kee, C. C., Harris, S., Booth, L. A., et al. (1998). Perspectives on the nursing management of osteoarthritis. *Geriatric Nursing-American Journal of Care for the Aging, 19*(1), 19–28.

Kellick, K. A., Martins-Richards, J., & Chow, C. (1998). Pharmacology update. Management of arthritis. *Lippincott's Primary Care Practice, 2*(1), 66–80.

Ling, S. M., & Bathon, J. M. (1998). Osteoarthritis in older adults. *Journal of the American Geriatrics Society, 46*(2), 216–225.

Lozada, C. J., & Altman, R. D. (1997). Osteoarthritis: A comprehensive approach to management. *Journal of Musculoskeletal Medicine, 14*(11), 26–28, 33–34, 36–38.

Ross, C. (1997). A comparison of osteoarthritis and rheumatoid arthritis: Diagnosis and treatment. The Nurse Practitioner, 22 *(9), 20, 23–24, 27–28.*

Sorensen, L. B., & Blair, J. M. (1997). Rheumatologic diseases. In C. K. Cassel, H. J. Cohen, E. B. Larson, et al. (Eds.), *Geriatric medicine* (3rd ed., pp. 449–479). New York: Springer.

Wasti, S. A., & Chamberlain, M. A. (1996). Rheumatological rehabilitation in older adults. *Reviews in Clinical Gerontology, 6*(3), 255–271.

Rheumatoid Arthritis (RA)

Baum, J. (1998). Rheumatoid arthritis: How to make the most of laboratory tests in the work-up. *Consultant, 38*, 1341–1344, 1347–1348.

Bennett, J. C., & Moreland, L. W. (1997). Rheumatoid arthritis. In T. E. Andreoli, J. C. Bennett, C. C. Carpenter, & F. Plum, *Cecil essentials of medicine* (4th ed., pp. 594–597). Philadelphia: W. B. Saunders.

Biundo, J. J., & Hughes, G. M. (1997). Rheumatoid arthritis: Part 1: Practical guidelines on rest, ambulatory aids, and exercise programs. *Consultant, 37*, 2958–2960, 2962–2963, 2967–2969.

Biundo, J. J., & Hughes, G. M. (1997). Rheumatoid arthritis: Part 2: Thermal modalities, occupational therapy, and psychological help. *Consultant, 37*, 3123–3124, 3129–3130.

Gremillion, R. B., & van Vollenhoven, R. F. (1998). Rheumatoid arthritis: Designing and implementing a treatment plan. *Postgraduate Medicine, 103*, 103–106, 110, 116–118, 121–123.

Miller-Blair, D. J., & Robbins, D. L. (1993). Rheumatoid arthritis: New science, new treatment. *Geriatrics, 48*, 28–31, 35–38.

Puri, S. (1998). End-stage rheumatoid arthritis. *Consultant, 38*, 177.

Polymyalgia Rheumatica (PR)

Bennett, J. C., & Moreland, L. W. (1997). Vasculitides. In T. E. Andreoli, J. C. Bennett, C. C. Carpenter, & F. Plum, *Cecil essentials of medicine* (4th ed., pp. 614–619). Philadelphia: W. B. Saunders.

Dwolatzky, T., Sonnenblick, M., & Nesher, G. (1997). Giant cell arteritis and polymyalgia rheumatica: Clues to early diagnosis. *Geriatrics, 52*(6), 38–40, 43–44.

Sack, K. E. (1996). Musculoskeletal disease. In E. T. Lonergan (Ed.), *Geriatrics* (pp. 207–234). Stamford, CT: Appleton & Lange.

Hip Fracture

Birge, S. J., Morrow-Howell, N., & Proctor, E. K. (1994). Hip fracture. *Clinics in Geriatric Medicine, 10*(4), 589–603.

Borgquist, L., Ceder, L., & Thorngren, K. G. (1990). Function and social status 10 years after hip fracture: Prospective follow-up of 103 patients. *Acta Orthopaedica Scandinavica, 61*, 404–410.

Cummings, S. R., Phillips, S. L., Wheat, M. E., Black, D., Goosby, E. Wlodarczyk, D., et al. (1988). Recovery of function after hip fracture: The role of social supports. *Journal of the American Geriatrics Society, 36*(9), 801–806.

Elton, R. D. (1996). Geriatric medicine. *British Medical Journal, 312*, 561–563.

Ethans, K. D., & MacKnight, C. (1998). Hip fracture in the elderly. *Postgraduate Medicine, 103*, 157–158, 163–164, 167, 169–170.

Fitzgerald, J. F., Moore, P. S., & Dittus, R. S. (1988). The care of elderly patients with hip fracture: Changes since implementation of the prospective payment system. *New England Journal of Medicine, 319*, 1392–1397.

Grisso, J. A., Kelsey, J. L., Strom, B. L., O'Brien, L. A., Maislin, G. LaPann, K., et al. (1994). Risk factors for hip fracture in black women. The Northeast Hip Fracture Study Group. *New England Journal of Medicine, 330*(22), 1555–1559.

Koval, K. J., & Zuckerman, J. D. (1994). Current concepts review: Functional recovery after fracture of the hip. *Journal of Bone and Joint Surgery, 76*(5), 751–758.

Mehta, A. J., & Nastasi, A. E. (1993). Rehabilitation of fractures in the elderly. *Clinics in Geriatric Medicine 9*(4), 717–727.

Stinnett, K. A. (1996). Occupational therapy intervention for the geriatric client receiving acute and subacute services following total hip replacement and femoral fracture repair. *Topics in Geriatric Rehabilitation, 12*(1), 23–31.

Tinetti, M. E., Baker, D. I., Gottschalk, M., Garrett, P., McGeary, S., Pollack, D., & Charpentier, P. (1997). Systematic home-based physical and functional therapy for older persons after hip fracture. *Archives of Physical Medicine and Rehabilitation, 78*, 1237–1247.

Chapter 9: Neurological System

Dizziness

Burke, M. (1995). Dizziness in the elderly: Etiology and treatment. *Nurse Practitioner, 20*(12), 28, 31–35.

Davis, L. E. (1994). Dizziness in elderly men. *Journal of the American Geriatrics Society, 42*(11), 1184–1188.

Dewane, J. A. (1995). Dealing with dizziness and disequilibrium in older patients: A clinical approach. *Topics in Geriatric Rehabilitation, 11*(1), 30–38.

Lilley, M. D. (1997). Postprandial blood pressure changes in the elderly. *Journal of Gerontological Nursing, 23*(12), 17–25.

Sloane, P. D. (1996). Evaluation and management of dizziness in the older patient. *Clinics of Geriatric Medicine, 12*(4), 785–801.

Sloane, P. D., Hartman, M., & Mitchell, C. M. (1994). Psychological factors associated with chronic dizziness in patients aged 60 and older. *Journal of the American Geriatrics Society, 42*(8), 847–852.

Weinstein, B. E., & Devons, C. A. J. (1995). The dizzy patient: Stepwise workup of a common complaint. *Geriatrics, 50*(6), 42–46, 49–51.

Yardley, L., & Luxon, L. (1994). Treating dizziness with vestibular rehabilitation: Exercises provide physical and psychological benefits. *British Medical Journal, 308*(6939), 1252–1253.

Seizures

Delanty, N., Vaughn, C. J., & French, J. A. (1998). Medical causes of seizures. *Lancet, 352*(9125), 383–390.

Drury, I., & Beydoun, A. (1993). Seizure disorders of aging: Differential diagnosis and patient management. *Geriatrics, 48*(5), 52–54, 57–58.

Haideer, A, Tuchek, J. M., & Haider, S. (1996). Seizure control: How to use the new anti-epileptic drugs in older patients. *Geriatrics, 51*(9), 42–45.

Hartshorn, J. C. (1996). Seizures and the elderly. *Critical Care Nursing Clinics of North America, 8*(1), 71–78.

Hilton, G. (1997). Seizure disorders in adults: Evaluation and management of new onset seizures. *The Nurse Practitioner, 22*(9), 42, 45, 49–50.

Reith, J., Jorgensen, H. S., Nakayama, H., et al. (1997). Seizures in acute stroke: Predictors and prognostic significance: The Copenhagen Stroke Study. *Stroke, 28*(8), 1585–1589.

Transient Ischemic Attack (TIA)/Cerebrovascular Accident (CVA)

Burvill, P., Johnson, G., Jamrozik, K., Anderson, C., & Stewart-Wynne, E. (1997). Risk factors for post-stroke depression. *International Journal of Geriatric Psychiatry, 12*, 219–226.

Chrzanowski, D. D. (1998). Managing atrial fibrillation to prevent its major complication: Stroke. *The Nurse Practitioner, 23,* 26, 32–34, 36–37, 41–42.

Goldman, L. (Ed.). (1994). Neurology. *Medical knowledge self-assessment program, Book 3, Book 5.* American College of Physicians.

Kelley, R. E. (1998). Stroke prevention and intervention. *Postgraduate Medicine, 103,* 43–45, 49–50, 56–58, 61.

Langhorne, P., & Stott, D. J. (1995). Acute cerebral infarction: Optimal management in older patients. *Drugs and Aging, 6,* 445–455.

National Institute of Neurological Disorders and Stroke. (1991). Benefit of carotid endarterectomy for patients with high-grade stenosis of the internal carotid artery [On-line]. Available: http://www.nlm.nih.gov/databases/alerts/stenosis.html.

Plum, F., & Posner, J. B. Cerebrovascular disease. (1997). In T. E. Andreoli, J. C. Bennett, C. C. Carpenter, & F. Plum, *Cecil essentials of medicine* (4th ed., pp. 858–873). Philadelphia: W. B. Saunders.

Poole, R. M., & Chimowitz, M. I. (1994). Ischemic stroke and TIA: Clinical clues to common causes. *Geriatrics, 49,* 37–40, 42.

Ross, M. E. Cerebrovascular disease. In K. J. Isselbacher, E. Braunwald, J. D. Wilson, J. B. Martin, A. S. Fauci, & D. L. Kasper (Eds.), *Harrison's principles of internal medicine companion handbook* (13th ed., pp. 703–710). New York: McGraw-Hill.

Sasaki, H., Sekizawa, K., Yanai, M., Arai, H., Yamaya, M., & Ohrui, T. (1997). New strategies for aspiration pneumonia. *Internal Medicine, 36,* 851–855.

Van Damme, H., Lacroix, H., Desiron, Q., Nevelsteen, A., Limet, R., & Suy, R. (1996). Carotid surgery in octogenarians: Is it worthwhile? *Acta Chirurgica Belgica, 96*(2), 71–77.

Parkinson's Disease (PD)

Aminoff, M. J., Burns, R. S., & Silverstei, P. M. (1997). Update on Parkinson's disease. *Patient Care, 31*(10), 12–25.

Brod, M., Mendelsohn, G. A., & Roberts, B. (1998). Patients' experiences of Parkinson's disease. *Journals of Gerontology Series B, psychological sciences and social sciences, 53*(4), 213–222.

Duvoisin, R. C., & Sage, J. (1996). *Parkinson's disease: A Guide for patient and family* (4th ed.). Philadelphia: Lippincott-Raven.

Fernandez, H. H., & Durso, R. (1998). Clozapine for dopaminergic-induced paraphilias in Parkinson's disease. *Movement Disorders, 13*(3), 597–598.

Menza, M. A., & Liberatore, B. I. (1998). Psychiatry in the geriatric neurology practice. *Neurologic Clinics,* 16(3), 611–633.

Nadeau, S. E. (1997). Clinical decisions: Parkinson's disease. *Journal of the American Geriatrics Society, 45*(2), 233–240.

Nagaya, M., Kachi, T., Yamada, T., et al. (1998). Videofluorographic study of swallowing in Parkinson's disease. *Dysphagia, 13*(2), 95–100.

Silver, D. E., & Ruggieri, S. (1998). Initiating therapy for Parkinson's disease. *Neurology, 50*(6 Suppl 6), S18–22, 44–48.

Uitti, R. J. (1998). Tremor: How to determine if the patient has Parkinson's disease. *Geriatrics, 53*(5), 30–34.

Valldeoriola, F., Nobbe, F. A., & Tolosa, E. (1997). Treatment of behavioural disturbances in Parkinson's disease. *Journal of Neural Transmission, 51*(Suppl.), 175–204.

Falls

Kiely, D. K., Kiel, D. P., Burrows, A. B., & Lipsitz, L. A. (1998). Identifying nursing home residents at risk for falling. *Journal of The American Geriatrics Society, 46*(5), 551–555.

Lawrence, J. I., & Maher, P. L. (1992). An interdisciplinary falls consult team: A collaborative approach to patient falls. *Journal of Nursing Care Quality, 6*(3), 21–29.

Lundin-Olsson, L., Nyberg, L., & Gustafson, Y. (1997). "Stops walking when talking" as a predictor of falls in elderly people. *The Journal of Musculoskeletal Medicine, 14*(10), 46.

Neufeld, R. R., Tideiksaar, R., Yew, E., Brooks, F., Young, J., Brown, G., & Hsu, M. (1991). A multidisciplinary falls consultation service in a nursing home. *Gerontologist, 31*(1), 120–123.

Nevitt, M. C., Cummings, S. R., & Hudes, E. S. (1991). Risk factors for injurious falls: A prospective study. *Journal of Gerontology, 46*(5), 164–170.

Ray, W. A., Griffin, M. R., Schaffner, W., Baugh, D. K., & Melton, L. J. (1987). Psychotrophic drug use and the risk of hip fracture. *New England Journal of Medicine, 316*(7), 363–369.

Redford, J. B. (1991). Preventing falls in the elderly. *Hospital Medicine, 27*(2), 57–71.

Rubenstein, L. Z., Josephson, K. R., & Robbins, A. S. (1996). Falls and their prevention. In R. W. Besdine, L. Z. Rubenstein, & L Snyder (Eds.), *Medical care of the nursing home resident: What physicians need to know* (pp. 103–115). Philadelphia: American College of Physicians.

Schulman, B. K., & Acquaviva, T. (1987). Falls in the elderly. *The Nurse Practitioner, 12*(11), 30–37.

Spellbring, A. M. (1992). Assessing the elderly patients at high risk of falls: A reliability study. *Journal of Nursing Care Quality, 6*(3), 30–35.

Sudarsky, L. (1990). Geriatrics: Gait disorders in the elderly. *New England Journal of Medicine, 322*(20), 1441–1446.

Tideiksaar, R. (1988). Falls in the elderly: An approach to management. *Physicians Assistant, 12*(10), 114, 117–118, 120, 123–126, 128, 130, 132.

Tideiksaar, R., & Kay, A. D. (1986). What causes falls?: A logical diagnostic procedure. *Geriatrics, 41*(12), 32–50.

Tinetti, M. E., Liu, W. L., & Ginter, S. F. (1992). Mechanical restraint use and fall-related injuries among residents of skilled nursing facilities. *Annals of Internal Medicine, 116*(5), 369–374.

Tinetti, M. E., & Speechley, M. (1989). Prevention of falls among the elderly. *The New England Journal of Medicine, 320*(16), 1055–1059.

Tinetti, M. E., Williams, T. F., & Mayewski, R. (1986). Fall risk index for elderly patients based on number of chronic disabilities. *The American Journal of Medicine, 80*(3), 429–434.

Turkoski, B., Pierce, L. L., Schreck, S., Salter, J., Radziewicz, R., Guhde, J., & Brady, R. (1997). Clinical nursing judgment related to reducing the incidence of falls by elderly patients. *Rehabilitation Nursing, 22*(3), 124–130.

Delirium

Buckwalter, K. C., & Buckwalter, J. A. (1998). Acute cognitive dysfunction (delirium). *Archives of the American Academy of Orthopaedic Surgeons, 2*(1), 9–19.

Foreman, M. D. (1996). Delirium in the emergency department. In C. W. Bradway, *Nursing Care of Geriatric Emergencies* (pp. 252–282). New York: Springer.

Foreman, M. D., & Zane, D. (1996). Nursing strategies for acute confusion in elders. *American Journal of Nursing, 96*(4), 44–52.

Francis, J. (1997). Delirium. In C. D. Cassel, H. J. Cohen, E. B. Larson, et al. (Eds.), *Geriatric medicine* (3rd ed., pp. 917–922). New York: Springer.

Meredith, L. A., & Filley, C. M. (1996). Acute confusional state. In D. Jahnigen & R. Schrier (Eds.), *Geriatric medicine* (2nd ed., pp. 283–291). Cambridge: Blackwell Science.

Milisen, K., Foreman, M. D., Godderis, J., et al. (1998). Delirium in the hospitalized elderly: Nursing assessment and management. *Nursing Clinics of North America, 33*(3), 417–439.

Musselman, D. L., Hawthorne, C. N., & Stoudemire, A. (1997). Screening for delirium: A means to improved outcome in hospitalized elderly patients. *Reviews in Clinical Gerontology, 7*(3), 235–256.

Patkar, A. A., & Kunkel, E. J. S. (1997). Practical geriatrics. Treating delirium among elderly patients. *Psychiatric Services, 48*(1), 46–48.

Weissmen, C. (1996). Strategies for managing delirium in critically ill patients. *Journal of Critical Illness, 11*(5), 295–297, 301–302, 307.

Dementia

Allardyce, J., & McKeeith, I. G. (1997). Dementia with lewy bodies. *Reviews in Clinical Gerontology, 7*(2), 163–170.

Buckwalter, K. C., & Buckwalter, J. A. (1998). Chronic cognitive dysfunction (dementia). *Archives of the American Academy of Orthopaedic Surgeons, 2*(1), 20–32.

Early identification of Alzheimer's disease and related dementias: *Clinical practice guideline.* (1996). United States Department of Health & Human Services Publications. Public Health Service AHCPR 97-0703.

McCarten, J. R. (1997). Recognizing dementia in the clinic: Whom to suspect, whom to test. *Geriatrics, 52*(Suppl. 2), S17–S21.

O'Brien, M. E. (1994). The dementia syndromes: Distinguishing their clinical differences. *Postgraduate Medicine, 95*(5), 91–93, 97–99, 101 passim.

Robinson, B. E. (1997). Guideline for initial evaluation of the patient with memory loss. *Geriatrics, 52*(12), 30–32, 35–36, 39.

Robinson, B. E. (1998). Dementia in primary care. Diagnosis of irreversible dementia: How extensive the evaluation? *Geriatrics, 53*(1), 49–50, 52, 55.

Chapter 10: Endocrine System

Diabetes Mellitus

American Diabetes Association. (1997). Diabetes mellitus and exercise. *Diabetes Care, 20*(Suppl. 1), S51.

American Diabetes Association. (1997). Nutrition recommendations and principles for people with diabetes mellitus. *Diabetes Care, 20*(Suppl. 1), S14–S17.

Brody, G. M. (1992). Diabetic ketoacidosis and hyperosmolar hyperglycemic nonketotic coma. *Topics in Emergency Medicine, 14*(1), 12–22.

Brown, D. F., & Jackson, T. W. (1994). Diabetes: "Tight control" in a comprehensive treatment plan. *Geriatrics, 49*(6), 24–27, 29, 33–34.

Diabetes Control and Complications Trial (DCCT). (1987). Results of feasibility study. *Diabetes Care, 10*, 1–19.

Morrow, L. A., & Minaker, M. D. (1995). Treatment of diabetes mellitus in the elderly. In R. N. Winickoff (Ed.), *Strategies in Geriatrics, 2*(4), 1–5. Department of Veterans Affairs.

Ohkubo, Y., Kishikawa, H., Araki, E., Miyata, T., Isami, S., Motoyosyi, S., Kojima, Y., Furuyoshi, N., & Shichiri, M. (1995). Intensive insulin therapy prevents the progression of diabetic microvascular complications in Japanese patients with non-insulin dependent diabetes mellitus: A randomized prospective 6-year study. *Diabetes Research and Clinical Practice, 28*, 103–117.

Hypothyroidism

Helfand, M., & Redfern, C. C. (1998). Screening for thyroid disease: An update. *Annals of Internal Medicine, 129*, 144–158.

Hurley, D. L., & Gharib, H. (1995). Detection and treatment of hypothyroidism and Graves' disease. *Geriatrics, 50*, 41–44.

Johnson, J. L., & Felicetta, J. V. (1992). Hypothyroidism: A comprehensive review. *Journal of the American Academy of Nurse Practitioners, 4*, 131–138.

Martinez, M., Derksen, D., & Kapsner, P. (1993). Making sense of hypothyroidism: An approach to testing and treatment. *Postgraduate Medicine, 93*, 135–138, 141–145.

Shetty, K. R., & Duthie, E. H. (1995). Thyroid disease and associated illness in the elderly. *Clinics in Geriatric Medicine, 11*(2), 311–325.

Shoback, D. (1996). Thyroid disease and disorders of calcium and phosphorous balance. In E. T. Lonergan (Ed.), *Geriatrics* (pp. 166–182). Stamford, CT: Appleton & Lange.

Yeomans, A. C. (1990). Assessment and management of hypothyroidism. *Nurse Practitioner, 15*(11), 8, 11–12, 14, 16.

Hyperthyroidism

Gambert, S. R. (1995). Hyperthyroidism in the elderly. *Clinics in Geriatric Medicine, 11*(2), 181–188.

Haddad, G. (1998). Is it hyperthyroidism? You can't always tell from the clinical picture. *Postgraduate Medicine, 104*(1), 42–44, 53–55, 59.

Isley, W. L. (1993). Thyroid dysfunction in the severely ill and elderly: Forget the classic signs and symptoms. *Postgraduate Medicine, 94*(3), 111–118, 127–128.

Kennedy, J. W., & Caro, J. F. (1996). The ABCs of managing hyperthyroidism in the older patient. *Geriatrics, 51*(5), 22–24, 27, 31–32.

Shoback, D., & Jaffe, M. (1996). Thyroid disease and disorders of calcium and phosphorus balance. In E. T. Lonergan (Ed.), *Geriatrics* (pp. 166–182). Stamford, CT: Appleton & Lange.

Hyperlipidemia

Abrams, J., Vela, B. S., Coultas, D. B., Samaan, S. A., Malhotra, D., & Roche, R. J. (1995). Coronary risk factors and their modification: Lipids, smoking, hypertension, estrogen, and the elderly. *Current Problems in Cardiology, 20*(8), 533–610.

American Heart Association. (1994). *Heart and stroke facts: 1994 Statistical supplement.* Dallas, TX: American Heart Association.

Avorn, J., Monette, J., Lacour, A., Bohn, R. L., Monane, M., Mogun, H., et al. (1998). Persistence of use of lipid-lowering medications: A cross-national study. *Journal of American Medical Association, 279*(18), 1458–1462.

Garber, A. M., Littenberg, B., Sox, H. C., Wagner, J. L., & Gluck, M. (1991). Costs and health consequences of cholesterol screening for asymptomatic older Americans. *Archives of Internal Medicine, 151*, 1089–1095.

LaRosa, J. C. (1993). Estrogen: Risk versus benefit for the prevention of coronary artery disease. *Coronary Artery Disease, 4*(7), 588–594.

LaRosa, J. C. (1996). Dyslipidemia and coronary artery disease in the elderly. *Clinics in Geriatric Medicine, 12*(1), 33–40.

Leaf, D. A. (1994). Lipid disorders: Applying new guidelines to your older patients. *Geriatrics, 49*(5), 35–38, 40–41.

Nolan, L., & O'Malley, K. (1988). Prescribing for the elderly, I: Sensitivity of the elderly to adverse drug reactions. *Journal of the American Geriatrics Society, 36*, 142–149.

Wones, R. G. (1989). Screening, diagnosis, and treatment of hypercholesterolemia. *Primary Care, 16*(1), 63–82.

Fluid and Electrolyte Abnormalities

Abul-Ezz, S. R., Bunke, C. M., Singh, H., Shah, S. V. (1997). Fluid and electrolyte disorders. In T. E. Andreoli, J. C. Bennett, C. C. Carpenter, & F. Plum (Eds.), *Cecil essentials of medicine* (4th ed., pp. 188–203). Philadelphia: W. B. Saunders.

Chou, S., & Lindeman, R. D. (1995). Structural and functional changes of the aging kidney. In H. R. Jacobson, G. E. Striker, & S. Klahr (Eds.), *The principles and practice of nephrology* (2nd ed., pp. 510–514). St. Louis: Mosby.

Faubert, P. F., & Porush, J. G. (1995). Disorders of water, sodium, and divalent-ion metabolism. In H. R. Jacobson, G. E. Striker, & S. Klahr (Eds.), *The principles and practice of nephrology* (2nd ed., pp. 515–518). St. Louis: Mosby.

Hobbs, J. (1986). Office laboratory evaluation of fluid, electrolyte, and acid-base disorders. *Primary Care, 13*(4), 761–782.

Sica, D. A. (1994). Renal disease, electrolyte abnormalities, and acid-base imbalance in the elderly. *Clinics in Geriatric Medicine, 10*(1), 197–211.

Osteoporosis

Baran, R. W., Kiel, D. P., Patterson, H., et al. (1998). Diagnosis and treatment of osteoporosis in long-term care facilities. *The Consultant Pharmacist, 13*(6), 685–689.

Barrett-Connor, E. (1998). Rationale for later and less postmenopausal estrogen. *Aging, 10*(2), 158.

Blanchard, F., Papapoulos, S., Compston, J., & Maggi, S. (1998). Osteoporosis: Strategies for prevention. *Aging, 10*(2), 161–162.

Bellantoni, M. R. (1996). Osteoporosis prevention and treatment. *American Family Physician, 54*(3), 986–992.

Eastell, R. (1998). Drug therapy: Treatment of postmenopausal osteoporosis. *New England Journal of Medicine, 338*(11), 736–746.

Girvin, J. (1998). Established osteoporosis. *Elderly Care, 10*(2), 23–28.

Kroger, H., & Reeve, J. (1998). Diagnosis of osteoporosis in clinical practice. *Annals of Medicine, 30*(3), 278–287.

Notelovitz, M. (1997). Osteoporosis: Alternatives for keeping bone strong. *Contemporary Nurse Practitioner, 2(1), 7–19.*

Rosenthal, R. E. (1998). Osteoporosis. *Archives of the American Academy of Orthopaedic Surgeons, 2*(1), 52–59.

Taxel, P. (1998). Osteoporosis: Detection, prevention, and treatment in primary care. *Geriatrics, 53*(8), 22–23, 27–28, 33 passim.

Erectile Dysfunction

Ackerman, M. D., Montague, D. K., & Morganstern, S. (1994). Impotence: Help for erectile dysfunction. *Patient Care, 28*(5), 22–25, 29–30, 32.

Federman, D. D. (1999). Viagra: A major advance. *The Clinical Advisor, 78.*

Goldstein, I., Lue, T. F., Padma-Nathan, H., et al. (1998). Oral sildenafil in the treatment of erectile dysfunction. *New England Journal of Medicine, 338,* 1397–1404.

Johnson, L. E., & Morley, J. E. (1988). Impotence in the elderly. *American Family Physician, 38*(5), 225–240.

LoPiccolo, J. (1991). Counseling and therapy for sexual problems in the elderly. *Clinics in Geriatric Medicine, 7*(1), 161–179.

McCracken, A. L. (1988). Sexual practice by elders: The forgotten aspect of functional health. *Journal of Gerontological Nursing, 14*(10), 13–18.

Hahn, K. (1989). Sexuality and COPD. *Rehabilitation Nursing, 14,* 191–195.

Morley, J. E., Korenman, S. G., Mooradian, A. D., & Kaiser, F. E. (1987). UCLA geriatric grand rounds: Sexual dysfunction in the elderly male. *Journal of the American Geriatrics Society, 35*(11), 1014–1022.

Mulligan, T., & Modigh, A. (1991). Sexuality in dependent living situations. *Clinics in Geriatric Medicine, 7*(1), 153–160.

Rousseau, P. (1988). Impotence in elderly men. *Postgraduate Medicine, 83*(6), 212–219.

Singer, C., Weiner, W. J., Sanchez-Ramos, J., & Ackerman, M. (1991). Sexual function in patients with Parkinson's disease. *Journal of Neurology, Neurosurgery & Psychiatry, 54*(10), 942.

Zeiss, R. A., Delmonico, R. L., Zeiss, A. M., & Dornbrand, L. (1991). Psychologic disorder and sexual dysfunction in elders. *Clinics in Geriatric Medicine, 7*(1), 133–151.

Chapter 11: Hematologic System

Anemia

Barkin, J. S., Green, R., Johnson, B., & Krantz, S. (1998). A practical workup for the patient with anemia. *Patient Care Nurse Practitioner, 1,* 30–36, 39–42.

Bushnell, F. K. (1992). A guide to primary care of iron-deficiency anemia. *Nurse Practitioner, 17,* 70–74.

Fairbanks, V. F. (1997). Iron therapy in older women: When to use, when to eschew? *Consultant, 37,* 3024.

Lipschitz, D. A. (1988). *Current issues: Anemia in the elderly.* Raritan, NJ: Ortho Pharmaceuticals/Toltzis Communications.

Massey, A. C. (1992). Microcytic anemia: Differential diagnosis and management of iron deficiency anemia. *The Medical Clinics of North America, 76*(3), 549–565.

Moses, P. L., & Smith, R. E. (1995). Endoscopic evaluation of iron deficiency anemia: A guide to diagnostic strategy in older patients. *Postgraduate Medicine, 98*(2), 213–216, 219, 222–224.

Scott, R. B. (1993). Common blood disorders: A primary care approach. *Geriatrics, 48*(4), 72–76, 79–80.

Semla, T. P., Beizer J. L., & Higbee M. D. *Geriatric dosage handbook* (4th ed., p. 258). Hudson, OH: Lexi-Comp.

Small, E., & Damon, L. (1996). Blood. In E. Lonergan (Ed.), *Geriatrics* (pp. 262–287). Stamford, CT: Appleton & Lange.

Vitamin B12 deficiency. 1998. *The Clinical Advisor, 47.*

Leukemia

Champlin, R. E., Gajewski, J. L., & Golde, D. W. (1989). Treatment of acute myelogenous leukemia in the elderly. *Seminars in Oncology, 16*(1), 51–56.

Dagg, J. (1990). Leukaemias and malignant lymphoma. In F. I. Caird & T. B. Brewin (Eds.), *Cancer in the elderly* (pp. 203–225). London: Wright.

DeVita, T., Jr., Hellman, S., & Rosenberg, S. (Eds.). (1997). *Cancer principles and practice of oncology* (5th ed.). Philadelphia: J. B. Lippincott.

Freedman, M. L. (1992). Blood disorders and their management in old age. In J. C. Brocklehurst, R. C. Tallis, & H. M. Fillit (Eds.), *Textbook of geriatric medicine and gerontology* (4th ed., pp. 873–886). London: Churchill Livingston.

Gibbins, F. J. (1975). Haematological problems in the older patient. *The Practitioner, 215*(1289), 606–609.

Hayhoe, F. G. J., & Reese, J. (1985). The leukemias. In M. J. M. Denham & I. Chanarin (Eds.), *Blood disorders in the elderly* (pp. 188–207). London: Churchill Livingston.

Lundquist, D. M., & Stewart, F. M. (1994). An update on non-Hodgkin's lymphomas. *The Nurse Practitioner, 19*(10), 41–54.

Mitus, A. J., & Rosenthal, D. S. (1991). Adult leukemias. In A. I. Holleb, D. J. Fink, & G. P. Murphy (Eds.), *American cancer society textbook of clinical oncology.* Atlanta: The American Cancer Society, Inc.

Mortimer, J. E., Blinder, M. A., & Arguette, M. A. (1992). Approach to the cancer patient. In M. Woodley & A. Whelan (Eds.), *Manual of medical therapeutics: The Washington manual* (27th ed., pp. 356–374). Boston: Little, Brown, & Company.

Silber, R. (1982). Chronic lymphocytic leukemia in the elderly. *Hospital Practice, 17*(6), 131–141.

Stone, R. M., & Mayer, R. J. (1993). The approach to the elderly patient with acute myeloid leukemia. *Hematology/Oncology Clinics of North America, 7*(1), 65–79.

Wachtel, T. J. (1997). Hematologic malignancies. In F. F. Ferri, M. D. Fretwell, & T. J. Wachtel (Eds.), *Practical guide to the care of the geriatric patient* (2nd ed., pp. 318–323). St. Louis: Mosby.

Chapter 12: Psychiatric Disorders

Depression

Blazer, D. G., & Koenig, H. G. (1996). Mood disorders. In E. W. Busse & D. G. Blazer (Eds.), *Textbook of geriatric psychiatry* (2nd ed., pp. 235–263). Washington, D.C.: American Psychiatric Press, Inc.

Davis, K. M., & Mathew, E. (1998). Pharmacologic management of depression in the elderly. *The Nurse Practitioner, 23*(6), 16, 18, 26 passim.

Diamond, P. T., Holroyd, S., Macciocchi, S. N., et al. (1995). Prevalence of depression and outcome on the geriatric rehabilitation unit. *American Journal of Physical Medicine & Rehabilitation, 74*(3), 214–217.

Kurlowiez, L. H., & Streim, J. E. (1998). Measuring depression in hospitalized, medically ill, older adults. *Archives of Psychiatric Nursing, 12*(4), 209–218.

Meldon, S. W., Emerman, C., Schubert, D. S. P., et al. (1997). Depression in geriatric ED patients: Prevalence and recognition. *Annals of Emergency Medicine, 30*(2), 141–145.

Onega, L. L., & Abraham I. L. (1998). Differentiated nursing assessment of depressive symptoms in community-dwelling elders. *Nursing Clinics of North America, 33*(3), 407–416.

Robinson, B. E. (1998). Depression. *Archives of the American Academy of Orthopaedic Surgeons, 2*(1), 33–38.

Anxiety

Koder, D. (1998). Treatment of anxiety in the cognitively impaired elderly: Can cognitive-behavior therapy help? *International Psychogeriatrics, 10*(2), 173–182.

Schneider, L. S. (1996). Overview of generalized anxiety disorder in the elderly. *Journal of Clinical Psychiatry, 7*(57 Suppl.), 34–45, 52–54.

Sheikh, J. I. (1996). Anxiety and panic disorders. In E. W. Busse & D. G. Blazer (Eds.), *Textbook of geriatric psychiatry* (2nd ed., pp. 279–289). Washington, D.C.: American Psychiatric Press, Inc.

Chapter 13: The Frail Elderly

Ebersole, P. (1976). Developmental tasks in late life. In I. M. Burnside (Ed.), *Nursing and the aged.* New York: McGraw-Hill.

Jacob, G. M., & Palmer, R. M. (1998). Tools for assessing the frail elderly: Geriatric evaluation focuses on improving quality of life. *Postgraduate Medicine, 104*(1), 135–138, 143–146, 152–153.

Ham, R. J. (1994). The signs and symptoms of poor nutritional status. *Primary Care, 21*(1), 33–54.

Havighurst, R. J. (1972). *Developmental tasks and education.* New York: D. McKay Co.

Horwarth, C. C. (1991). Nutrition goals for older adults: A review. *The Gerontologist, 31*(6), 811–821.

Markson, E. W. (1997). Functional, social, and psychological disability as causes of loss of weight and independence in older community-living people. *Clinics in Geriatric Medicine, 13*(4), 639–651.

Rudman, D., & Cohan, M. E. (1992). Nutrition in the elderly. In E. Calkins, A. B. Ford, & P. R. Katz (Eds.), *Practice of geriatrics* (2nd ed., pp. 19–32). Philadelphia: W. B. Saunders Company.

Verdery, R. B. (1997). Clinical evaluation of failure to thrive in older people. *Clinics in Geriatric Medicine, 13*(6), 769–778.

Zawada, E. T. (1996). Malnutrition in the elderly: Is it simply a matter of not eating enough? *Postgraduate Medicine, 100*(1), 207–208, 211–212, 214, 220–222, 225.

Chapter 14: Pressure Ulcers

Baranoski, S. (1995). Wound assessment and dressing selection. *Ostomy/Wound Management, 41*(Suppl. 7A), S 7–14.

Bergstrom, N. I. (1997). Strategies for preventing pressure ulcers. *Clinics in Geriatric Medicine, 13*(3), 437–454.

Burdette-Taylor, S., & Taylor, T. G. (1993). Wound cultures: What, when and how. *Ostomy/Wound Management, 39*(8), 26–32.

Cerrato, P. L. (1986). How diet helps the skin fight pressure sores. *RN, 49*(1), 67–68.

Findlay, D. (1996). Practical management of pressure ulcers. *American Family Physician, 54*(50), 1519–1528.

Fowler, E., & vanRijswijk, L. (1995). Using wound debridement to help achieve the goals of care. *Ostomy/Wound Management, 41*(Suppl. 7A), S 23–35.

Goode, P. S., & Thomas, D. R. (1997). Pressure ulcers: Local wound care. *Clinics in Geriatric Medicine, 13*(3), 543–552.

Krainski, M. M. (1992). Pressure ulcers and the elderly. *Ostomy/Wound Management, 38*(5), 22–37.

Krasner, D. (1991). Resolving the dressing dilemma: Selecting wound dressings by category. *Ostomy/Wound Management, 35*(4), 62–69.

Levine, J. M., Simpson, M. A., & McDonald, R. J. (1989). Pressure sores: A plan for primary care prevention. *Geriatrics, 44*(4), 75–90.

Maklebust, J. (1997). Pressure ulcer assessment. *Clinics in Geriatric Medicine, 13*(3), 455–481.

Niazi, Z. B. N., & Salzberg, C. A. (1997). Operative repair of pressure ulcers. *Clinics in Geriatric Medicine, 13*(3), 587–597.

Rook, J. L. (1997). Wound care pain. *The Nurse Practitioner, 22*(3), 122–136.

Stotts, N. A., & Hunt, T. K. (1997). Managing bacterial colonization and infection. *Clinics in Geriatric Medicine, 13*(3), 565–597.

Thomas, D. R. (1997). The role of nutrition in prevention and healing of pressure ulcers. *Clinics in Geriatric Medicine, 13*(3), 497–511.

U.S. Department of Health and Human Services. (1992). *Pressure ulcers in adults: Prediction and prevention* (AHCPR Publication No. 92-0047). Rockville, MD: Author.

White, G. L., & Forsythe, W. A., III. (1993). Tobacco use and wound healing: Understanding the mechanisms. *Clinician Reviews, 3*(9), 42–48.

Willey, T. (1992). Use a decision tree to choose wound dressings. *AJN, 92*(2), 43–46.

Chapter 15: Special Hygiene Needs

Skin, Nail and Foot Hygiene

Edelstein, M. A. (1987). If the shoe fits: Footwear considerations for the elderly. *Physical and Occupational Therapy in Geriatrics, 5*(4), 1–16.

Heckheimer, E. F. (1989). *Health promotion of the elderly in the community.* Philadelphia: W. B. Saunders Company.

Helfand, A. D. (1989). Nail and hyperkeratotic problems in the elderly foot. *American Family Physician, 39*(2), 101–110.

Hoop, R. A., & Sundberg, S. (1974). The effects of soaking and lotion on dryness of the skin in the feet of the elderly patient. *Journal of the American Podiatry Association, 64*(10), 747–760.

Kosinski, M., & Ramsharitar, S. (1994). In-office management of common geriatric foot problems. *Geriatrics, 49*(15), 43–48.

Dental Hygiene

Heckheimer, E. F. (1989). *Health promotion of the elderly in the community.* Philadelphia: W. B. Saunders Company.

Replogle, W. H., & Beebe, D. K. (1996). Halitosis. *American Family Physician, 53*(4), 1215–1224.

Sleep Hygiene

Ancoli-Israel, S. (1997). Sleep problems in older adults: Putting myths to bed. *Geriatrics, 52*(1), 20–28.

Brown, L. K. (1997). Sleep and sleep disorders in the elderly. *Nursing Home Medicine, 5*(10), 346–353.

Johnston, J. E. (1994). Sleep problems in the elderly. *Journal of the American Academy of Nurse Practitioners, 6*(4), 161–166.

Maggi, S., Langlois, J. A., Minicuci, N., Grigoletto, F., Pavan, M., Foley, D. J., & Enzi, G. (1998). Sleep complaints in community-dwelling older persons: Prevalence, associated factors, and reported causes. *Journal of the American Geriatrics Society, 46*(2), 161–168.

Nakra, B. R., Brassbery, G. T., & Peck, B. (1991). Insomnia in the elderly. *American Family Physician, 43*(2), 477–483.

National Institutes of Health. (1991). Consensus development conference statement: The treatment of sleep disorders of older people. Association of Professional Sleep Societies. *Sleep, 14*(2), 169–177.

Chapter 16: Pain Management

American Geriatrics Society. The management of chronic pain in older persons. *The Journal of the American Geriatrics Society, 46*(5), 635–651.

Cherney, N. I., & Portenoy, R. K. (1993). Cancer pain management: Current strategy. *Cancer, 72*(Suppl. 11), 3393–3415.

Cicala, R. S., & Wright, H. (1991). Transcutaneous electrical nerve stimulation in the elderly. *Pain Management, 4*(2), 22–26.

Ferrell, B. A. (1991). Pain management in elderly people. *Journal of the American Geriatric Society, 39*(1), 64–73.

Ferrell, B. A. (1996). Pain evaluation and management. In R. W. Besdine, L. Z. Rubenstein, & L. Snyder (Eds.), *Medical care of the nursing home resident: What physicians need to know* (pp. 91–99). Philadelphia: American College of Physicians.

Ferrell, B. A., Ferrell, B. R., & Rivera, L. (1995). Pain in cognitively impaired nursing home patients. *Journal of Pain and Symptom Management, 10*(8), 591–598.

Ferrell, B. R., & Ferrell, B. A. (1990). More research needed on geriatric pain management. *Provider, 16*(7), 31–32.

Ho, K., Spence, J., & Murphy, M. F. (1996). Review of pain- measurement tools. *Annals of Emergency Medicine, 27*(4), 427–439.

Hurley, A. C., Volicer, B. J., Hanrahan, P. A., Houde, S., & Volicer, L. (1992). Assessment of discomfort in advanced alzheimer patients. *Research in Nursing and Health, 15*(5), 369–377.

Lipman, A. G. (1991). Opioid use in the treatment of pain: Refuting 10 common myths. *Pain Management, 4*(4), 13–17.

Mace, N. (1989). A new method for studying the patient's experience of care. *The American Journal of Alzheimer's Care and Related Disorders & Research, 9*(10), 4–6.

McCaffery, M., & Beebe, R. (1989). *Pain: Clinical manual for nursing practice.* St. Louis: Mosby.

McCaffery, M., & Ferrell, B. R. (1991). Patient age: Does it affect your pain-control decisions? *Nursing '91, 21*(9), 44–48.

Middaugh, S. J., Levin, R. B., Kee, W. G., Barchiesi, F. D., & Roberts, J. M. (1988). Chronic pain: Its treatment in geriatric and younger patients. *Archives in Physical Medicine Rehabilitation, 69*(12), 1021–1026.

Parmelee, P. A., Smith, B., & Katz, I. R. (1993). Pain complaints and cognitive status among elderly institution residents. *Journal of the American Geriatric Society, 41*(5), 517–522.

Portenoy, R. K., & Farkash, A. (1988). Practical management of non-malignant pain in the elderly. *Geriatrics, 43*(5), 29–47.

Portenoy, R. K., & Waldman, S. D. (1991). Recent advances in the management of can pain: Part II—Nonpharmacologic approaches. *Pain Management, 4*(4), 18–24.

Romano, J. M., Turner, J. A., & Sullivan, M. D. (1991). Pain management update. *Pain Management, 4*(2), 10–11.

Rudy, T. E., Kerns, R. D., & Turk, D. C. (1988). Chronic pain and depression: Toward a cognitive–behavioral mediation model. *Pain, 35*(2), 129–140.

Savage, S. R. (1996). Long-term opioid therapy: Assessment of consequences and risks. *Journal of Pain and Symptom Management, 11*(5), 274–285.

Simington, J. A., & Laing, G. P. (1993). Effects of therapeutic touch on anxiety in the institutionalized elderly. *Clinical Nursing Research, 2*(4), 438–450.

Tollison, J. W., & Longe, R. L. (1991). Special considerations in pharmacologic pain management. Part II: The elderly. *Pain Management, 4*(3), 29–34.

The American Academy of Pain Medicine and the American Pain Society. (1996). *The use of opioids for the treatment of chronic pain*. Glenview, IL: American Academy of Pain Medicine, American Pain Society.

U.S. Department of Health and Human Services. (1992). *Acute pain management* (AHCPR Publication No. 92-0032). Rockville, MD: Author.

U.S. Department of Health and Human Services. (1994). *Management of cancer pain* (AHCPR Publication No. 94-0592). Rockville, MD: Author.

Walco, G. A., & Dowite, N. T. (1991). Vertical versus horizontal visual analogue scales of pain intensity in children. *Journal of Pain and Symptom Management, 6*(3), [Abstract], 200.

Chapter 17: Management of the Post-Menopausal Woman

Berardicci, A., & Lengacher, C. A. (1998). Osteoporosis in perimenopausal women: Current perspectives. *American Journal for Nurse Practitioners, 2*(9), 9–14.

Bidikov, I., & Meier, D. E. (1997). Clinical decision-making with the woman after menopause. *Geriatrics, 52*(3), 28–30, 32, 34–35.

Cadelago, L. G. (1994). Coronary artery disease: Are there differences between women and men? *Clinician Reviews, 4*, 57–58, 60–62, 65, 68–70, 72, 75–76, 78.

Cumming, D. C., & Cumming, C. E. (1998). Hormone replacement therapy: Part 1: Should your patient do with—or without—it? *Consultant, 38*, 2417–2420, 2425–2427, 2431.

Cumming, D. C., & Cumming, C. E. (1998). Hormone replacement therapy: Part 2: Should your patient do *without* it? *Consultant, 38*, 2435–2438, 2441–2442.

Eli Lilly and Company. (1997). *Beyond menopause: Taking charge of your health* [Brochure]. Indianapolis, IN: Eli Lilly and Company.

Greendale, G. A., & Judd, H. L. (1993). The menopause: Health implications and clinical management. *Journal of the American Geriatrics Society, 41*(4), 426–434.

Hammond, C. B. (1997). Management of menopause. *American Family Physician, 55*(5), 1667–1674, 1679–1680.

Jensen, J., Nilas, L., & Christiansen, C. (1986). Cyclic changes in serum cholesterol and lipoproteins following different dosages of combined postmenopausal hormone replacement therapy. *British Journal of Obstetrics and Gynaecology, 93*, 613–618.

LaRosa, J. C. (1997). Cholesterol management in women and the elderly. *Journal of Internal Medicine, 241*, 307–316.

Murphy, J. L. (Ed.), (1998). *Nurse Practitioner's Prescribing Reference.* New York: Prescribing Reference, Inc.

Schwartz, L. B. (1998). Hormone replacement therapy: Weighing the pros and cons in women with a history of hypercoagulability. *Consultant, 38*, 846, 848.

Speroff, L. (1993). Menopause and hormone replacement therapy. *Clinics in Geriatric Medicine, 9*(1), 33–51.

Warner, S. L. (1995). Preventive health care for the menopausal woman. *Infertility and Reproductive Medicine Clinics of North America, 6*(4), 675–696.

Chapter 18: Palliative Care

Abrahm, J. L. (1998). Promoting symptom control in palliative care. *Seminars in Oncology Nursing, 14*(2), 95–109.

Brant, J. M. (1998). The art of palliative care: Living with hope, dying with dignity. *Oncology Nursing Forum, 25*(6), 995–1004.

Catterall, R. A., Cox, M., Greet, B. et al. (1998). Spiritual care. The assessment and audit of spiritual care. *International Journal of Palliative Nursing, 4*(4), 162–168.

O'Donnell, V. (1998). Symptom management: The pharmacological management of respiratory tract secretions. *International Journal of Palliative Nursing, 4*(4), 199–203.

Rousseau, P. (1996). Non-pain symptom management in terminal care. *Clinics of Geriatric Medicine, 12*(2), 313–327.

Schonwetter, R. S. (1996). Care of the dying geriatric patient. *Clinics of Geriatric Medicine, 12*(2), 253–265.

Sheehan, D. C., & Forman, W. B. (1997). Symptomatic management of the older person with cancer. *Clinics in Geriatric Medicine, 13*(1), 203–219.

Tierney, J., & Wilson, D. (1994). Hospice care versus home health care: Regulatory distinctions and program intent. *American Journal of Hospice & Palliative Care, 11*(2), 14–19, 22.

Von Guten, C. F., & Twaddle, M. L. (1996). Terminal care for non-cancer patients. *Clinics of Geriatric Medicine, 12*(2), 349–358.

Chapter 19: Management of the Alzheimer's Patient

Adler, G. (1997). Driving and dementia: Dilemmas and decisions. *Geriatrics, 52*(Suppl. 2), S26–S29.

Lehninger, F. W., Ravindran, V. L., & Stewart, J.T. (1998). Management strategies for problem behaviors in the patient with dementia. *Geriatrics, 53*(4), 55–56, 66, 68 passim.

Lesseig, D. Z. (1998). Pharmacotherapy for long-term care residents with dementia-associated behavioral disturbance. *Journal of Psychosocial Nursing & Mental Health Services, 36*(2), 27–31.

Morris, J. C. (1997). Alzheimer's disease: A review of clinical assessment and management issues. *Geriatrics, 52*(Suppl. 2), S22–S25.

Practice guidelines for the treatment of patients with Alzheimer's disease and other dementias of late life. (1997). *American Journal of Psychiatry, 154*(5, Suppl).

Salzman, C. (Ed.), (1998). *Clinical geriatric psychopharmacology* (3rd ed.). Baltimore: Williams and Wilkins.

Watson, R. (1997). Under-nutrition, weight loss and feeding difficulty in elderly patients with dementia: A nursing perspective. *Reviews in Clinical Gerontology, 7*(4), 317–326.

Chapter 20: Alternatives to Living Alone

Cannava, E. (1994). "Gerodesign": Safe and comfortable living spaces for older adults. *Geriatrics, 49*(11), 45–46, 48–49.

Capitman, J., Abrahams, R., & Ritter, G. (1997). Measuring the adequacy of home care for frail elders. *Gerontologist, 37*(3), 303–313.

Hammer, B. J. (1998). Community resources. In A. S. Luggen et al., *NGNA Core Curriculum for Gerontological Advanced Practice Nurses* (pp. 324–327). Thousand Oaks, CA: Sage.

Lee, W., Eng, C., Fox, N., et al. (1998). PACE: A model for integrated care of frail older patients. *Geriatrics, 53*(6), 65–66, 69 passim.

Meiner, S. (1998). Community living/life care centers. In A. S. Luggen et al., *NGNA Core Curriculum for Gerontological Advanced Practice Nurses* (pp. 332–325). Thousand Oaks, CA: Sage.

Meyer, H. (1998). The bottom line on assisted living. *Hospitals & Health Networks, 72*(14), 22–26.

Ross, M. E. T., & Wright, M. F. (1998). Long-term care for elderly individuals and methods for financing. *Journal of Community Health Nursing, 15*(2), 77–89.

Tellis-Nayak, M. (1998). The post-acute continuum of care: Understanding your patient's options. *American Journal of Nursing, 98*(8), 44–49.

Tinker, A. (1997). Housing for elderly people. *Reviews in Clinical Gerontology, 7*(2), 171–176.

Chapter 21: Legal and Ethical Issues

High, D. M. (1994). Surrogate decision making: Who will make decisions for me when I can't? *Clinics in Geriatric Medicine, 10*(3), 445–462.

Hodges, M. O., & Tolle, S. W. (1994). Tube feeding decisions in the elderly. *Clinics in Geriatric Medicine, 10*(3), 475–488.

Kapp, M. B. (1994). Ethical aspects of guardianship. *Clinics in Geriatric Medicine 10*(3), 501–512.

Kellogg, F. R., Brickner, P. W., & Crain, M. (1997). Ethical issues and concerns of the frail aged. In P. W. Brickner, F. R. Kellogg, A. J. Lechich, et al. (Eds.), *Geriatric home care* (pp. 59–78). New York: Springer.

Kellogg, F. R., Brickner, P. W., & Crain, M. (1997). Life-support therapies for the frail elderly: Strategies for discussion and making choices. In P. W. Brickner, F. R. Kellogg, A. J. Lechich, et al. (Eds.), *Geriatric home care* (pp. 79–99). New York: Springer.

Pearlman, R. A. (1997). Determination of decision-making capacity. In C. K. Cassel, H. J. Cohen, E. B. Larson, et al. (Eds.), *Geriatric medicine* (3rd ed., pp. 201–209). New York: Springer.

Smith, G. P. (1996). *Legal and healthcare ethics for the elderly.* Washington, D.C.: Taylor and Francis.

Chapter 22: Medication Issues

Beers, M. H. (1992). Medication use in the elderly. In E. Calkins, A. B. Ford, & P. R. Katz (Eds.), *Practice of geriatrics* (2nd ed., pp. 33–49). Philadelphia: W. B. Saunders Company.

Beers, M. H., Ouslander, J. G., Rollingher, I., Reuben, D. B., Brooks, J., & Beck, J. C. (1991). Explicit criteria for determining inappropriate medications use in nursing home residents. *Archives of Internal Medicine, 151*, 1825–1832.

Bennett, W. M. (1990). Geriatric pharmacokinetics and the kidney. *American Journal of Kidney Diseases, XVI*(4), 283–288.

Carty, M. A., & Everitt, D. E. (1989). Basic principles of prescribing for geriatric outpatients. *Geriatrics, 44*(6), 85–88, 90–92, 97–98.

Eliopoulos, C. (1998). Drugs: Special considerations in the elderly. In Eliopoulos, C. *Manual of gerontologic nursing* (pp. 337–347). St. Louis: Mosby.

French, D. G. (1996). Avoiding adverse drug reactions in the elderly patient: Issues and strategies. *Nurse Practitioner, 21*(9), 90, 96–97, 101–102, 104–105.

Hahn, K., & Wietor, G. (1992). Helpful tools for medication screenings. *Geriatric Nursing*, 160–166.

Hobson, M. (1992). Medications in older patients. *Western Journal of Medicine, 157*, 539–543.

Lindley, C. M., Tully, M. P., Paramsothy, V., & Tallis, R. C. (1992). Inappropriate medication is a major cause of adverse drug reactions in elderly patients. *Age and Ageing, 21*, 294–300.

Lowenthal, D. T. (1987). Drug therapy in the elderly: Special considerations. *Geriatrics, 42*(11), 77–82.

Palmieri, D. T. (1991). Clearing up the confusion: Adverse effects of medications in the elderly. *Journal of Gerontological Nursing, 17*(10), 32–35.

Piraino, A. J. (1997). Drug use in the elderly: Tips for avoiding adverse effects and interactions. *Consultant, 37*, 2825–2827, 2830–2834.

Sloan, R. W. (1992). Principles of drug therapy in geriatric patients. *American Family Physician, 45*(6), 2709–2718.

Stolley, J. M., Buckwalter, K. C., & Fjordbak, B. (1991). Iatrogenesis in the elderly: Drug-related problems. *Journal of Gerontological Nursing, 17*(9), 12–17.

Williams, P., & Rush, D. R. (1986). Geriatric polypharmacy. *Hospital Practice 21*(2), 109–120.

Chapter 23: Rehabilitation Issues

Brummel-Smith, K. (1998). Rehabilitation. In T. T. Yoshikawa, E. L. Cobbs, & K. Brummel-Smith (Eds.), *Practical ambulatory geriatrics* (2nd ed., pp. 26–34). St. Louis: Mosby.

Caird, F. I., & Evans, J. G. (1996). Medicine in old age. In D. J. Weatherall, J. G. Ledingham, & D. A. Warrell (Eds.), *Oxford textbook of medicine* (3rd ed., Vol. 3, pp. 4331–4396). New York: Oxford University Press.

Clothier, J., & Grotta, J. (1991). Recognition and management of post-stroke depression in the elderly. *Clinics in Geriatric Medicine, 7*(3), 493–506.

Cordts, G. A. (1996). Exercise in the elderly: Can it improve function? In M. A. Forciea & R. Lavizzo-Mourey (Eds.), *Geriatric secrets* (pp. 68–72). Philadelphia: Hanley & Belfus, Inc.

Erickson, R. V. (1996). Rehabilitation. In R. W. Besdine, L. Z. Rubenstein, & L. Snyder (Eds.), *Medical care of the nursing home resident: What physicians need to know* (pp. 131–142). Philadelphia: American College of Physicians.

Ferri, F. E. (1997). Geriatric rehabilitation. In F. F. Ferri, M. D. Fretwell, & T. J. Wachtel (Eds.), *Practical guide to the care of the geriatric patient* (2nd ed., pp. 429–457). St. Louis: Mosby.

Harper, C. M., & Lyles, Y. M. (1988). Physiology and complications of bed rest. *Journal of the American Geriatrics Society, 36*(11), 1047–1054.

Kelly-Hayes, M. (1996). Functional evaluation. In S. P. Hoeman (Ed.), *Rehabilitation nursing: Process and application* (2nd ed., pp. 144–155). St. Louis: Mosby.

Marsiglio, A., & Holm, K. (1988). Physical conditioning in the aging adult. *The Nurse Practitioner, 13*(9), 33–41.

Radwanski, M. B., & Hoeman, S. P. (1996). Geriatric rehabilitation nursing. In S. P. Hoeman (Ed.), *Rehabilitation nursing: Process and application* (2nd ed., pp. 683–699). St. Louis: Mosby.

Resnick, B. (1996). Motivation in geriatric rehabilitation. IMAGE: *Journal of Nursing Scholarship, 28*(1), 41–45.

Chapter 24: Substance Abuse

Danis, P. G., & Seaton, T. L. (1997). Helping your patients to quit smoking. *American Family Physician, 55*(4), 1207–1214.

Fitzgerald, J. L., & Mulford, H. A. (1992). Elderly vs younger problem drinker "treatment" and recovery experiences. *British Journal of Addiction, 87*(9), 1281–1291.

Gambert, S. R. (1997). Alcohol abuse: Medical effects of heavy drinking in late life. *Geriatrics, 52*(6), 30–37.

Joseph, C. L. (1995). Alcohol and drug misuse in the nursing home. *The International Journal of Addictions, 30*(13 & 14), 1953–1984.

Kappas-Larson, P., & Lathrop, L. (1993). Early detection and intervention for hazardous ethanol use. *The Nurse Practitioner, 18*(7), 50–55.

Marcus, M. T. (1993). Alcohol and other drug abuse in elders. *Journal of ET Nurses, 20*(3), 106–110.

McLoughlin, D. M., & Farrell, M. (1997). Substance misuse in the elderly. In I. J. Norman & S. J. Redfern (Eds.), *Mental health care for elderly people* (pp. 205–221). New York: Churchill-Livingston.

McMahon, A. L. (1993). Substance abuse among the elderly. *Nurse Practitioner Forum, 4*(4), 231–238.

Reid, M. C., & Anderson, P. A. (1997). Geriatric substance use disorders. *Medical Clinics of North America, 81*(4), 999–1016.

Scott, R. E. (1998). Substance abuse continuum of care: Guidelines, clinical pathway and performance improvement. *Federal Practitioner, 15*(Suppl. 3), 17–23.

Scripps Howard News Service. (June 5, 1998). Mature women hiding addictions, study says. *The Tennessean*, p. A11.

Soloman, K., Manepalli, J., Ireland, G. A., & Mahon, G. M. (1993). Alcoholism and prescription drug abuse in the elderly: St. Louis University grand rounds. *Journal of the American Geriatrics Society, 41*(1), 57–69.

Thibault, J. M., & Maly, R. C. (1993). Recognition and treatment of substance abuse in the elderly. *Primary Care: Clinics in Office Practice, 20*(1), 155–165.

U.S. Department of Health and Human Services. (1996). *Smoking cessation: Information for specialist* (AHCPR Publication No. 96-0694). Rockville, MD: Author.

Chapter 25: Special Issues

Allan, M. A. (1998). Elder abuse: A challenge for home care nurses. *Home Healthcare Nurse, 16*(2), 103–110.

Buchanan, D., Farran, C., & Clark, D. (1995). Suicidal thought and self-transcendence in older adults. *Journal of Psychosocial Nursing and Mental Health Services, 33*(10), 31–34.

Capezuti, E., Brush, B. L., & Lawson, W. T. (1997). Reporting elder mistreatment. *Journal of Gerontological Nursing, 23*, 24–32.

Conwell, Y., & Brent, D. (1995). Suicide and aging, I: Patterns of psychiatric diagnosis. *International Psychogeriatrics, 7*(2), 149–164.

Conwell, Y., Raby, W. N., & Caine, E. D. (1995). Suicide and aging, II: The psychobiological interface. *International Psychogeriatrics, 7*(2), 165–181.

Costa, A. J. (1993). Elder abuse. *Primary Care, 20*(2), 375–389.

Devons, C. A. (1996). Suicide in the elderly: How to identify and treat patients at risk. *Geriatrics, 51*(3), 67–72.

Emick, M. A., & Hayslip, B. (1996). Custodial grandparenting: New roles for middle-aged and older adults. *International Journal of Aging and Human Development, 43*(2), 135–154.

Florio, E. R., Hendryx, M. S., Jensen, J. E., Rockwood, T. H., Raschko, R., & Dyck, D. G. (1997). A comparison of suicidal and nonsuicidal elders referred to a community mental health center program. *Suicide and Life-Threatening Behavior, 27*(2), 182–193.

Fuller-Thomson, E., Minkler, M., & Driver, D. (1997). A profile of grandparents raising grandchildren in the United States. *The Gerontologist, 37*(3), 406–411.

Greenberg, E. M. (1996). Violence and the older adult: The role of the acute care nurse practitioner. *Critical Care Nursing Quarterly, 19*(2), 76–84.

Hayden, M. F., & Heller, T. (1997). Support, problem-solving/coping ability, and personal burden of younger and older caregivers of adults with mental retardation. *Mental Retardation, 35*(5), 364–372.

Heller, T., & Factor, A. (1991). Permanency planning for adults with mental retardation living with family caregivers. *American Journal of Mental Retardation, 96*(2), 163–176.

Kelley, S. J. (1993). Caregiver stress in grandparents raising grandchildren. *IMAGE: Journal of Nursing Scholarship, 25*(4), 331–337.

Lachs, M. S., Williams, C. S., O'Brien, S., et al. (1998). The mortality of elder mistreatment. *Journal of American Medical Association, 280*, 428–432.

Lavrisha, M. (1997). What can nurses do about financial exploitation of elders? *Journal of Gerontological Nursing, 23*, 49–50.

McCarthy, J. M., & Mullan, E. (1996). The elderly with a learning disability (mental retardation): An overview. *International Psychogeriatrics, 8*(3), 489–501.

Mengel, M. H., Marcus, D. B., & Dunkle, R. E. (1996). "What will happen to my child when I'm gone?": A support and education group for aging parents as caregivers. *The Gerontologist, 36*(6), 816–820.

Paris, B. E., Meier, D. E., Goldstein, T., Weiss, M., & Fein, E. D. (1995). Elder abuse and neglect: How to recognize warning signs and intervene. *Geriatrics, 50*(4), 47–51.

Pursell, J. C. (1997, December). Harrington bangs gavel against elder abuse. *Active Times*, 6–8.

Ridenour, N., & Norton, D. (1997). Community-based persons with mental retardation: Opportunities for health promotion. *Nurse Practitioner Forum, 8*(2), 45–49.

Smith, G. C. (1997). Aging families of adults with mental retardation: Patterns and correlates of service use, need, and knowledge. *American Journal on Mental Retardation, 102*(1), 13–26.

Sullivan, M. D. (1997). Maintaining good morale in old age. *Western Journal of Medicine, 167*(4), 276–284.

Valente, S. M. (1997). Preventing suicide among elderly people. *American Journal for Nurse Practitioners, 1*(4), 15–19, 23–24, 31.

Watson, J. A., & Koblinsky, S. A. (1997). Strengths and needs of working-class African-American and Anglo-American grandparents. *International Journal of Aging and Human Development, 44*(2), 149–165.

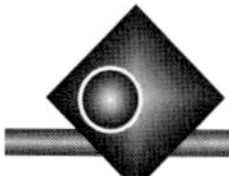

Index

The letter *t* after a page number indicates a table; the letter *f* indicates a figure.